THE NEO DIET

FIND YOUR SUPERHUMAN HEALTH
BY EATING THE "WRONG" FOODS

KEVIN AVENTURA

UNBOXING CHALLENGE

Join our Unboxing Challenge contest and win a 1-on-1 Strategy Session.

We know that if you are reading this, you already unboxed the book. But, why not relive that excitement one more time? ☺

Every month we will randomly select one winner. To participate, please follow the steps below.

RULES FOR THE CONTEST
- Film yourself unboxing The Neo Diet book or make a video sharing with your friends how excited you are about reading it.

- Use the hashtags:
  #NeoDietUnboxingChallenge #NeoHacker #NeoDiet

- Post the video on your public profile (instagram, facebook, youtube).

- Videos must not contain music in the background and must be shorter than 4 minutes in length.

- Submit the link to your video accessing my.neodiet.co/unboxing or by scanning the QR code below.

Good luck. We'll keep our fingers crossed!

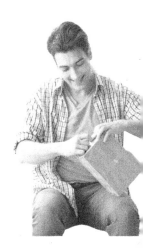

The information contained in this book is not designed to replace or take the place of any form of medicine or professional medical advice. The intent of the author is only to offer information of an anecdotal and general nature that may be part of your quest for physical, emotional, and spiritual well-being. The information in this book has been provided for educational and entertainment purposes only.

The information contained in this book has been compiled from sources deemed reliable, and it is accurate to the best of the Author's knowledge; however, the author cannot guarantee its accuracy and validity and cannot be held liable for any errors or omissions. Changes are periodically made to this book.

The author is not a licensed physician and offers no medical diagnoses, treatments, suggestions, or counseling. The information presented herein has not been evaluated by the U.S. Food and Drug Administration, and it is not intended to diagnose, treat, cure, or prevent any disease.
Exercise is also discussed in this book. All forms of exercise pose some inherent risks. The author advises readers to take full responsibility for their own safety and know their limits. Before following any advice in this book, be sure that your equipment is well maintained, and do not take risks beyond your level of experience, aptitude, training, and fitness.

Full medical clearance from a licensed physician should be obtained before beginning or modifying any diet, exercise, or lifestyle program, and physicians should be informed of all nutritional changes. The author claims no responsibility to any person or entity for any liability, loss, or damage caused or alleged to be caused directly or indirectly as a result of the use, application, or interpretation of the information presented herein.

For each e-book, paperback and hardcover book sale, $1 will be donated to help fight child hunger. Learn more about the organizations the author is partnering with by visiting neohacker.co/neodiet.

Published by Neo Press.
Illustrations by Hugo Machado.

ISBN (e-Book): 978-1-957602-00-4
ISBN (Paperback): 978-1-957602-01-1
ISBN (Hardcover): 978-1-957602-02-8

First Edition

Feeling like a superhuman!

Imagine waking up early in the morning feeling full of energy and pumped up for the day ahead. You feel so good, you don't even need your usual coffee.

You start getting dressed and . . . yeah, you're looking hot. *Wheet wheoo*! Not only are you feeling good, but you're looking good, and you know it.

During the workday, you are crushing it. Your Adderall-hooked colleagues are no competition for you. There is no procrastination, just productivity. And you finish all your daily tasks in half the time you usually need. That mental sharpness stays with you throughout the day, and you don't crash.

Somehow, people around you are nicer. Okay, this part is a lie. Idiots will continue to be idiots. You, on the other hand, are in such a good mood that everyone just seems nicer.

Done with work, time to go to the gym. Not because you need to, but because you want to. You need to burn some of that extra energy. Boom, another amazing workout!

You get home and eat nourishing food you like. There is no counting calories or eating cardboard food.

Before you go to bed, you put on some Marvin Gaye, and the rest I don't need to explain. There are no off days, and no need for excuses. Your hormones kick in, every day!

Sound too good to be true?

This is no fairy tale, no alternate reality in the metaverse. This can be you. Let me correct myself. This *will* be you if you are ready to leave your comfort zone and come with me on this journey.

It's not an easy road. I will challenge many of your beliefs. But I will teach you how to hack your biology and take control over your health and performance. You will become the superhuman that Mother Nature designed you to be!

TABLE OF CONTENTS

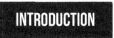

Welcome to the Matrix

"When I let go of what I am, I become what I might be."
Lao Tzu

DECISION TIME
This is your last chance. After this, there is no turning back.

Take the blue pill, and the story ends. You put down this book and go on with your life. You accept that there's nothing you can do. After all, what you just read is all "rainbows and butterflies," right? There is nothing one can do to fight the "bad genes." Why waste time on a losing battle?

Or . . .

You take the red pill and I will *show you how deep the rabbit hole goes.*

What you are going to read in the next few chapters will go against most of the things you have learned about health and nutrition. This is going to be controversial, and many critics will get all worked up. I honestly couldn't care less, because I know how this book is going to help you, and so many others.

As someone once said, insanity is doing the same thing over and over again but expecting different results. Enough of this. You deserve better. You deserve the truth.

After I'm finished with you, you will never be the same. And that will be my greatest gift to you.

The time has come. Swallow the red pill and take the first step toward achieving your full potential!

YOU HAVE BEEN LIED TO
The most accepted definition of *health* is the "absence of disease." According to this definition, if you haven't been diagnosed with any disease, congratulations, you are "healthy"!

This concept is pure BS. You can live your entire life without ever being diagnosed with anything, but still experience indigestion, headaches, weight gain, joint pain, brain fog, low libido, poor immunity, and an utter lack of motivation to do anything.

This is not healthy, nor is it normal. Because so many people feel just okay, we've somehow accepted this as the normal adult life. But it's not how it should be.

You are not to blame for this reality we live in. Our culture is full of health "facts" that we all blindly follow because everybody knows they're true. But how are these "truths" working for us? Is it possible that we've been fed convenient lies?

I'm not suggesting that there's this huge conspiracy in which the food industry, Big Pharma, and health institutions are doing this on purpose, but let's just say their profits have not been going *down*. As Dr. Andrew Saul said, *"Good health makes a lot of sense but does not make a lot of dollars."*

Please note, I have several friends who are doctors, nurses, therapists, and other health professionals. And they are the most loving people I know. They truly want the best for their patients and try to advise people to the best of their ability and knowledge. However, our medical system is broken.

We are superb at dealing with acute issues, but for chronic illness, we have held on to outdated science, and our approach is just wrong. Think about it. The current approach is to prescribe drugs for every single symptom the patient complains about, but there isn't much effort to really find and solve the actual cause of the problem.

If your roof is leaking, putting a bucket there to collect the water drops is not the solution. The solution is to fix the roof.

Being a chronic pill popper is not the solution.

I get it, taking a painkiller to ease a headache is a lot less work than trying to ferret out the cause of the headache. However, we are getting to a point where this approach is making us sicker. Reports show that prescription drugs now kill more people than cocaine and heroin combined. As crazy as this may sound, children today might have shorter life spans than their parents. This scary scenario results from the epidemic of mismanaged chronic diseases that are affecting the world's population.

So, what is the solution?

The solution has been in front of us all along. We have known this for millennia, but somewhere along the road we forgot the basics and focused on the new shiny toys. But there is no shiny toy that can beat a healthy diet.

Instead of medication, we need more diet education.

DO WE NEED "ANOTHER" NUTRITION BOOK?

As soon as the world was hit with the COVID-19 pandemic, my mother asked me what she should eat. Not only was she concerned about that unknown disease plaguing us, but this disease made her realize she needed to take better care of herself in order to preserve her quality of life for years to come.

She knew that I would have an answer for her, since I had been obsessed with studying nutrition since college. *What book do you recommend, son?*

After reflecting on this question for a while, I realized I could not think of a single book that addressed all the concepts I felt were essential. Sure, there are many excellent books that do a brilliant job of covering certain points, but sadly, they also completely miss other important aspects of your diet and health. The truth is that a great many health experts have been turning nutrition concepts into religions. Nutrition has become a place of skyscraper egos and fanaticism—not to mention the multi-billion-dollar industry that it is. There is no attempt to find middle ground or the best of all perspectives. Either you know the "truth" or you are the blind person who refuses to see the light. All sides of the diet world insult each other. Vegans versus carnivores, high carb versus keto, high fiber versus low FODMAP, and so on. Truly, all have significant arguments, but all miss the bigger picture.

Any marketer will tell you it's a lot easier to sell a diet with which, if everyone follows a single magic formula, all get healed. Unfortunately, *that does not exist in real life.* We all have individual physiological responses to food. We all have different lifestyles, genetics, gut microbiomes, and so on. These differences make you process food in your unique way. Just because your friend feels amazing with diet X does not mean that is the best approach for you. By following a one-size-fits-all approach, you may restrict yourself from foods you love that are actually amazing for you. Heck, some radical diets promote such a sense of restriction that people develop eating disorders like orthorexia and even full-blown anorexia nervosa.

Through permanent restriction, most diets are making us fragile. As long as you stay within that diet and supplement, you can indeed have a reasonably healthy life. But as soon as you slightly deviate from the plan, you will suffer. I don't know about you, but I refuse to become a fragile greenhouse flower. Being able to enjoy life, with the occasional excess, and still feel healthy and strong sounds like a better alternative.

This is where the Neo Diet is different. It does not aim to restrict with a single path that does not exist in real life. Instead, it acknowledges that you need to understand your own physiology and, while still following some basic principles, adjust them and personalize them to match your own situation.

Even though this is a book about diet, please do not see it as just another diet book. This is my personal quest for answers for my mother, for myself, for my friends and clients.

This book is not meant to restrict but rather to empower you with the information you need in order to make educated decisions, improve your health, and level up your quality of life. Ultimately, this is a guide, not a rule book. At the end of the day, this is your journey. Armed with the right knowledge, you'll be able to use this guide to regain control over your health and start feeling amazing every single day.

ABOUT THE AUTHOR

Let's get this out of the way. I am not a medical doctor, nutritionist, dietitian, or even a celebrity healing psychic. Why should you believe anything I have to say?

Actually, you shouldn't! You should never blindly believe anything presented to you by someone who supposedly is an expert. You should always take everything you read with a grain of salt and verify the research. Simply trusting everything we were told about nutrition has brought us to the mess we are in today.

That being said, here are a couple of reasons why you should read this book. Let me start by saying that I am an independent author, so I am writing what I want to write and not what anyone else thinks is commercially viable. As I'm writing this, barely anyone in the nutrition world knows me. I've never given interviews, never been on TV, never done podcasts, nada, zilch. If that changes in the future, I'll be glad—it'll mean I did a good job and helped some people. But for now, I am just a passionate guy whose mission has been to hear all sides of the story with an open mind and pin down the best they all offered. This allowed me to integrate the best research available in an unbiased and holistic approach.

Now that we've addressed the elephant in the room, let me briefly introduce myself. Hi, I'm Kevin. Nice to meet you. Please consider me your Morpheus (I hope you have watched *The Matrix*), a.k.a. your guide through this health journey. I studied physical therapy in college, and since then I have expanded my studies into areas such as osteopathy, naturopathy, and nutrition. I now work with people to help them achieve their best health and optimal levels of performance. But this whole health adventure began as an attempt to heal myself.

It all started when I was a newborn. I had all kinds of problems. If it had -*itis* in the name, I had it. It was so bad that my mother paid my pediatrician a monthly rate, not the usual fee per visit. No one really understood why I was so sick. After all, I was being raised on formula, which, according to all the doctors back then (and, sadly, many still today), was even better than mother's milk. My health issues, although "treatable" persisted as I grew up. In my teens, things got worse as I developed almost daily migraines. I did all kinds of exams, and nothing was ever found. My doctor's solution: *Take Tylenol whenever it hurts. Just make sure you eat something before you take it.*

During my college years, things didn't improve much. Let's just say my roommates and I did not have any idea about nutrition. Fried chicken and microwave pizza were our go-to meals. Favorite snack? Mayo sandwiches. I kid you not. You open a bread roll, you dump in a quarter of the mayonnaise jar, and you have a very filling snack. My health was not going in the right direction. My face had bigger craters than the moon, my brain was beyond foggy, and despite how much exercise I tried to do, the extra weight was accumulating.

After college, things got worse. I cleaned up my diet and became decently fit, but my mind was in a very dark place. It was like nothing in life could give me any pleasure, any joy. Life had lost its taste. I had no energy to get out of bed and face another day. Anytime I was alone, I felt like crying. There was this overwhelming sadness inside me, and I could not understand why. How was it possible that a young 25-year-old with an interesting job, a girlfriend who loved him, and family and friends who were always there for him was seriously considering ending his own life?

Honestly, I don't remember exactly what was the trigger, but I remember thinking that something had to be off with my physiology and that it was worth trying to find some answers. This sparked an obsession with healing myself, and I started to read all I could on mental health, biohacking, and functional medicine. As I read more and more, I noticed several similarities with the "old school" concepts I had picked up from naturopathic school. I had to understand how this "new science" was connected to the "old science." I spent months reading about Chinese traditional medicine, Ayurvedic medicine, and ancient foods and natural remedies from cultures all over the world. My goal was to find what the East and West had in common and use similar principles to experiment on myself. Through trial and error, I slowly started to heal myself, and that made me appreciate even more this precious thing we take for granted—our innate ability to heal if given the right tools.

My journey led to the development of this book. A meta-analysis of thousands of scientific articles, books, blog posts, podcasts, and interviews. I took the very best from all these opposing nutritional concepts and grouped them in a logical way anyone can follow.

This is the book I wish had existed 10 years ago, and it's also my way of paying it forward. The Neo Diet is for the ones I love but also for the people I have yet to meet. It's for doctors, therapists, nutritionists, coaches, athletes, and especially for you. I am truly honored you chose to read my work, and I'm incredibly excited to be your guide on this journey to achieve your superhuman potential.

UNDERSTANDING RESEARCH

Before we dive into all the information I have to share with you, I want to make a quick note on research.

Throughout this book, we're going to bust many myths that were supposedly backed by scientific research. How is that possible? Well, as in all professions, you get good and bad researchers, and, sadly, bad *research* also gets published often. Then we have the little detail that private companies fund a lot of research. This does not mean that all this research is fraudulent or biased, but one can see the obvious conflict of interests here. As studies show, industry-sponsored trials report positive outcomes significantly more often than trials financially backed by the government, nonprofits, or nonfederal organizations.

This is why you can go online and find completely contradictory research. Thus, it's essential to review it and assess its quality and funding.

Please also note that it is possible for so-called health experts to cherry-pick studies to support a preconceived belief they have. Sometimes, these health gurus already have high-profiting businesses based on a nutritional concept they're promoting. To support their business and reputation, they might need to choose studies that back up their claims, even if the studies are of questionable quality.

Finally, I just want to point out that there are different types of studies. Without going into excruciating detail, please know that the most valuable studies we can find are interventional ones. Ideally done with humans (but not always ethical or profitable), these studies analyze the effects of a specific intervention (i.e., eating blueberries) and measure the effects on a specific parameter or group of parameters (i.e., blood glucose). The other main type of study is the epidemiological study. These are population-based studies in which participants provide lifestyle data such as diet choices that researchers then use prospectively (forward) or retrospectively (backward) to correlate data patterns with health outcomes.

Epidemiological studies represent most studies, since they are significantly less expensive than interventional trials. But they have a major flaw. Correlation does not equal causation. Just because you eat bananas and have never had a stroke, it doesn't mean that it's the bananas that are preventing the stroke. Thousands of other factors in your life could be responsible.

As you can see, there's a lot to analyze, but I don't want to spend more time on this since I have bigger fish to fry. My point is to not believe everything you read just because it has a study associated with it. Even in this book, I still recommend that you look at the data and draw your own conclusions.

THE NEO DIET

Why do I call this book *The Neo Diet*? Based on some allusions I've worked in so far, it's easy to see that I am a big fan of the movie *The Matrix*. One could say I am drawing an analogy between your health journey and the journey of the movie's protagonist, Neo (Keanu Reeves), whose search for answers leads him to question everything he believes. His quest for the truth changes him radically and ultimately makes him incredibly powerful. While I humbly admit that this is a brilliant analogy, there is more to the book's title than that.

There are two key concepts behind this name.

1. Similarly to the concept of the Paleolithic (a.k.a. Paleo) diet, I want to refer back to the time when our lifestyle was more connected with nature. But I don't want to go all the way back to the Paleolithic era. Currently, we live in cities (settlements) and rely on agriculture and the raising of livestock for food. The era that marked the transition to this lifestyle is the Neolithic era. That is the one we have to explore and learn from. After all, 99 percent of people can't or won't live a hunter-gatherer lifestyle like folks in Paleolithic times. Even though I have much respect and admiration for many Paleo authors, it's time for Paleo 2.0, or, as I like to call it, the Neo Diet.

2. The second main concept behind this book's title has to do with the other meanings of the word *neo*. In English, *neo* is a prefix that comes from the Greek word *neos*, which means "new." In the Southern African language of Tswana, *neo* means "gift." Therefore, the Neo Diet is your new way of eating to change into a new self. And it's also the diet that keeps on giving.

WHAT TO EXPECT

What you are holding in your hands is the step-by-step blueprint you need to reach your full genetic potential and become the superhuman you were designed to be.

I tried to keep this book as light, informal, and entertaining as possible. Besides that, as I learned from Tim Ferriss and Tony Robbins, information without emotion isn't retained. So, by sharing some absurd, childish, or inappropriate jokes, I aim to momentarily throw you off and make you remember the information I was sharing. See, there is a science behind the madness.

Please don't be fooled. Despite my dry dad jokes, there are more than 3,000 scientific articles backing the information I am presenting to you. Starting in the next chapter, you'll find several footnotes linking the statements to their respective studies.

At times, I will get into detail in explaining certain concepts. Please bear with me. I wouldn't discuss these ideas if I didn't feel they were important. By understanding the "why," you will be a lot more successful in sticking to the "how" and getting the results you want.

Each chapter was built on the previous one. Skipping chapters might not provide the best experience, since you might miss concepts explained before. If any of the information presented feels overwhelming, don't panic. In chapters 17 to 19 we will integrate all these principles in an easy-to-follow way. Besides that, at the end of each chapter, you'll find a brief recap (Neo Summary) of what I discussed; actionable tasks (Neo Action) to put the concepts into practice; and a list of additional resources (Neo Recommendations) you can use to explore these topics further.

After we go through these chapters together, you will know more about nutrition and health than 99 percent of the population. Among many things you're going to learn:

- How your genetic code was programmed for the survival of the species and how, surprisingly, it might be making you sick. You will learn about epigenetics and how you can fight your bad genetics.

- The supposedly healthy foods that everyone tells you to eat that are secretly creating your brain fog, destroying your metabolism, wrecking your immune system, and compromising your mental health.

- Why our incredibly sanitized new world is killing the same organisms that can bring the very best out of your genetic potential. You'll also learn how man-made toxins are slowly killing us from the inside out, and what you can do to stop this.

- The biggest epidemic that you don't hear about on the news and how it is spreading inflammation and making most of the planet sick.

- How your body actually processes food for fuel and how health authorities worldwide still guide the masses using incorrect, more-than-60-year-old recommendations.

- How you can use meal timing to fix your metabolism and become antifragile.

- Who wins the carnivore-versus-vegan fight. The result might surprise you.

- How fiber is the sleeper secret agent that might save the world.

- What simple lifestyle changes will improve your shape and make you perform better everywhere—and I mean everywhere.

- And finally, how to do a complete system reboot. You're going to learn to reverse years of "intoxication" and start feeling like you've never felt before: healthy, vibrant, mentally sharp, full of stamina, and incredibly confident.

KILLER GENES, SELF-DESTROYING LIFESTYLES, AND TOXIC FOOD

How in the Heck Did We Get into This Mess?

"Those who do not remember the past are condemned to repeat it."
George Santayana

HUMAN CODE

If I had a quarter for every time I heard someone say there is no hope for them because they have "bad genes," I would be hanging out with Elon Musk and Jeff Bezos.

Please repeat after me: Bad genes don't mean poor health.

We were taught that all of us are born with this code inside us that dictates our destiny. Depending on the mix created by the genes from Mom and Dad, your genetic code is formed, and that dictates your future. Acne at 15, gastric reflux at 32, and stroke at 51. No point in fighting it. It has been written in the "code." As the Mandalorian says, "This is the way!"

Luckily for us, things are not this linear and there is plenty of hope for you, even if you have "bad genes."

Before we go into how this system works and how you can change your "destiny," it is important to understand what this genetic code and genes are.

DNA (deoxyribonucleic acid) is that "code," and it carries the hereditary material in your body's cells. DNA comprises four similar chemicals (bases):adenine, cytosine, guanine, and thymine, abbreviated as A, C, G, and T. The combination of these bases in distinct patterns makes up the DNA code that runs your operating system.

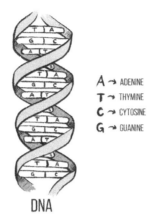

A → ADENINE
T → THYMINE
C → CYTOSINE
G → GUANINE

DNA

Genes are portions of your DNA that carry information regarding specific bodily processes or traits you have, like the color of your eyes and how big your nose is. These genes are grouped in bundles called chromosomes, which are contained within the nuclei of your cells.

To understand this, imagine your body as a book. Your DNA is the combination of all the written words. Your chromosomes are the chapters describing different functions in your body. And inside the chapters, your genes are the subsections about more specific traits.

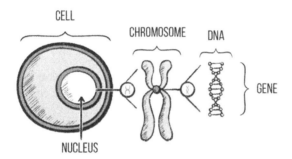

THE HUMAN GENOME PROJECT

After 1953, when Professors James Watson and Francis Crick described the structure of DNA for the first time, the scientific community was sure that genetics was the answer to understanding and even manipulating human health and disease. They believed that once we "cracked the code," we could avert all disease and change our DNA, designing upgraded humans.

The Human Genome Project (HGP) was created with the goal of sequencing the entire human genome (cracking the code). In 2000, after a massive coordinated effort across several institutions worldwide, the HGP announced that the human genetic code had been unlocked. This was huge for the scientific community. Finally, we were going to fix mutations and become disease-free. However, it's been more than a couple of years since then and we haven't gotten any healthier. What failed?

As expected, we found out that no two human individuals are genetically identical (except for identical, "real" twins, a.k.a. monozygotic twins), but the human species as a whole exhibits relatively little genetic diversity. Genetically, two people chosen at random are likely to be 99.9 percent identical. So then why do some people live long, healthy lives and others develop serious diseases early in life? The genetic code alone could not justify these differences.

To make this even more interesting, studies performed with identical twins revealed completely different health profiles even though they had the same genetic information.[1] Sure, there are diseases that have clear genetic origins, but they represent less than 20 percent of all disease.[2] In other words, 80 percent of your disease risk is determined by factors beyond your genes. Genes are only providers of possibility and not predictors of the future.

EPIGENETICS

While you cannot control your genetic heritage, now we know that the way you live your life will affect your gene expression.[3] On top of your DNA, you have a layer of molecules called epigenome. Depending on your lifestyle choices, the epigenome will work almost like a switch and will "turn on" and "turn off" your genes.[4] What this means is that even if you have so-called bad genes, you can still "turn them off" by making good lifestyle choices. This field of study is called epigenetics, and it has completely changed the narrative. Not only are these new findings great news because you can learn how to optimize your own health, but it has since been discovered that these effects are also carried forward into the next generation, where they can be magnified.[5] This means you can pass "better" or "worse" genes to your kids depending on the way you live. For example, researchers studied children of Holocaust survivors and uncovered that they presented altered profiles of stress hormones. The stress and tragedy their parents experienced predisposed their offspring to anxiety, depression, and post-traumatic stress disorder.[6]

Among all lifestyle influences, our diet is the most important one. Not only will our food become the building blocks for all our internal processes, but it will also interact with our DNA and guide our body positively or negatively. The science that studies how our food affects the way our genes express themselves is called nutrigenomics. In this book, you are going to learn how your genes are programmed and how you can use nutrigenomics to maximize the expression of your "best genes" while minimizing the expression of the ones making you fragile and sick.

GENETIC AUTOPILOT

The way we can use epigenetics in our favor is by having full knowledge of our "factory settings." Unfortunately, most people don't understand these settings. Similarly to all living organisms, we are programmed for the survival of the species. What this means is that if you are not living to help preserve the human species, your body will turn on what Dr. Steven Gundry calls your killer genes.

In his book *Dr. Gundry's Diet Evolution*, he explains how we all have a self-destruct mechanism with which our bodies will start attacking themselves so we don't become a liability to the human species.[7] Sounds strange, I know, but stay with me and you'll understand what this means.

We believe we are in control of our bodies. We decide to talk, to walk, to clap our hands, etc. But there are other processes you don't control, or can control only up to a certain point. For example, let's say that you decide to hold your breath. You can hold your breath for some time, but then you will get to a point when your "autopilot" kicks in, and it will force you to breathe.

The autopilot system is set so you can live long enough to perform your primary function—spreading the species. Your DNA is programmed so humans as a species can live as long as possible. Get one thing straight: Your genes don't care about you. To them, you are not special; you are just a host. If, through your lifestyle, you are not doing what they expect from you, you will be seen as an obstacle, and your genetic code will remove you from the equation. Your genes will turn on the self-destruct mode, and *hasta la vista*, baby!

It's kind of spooky, but on the positive side, by understanding your programming, you can trick your genes into keeping you here longer.

SURVIVAL PROGRAMMING

To understand your programming, consider an example using a female lion. Let's call her Patrice. Just like all other animals, Patrice has an innate instinct to seek pleasure. Biologically speaking, the stimuli producing the sensation of pleasure are the ones that promote the survival of the species. In other words, animals are wired to feel good while doing the things that will help their kin survive.

The first example that pops to mind is sex. When fully developed, Patrice will want to spend the night with Fred, not because she always dreamt of becoming a mother and Fred seems like a friendly lion, but because she has pleasure with sex. By being programmed to enjoy the procreation act, she will want to do it more, and the chances of having little lions increase. More lions, better chances of the species surviving.

Beyond sex, Patrice also gets pleasure through food. When she is starving, she will eat whatever she can put her paw on, but if she can choose, she will prefer some fatty meat. As animals, we find more pleasure with calorie-dense foods. That's no coincidence. We derive more pleasure from these foods because they will provide us with more calories (even if the foods are not good for us, per se). More calories mean more fuel. More fuel means more energy to live another day and to go make some babies. At the end, that's all that matters.

If I give you the choice between eating a head of lettuce or a slice of cake, you might fight your instincts and go for the lettuce because you know the cake will not help you with your goals. But inside, you know the cake will taste *soooooo* much better. Occasionally, even though you consciously know you should pick the lettuce, you feel you don't have any willpower and you end up eating the cake. This is your programming. And the longing for pleasure is more powerful than the other instincts. For example, in a lab setting, rats were connected to a device that allowed them to press a button to receive a pleasure sensation in their brains. They became so addicted to pleasure that they didn't care about water or food. They just kept pressing the button until they starved to death.[8] Likewise, given a choice between a pellet of food and a pellet of cocaine, a rat will opt for cocaine until it dies.[9] This is the perfect example of why sometimes cake wins.

Let's go back to Patrice for another of the basic settings: energy conservation. Patrice and her fellow lions are lazy. They hunt some food and then spend a couple of days relaxing until their hunger forces them to do a little more hunting. Why is that? The same way she is programmed to seek high-calorie foods, she is also programmed to keep her metabolism low. That way, she will be more fuel efficient. If she were running around all day, she would burn her fuel reserves quicker, and if there was no food around, she could starve to death. By being lazy, she saves energy and can handle a couple of days without eating. The programming incentivizes getting the most energy with the least amount of effort.

The same happens with us. If you are hungry and you already have something there waiting for you to eat it, you won't think twice. But if you have nothing in the house, you often won't bother to go out and get anything.[10]

GENETIC PLEIOTROPY

Your programming is also designed to take into consideration the different stages of life. For instance, during early life, a high-calorie food might be good for you because it is making you grow and become strong. Eventually, you reach adulthood and you don't need as many calories, since you're no longer growing. Thus, if you continue to eat that same food, you notice you get fat and sick, and even age faster. Genes that activate one sequence of events during part of the life cycle will activate the opposite events in a later stage. This phenomenon is called genetic pleiotropy.

Going back to Patrice one last time. When she's growing, her genes want her to consume as many calories as possible so she can develop at warp speed. While she is young and procreating, she is still an important part of the master plan. As she ages, she becomes less important, and nature can't have her competing with other, younger females for food. Time to flip the switch (genetic pleiotropy) and start making her fat, sick, and old. The same foods that were great for her before are now slowly killing her.

KNOWING THE RULES

Now that you know the rules, you understand how you have these primal instincts that will slowly get you killed. You also comprehend how this world we live in, offering easy access to high-calorie foods, is not helping you with your goal of being healthy.

Fear not. By understanding the rules, we can also adapt our diets and lifestyles so we stop being perceived as inefficient humans who need to be eliminated. Throughout this book, we are going to discuss several strategies to trick your genes into believing that you still have a purpose here and you are not ready for self-destruction yet.

GENE MUTATIONS

At the beginning of this chapter, we talked about DNA and genes, but we did not discuss how we get these bad genes. Taking into consideration what we just discussed, let me ask you a question: If we were born with bad genes, why does our autopilot let us live long enough to procreate and pass on defective DNA? Supposedly, this is putting the human species at risk, right?

To answer this question, we need to get a bit more scientific and discuss gene mutations. When talking about gene mutations, our first thought is of being exposed to radiation and becoming like the Hulk or the Ninja Turtles. Unfortunately, according to my former science teacher, that doesn't happen in real life. Bummer!

Gene mutations, or single nucleotide polymorphisms (SNPs), are small DNA code changes that occur in at least 1 percent of the population. Scientists who know a lot more about this subject than I say that if these SNPs are maintained in our gene pool, it's because they might have neutral or even beneficial effects on species preservation.[11] For example, it is commonly accepted that the gene mutation that originates some red blood cell disorders such as thalassemia and sickle-cell disease may provide resistance against malarial infections.[12] In areas where malaria is common, individuals with this mutation are at an advantage for survival, and that is why your autopilot has kept that "bad gene."

As we learned before, when discussing epigenetics, we also know that diet and lifestyle have a major influence on your health and can activate and deactivate these genes. The physiological process controlling your genetic expression and determining whether a particular gene will be turned on or off is called methylation. When methylation occurs effectively, your body can keep bad genes turned off. On the other hand, if this system is not working properly, bad genes will be in full force. As Dr. Ben Lynch suggests in his book *Dirty Genes*, depression, anxiety, heart disease, dementia, obesity, autoimmune conditions, and cancer all have a genetic component.[13] We need proper methylation to keep these diseases in check.

Please note that methylation goes beyond genetic expression. It occurs countless times each second all over your body, playing an important role in cellular protection, metabolism, brain and muscle health, detoxification, stress response, immunity, cardiovascular function, and DNA repair.

OPTIMIZING METHYLATION

The best way to optimize your methylation is through diet and lifestyle. *Seeing a pattern here?* We want to make sure we are eating the foods with the nutrients required for these processes. And we also want to adopt a lifestyle congruent with our internal programming. Dr. Lynch states that some of the most important nutrients necessary for efficient methylation are protein, riboflavin (vitamin B_2), folate (vitamin B_9), cobalamin (vitamin B_{12}), and magnesium. Don't worry about looking for foods rich in these nutrients. I designed the Neo Diet considering these nutritional needs.

> **Neo Note: Folic Acid**
> Vitamin B_9, in its natural form, is called folate. The active version of this natural form is called methylfolate. Conversely, the artificial form you find in vitamins and food additives is called folic acid. According to Dr. Ben Lynch, this synthetic form is not usable but still gets into your folate receptors, preventing your body from using the real deal, methylfolate. This is important to know because many foods, like bread, cereal, cornmeal, flour, pasta, and rice, are enriched with folic acid and might put you at risk of not having enough methylfolate for proper methylation.
>
> Also, if you ever need to supplement with B_9, please make sure you're supplementing with folate and not folic acid.

There are other factors that Dr. Lynch also identifies as blockers of methylation. These are alcohol consumption, antacid consumption, inflammation, exposure to heavy metals, oxidative stress (accumulation of toxic free radicals), exposure to nitrous oxide, small intestinal bacterial overgrowth (SIBO), and other intestinal disturbances. Once again, these issues are covered in this book. *I got you!*

In conclusion, you do not have to worry about having bad genes. For most of the population, by respecting certain nutritional guidelines and adopting a better lifestyle (all inside the Neo Diet), you will be able to facilitate proper methylation and change your genetic destiny. In my case, I know that I have a genetic profile (and family history) that favors the development of Alzheimer's disease and colon cancer. However, I am taking care of my methylation through nutrition and lifestyle, and I'm confident I will be the one breaking this link and passing better genes to my offspring. You can do the same.

THE QUEST FOR ANSWERS

I think we can all agree that technology has had a tremendous impact on how we live. Just in the past 100 years alone, our lifestyles have changed dramatically. We spend most of our time indoors, get our food from grocery stores, binge-watch Netflix, and even have food delivery apps that bring already-prepared meals straight to our doorsteps. Obviously, there are good and bad sides to these advancements, but what's important here is to recognize that in those 100 years, our genetic code could not keep up with these lifestyle changes. It takes time for genes to adapt, and 100 years or even 1,000 years is insignificant compared with our entire timeline here on earth. Several researchers blame this evolutionary discordance as the cause of all disease.[14-20]

Even though I tend to agree with this hypothesis, I also don't feel like leaving my house and going to the woods to adopt the hunter-gatherer lifestyle in order to be in sync with my genes. Nothing wrong with that, but it's just not for me. Besides, since the Neolithic era, we can find tribes and civilizations that learned how to live with their Paleolithic genes and exhibited great health. These civilizations did not have access to the technology we have today, but we should not let that fact underrate the information they possessed. For centuries, even millennia, these peoples would test what worked and didn't work and then would pass this knowledge down from generation to generation.

Because of our shiny-new-toy syndrome, we shifted our attention toward new fads and lost touch with these ancient secrets. Luckily, recent research has uncovered the science behind many of these ancient practices, and we can now ascertain why they worked.

We will explore much of this knowledge throughout this book, but the moral of the story here is that our past holds many answers for a better future. By knowing our genetic wiring and how our world has changed, we can understand (without judgments) why we've been getting fatter, dumber, lazier, and sicker. Most importantly, we can avert this terrible fate.

FROM SCAVENGERS TO HUNTERS

I wish we could go on a field trip to the past inside the magic school bus, like in the cartoons. Unfortunately, that is not possible. *At least not yet.* The best we can do is to look at some of the best available data from anthropologists. Without going into tiresome details, I will focus on what I believe are the most important changes in our evolution and the evolution of our diet.

Set your clock to about 4 million years ago. Our ancestors of that time, beautifully named *Australopithecus afarensis*, are roaming around on their two feet. They are almost like a hybrid between what we would consider a modern human and a chimpanzee, but they still have more chimp in them than human. Their diet is like what our modern-day chimps eat—a menu filled mainly with grass, leaves, and fruits. Yummy!

At this stage, our mega-great-grandparents have small brains (just slightly bigger than what a present-day chimpanzee has), and their digestive tracts are also similar to those of our ape friends—big colons to ferment all those leaves, grasses, and fruits.

Fast-forward another 2 million years and suddenly their brain size starts to grow more rapidly. This pace was maintained until about 40,000 years ago, when the brain reached an apex volume of 1,600 cubic centimeters. With this brain growth, our ancestors became more intelligent and developed communication and group behavior, things that were essential for our evolution.

Some theorize that this sudden change resulted from learning about fire and using it to cook. Cooking would have allowed them to eat foods that were too tough or too toxic to eat raw. It also would have permitted them to consume more parts of the dead animals they found. Makes sense, but many scientists believe that our MasterChef skills did not emerge until about 500,000 years ago, which would not match our math.[21]

Independently of whether the cooking theory is correct, most authors agree that about 2.5 million years ago, our distant ancestors started using stone tools. This allowed them to transition from scavengers to hunters. They moved from eating plenty of leaves and grasses, and some animal leftovers, to all-you-can-eat barbecue, or steak tartare, depending on who's right about cooking. Either way, instead of being limited to bone marrow and brain (not accessible to other animals because of being surrounded by bone), now our ancestors could eat visceral organs, fat, and muscle meat.[22,23]

The abundance of calories and nutrients in these foods allowed us to grow our brain size exponentially and start shifting our digestive system. Even back then, we were wired to prioritize calorie-dense foods and to save energy. Why bother spending all day eating leaves when you could just kill one animal and get all the nutrition and calories needed for a couple of days? With this dietary change, our predecessors no longer needed large guts to break down cellulose from plants. Instead, according to what's called the expensive tissue hypothesis, our colons got smaller, and the extra "energy" went into the development of the brain.

Independently of your current dietary beliefs, animal foods were essential to our development. As stated by UC Berkeley researcher Katherine Milton in her paper *The Critical Role Played by Animal Source Foods in Human Evolution*:

> Without routine access to animal source foods, it is highly unlikely that evolving humans could have achieved their unusually large and complex brain while simultaneously continuing their evolutionary trajectory as large, active and highly social primates. As human evolution progressed, young children in particular, with their rapidly expanding large brain and high metabolic and nutritional demands relative to adults would have benefited from volumetrically concentrated, high quality foods such as meat.[24]

The more carnivorous diet clearly made our species bloom. Fossil records show that our hunter-gatherer ancestors had bigger brains but were also taller and had a sturdier bone structure than earlier specimens.[25]

Our ancestors would roam the African plain as clans. They would walk for miles in order to locate their prey. Clearly in no position to compete in the 100-meter dash with gazelles and antelopes, they took advantage of their bigger brains and newly developed communication skills to outsmart these animals. Catching one of them would mean food for everyone. After feasting on game, they would have plenty of time to relax and be social. They would also eat a few seasonal edible plants in combination with their meat. Once they were hungry again, it was time to repeat the cycle.

THE NEOLITHIC REVOLUTION

After this transition from scavengers to hunter-gatherers, the next major evolutionary shift happened about 10,000 years ago when *Homo sapiens* settled and started farming. No one knows exactly what led to this shift, but the transition to the Neolithic era radically changed our diet and the way we interacted with our environment. Most importantly, it set the foundation for human life as we know it today.

We were no longer nomads wandering the savanna looking for our next meal. Now we were living in settlements around our farms and domesticated animals. For the first time in history, we could produce a surplus of food beyond our daily needs. This abundance marked an increased rate of growth of our primitive communities and also permitted the development of our technology and cultural expansion.[26]

Living in permanent settlements with our animals, combined with inadequate sanitary practices, led to the spread of waterborne and zoonotic diseases. Short-term, this was catastrophic for our health, but from an evolutionary standpoint, the humans living with domesticated mammals ended up building immunity against many infectious diseases. Within each generation, this increased their chances of survival.

Grains became an integral part of our diet and changed our social dynamics. People could now cultivate these calorie-dense foods when and where they wished. Grains could also be easily stored and transported, which made them rank high in our Neolithic diet. There is no doubt they were essential to feeding these peoples, but as argued by the Paleo diet community, they also made us sicker. As you are going to learn later in this book, if not properly prepared and if consumed in excess, most grains have several toxic components that can harm us.

What is important to clarify is that the Neolithic era does not mark the introduction of grains. We were already eating grains, but probably in lesser quantities. Research shows that our ancestors were possibly consuming grains as early as the Middle Paleolithic (105,000 years ago), based on grass seed residue on tools found in Mozambique.[27]

With the rise in grain consumption in the Neolithic era, we can see an increase in certain diseases, but these were not shared by the entire population. Studies defend that those less active, in a higher position in the societal hierarchy (like tribe leaders), might have had excess weight, cardiovascular disease, and even teeth decay.[28] This is easy to justify since they would have had a sedentary lifestyle and would have been more prone to commit dietary excesses because of their societal position. However, for the population working in the fields, their massive energy expenditure would have made this high-calorie diet less harmful.

Am I saying the Paleo advocates are wrong? Not at all; several studies conclude that the transition to grain-based diets reduced life expectancy and average height, and increased infectious diseases, chronic diseases, inflammatory diseases, multiple nutritional deficiencies, and even infant mortality.[29-32] What I am saying is that there are always several sides to one story. Having a simplistic vision of any event limits your understanding. Yes, our Paleo genes were not prepared for such drastic change, but with time, we also learned how to capitalize on this Neolithic lifestyle. Not only were we able to domesticate more and more animals for their meat and dairy, but we also used their manure for our soils and their wool for clothing.

Time and experience brought us more wisdom. All over the world, different cultures had different processes to achieve better nutrition and to minimize the toxic effects of some of these "non-Paleo" foods. As Dr. Catherine Shanahan mentions in her book *Deep Nutrition*, "This library of knowledge was not a tertiary aspect of these cultures. It was ensconced safely within the vaults of religious doctrine and ceremony to ensure its unending revival." Through trial and error, these traditional cultures were able not only to survive but to thrive in this Neolithic lifestyle.

THE INDUSTRIAL REVOLUTION

The transition between the late 18th century and the beginning of the 19th century marks the Industrial Revolution. As the name indicates, this represents the shift from hand labor to machine-powered industry. Not only did this constitute a change in our labor practices, but it also started a philosophical shift. Our past was no longer a source of wisdom. Now, the past was to be forgotten; the future held all the answers.

In the 1890s, technology brought us the steel-roller mill, which processed grains into flour without the oil-rich germ and fiber-rich bran. With this change in processing, you could no longer get any nutrition out of this food, and your body would digest it incredibly fast, similar to table sugar. Just in the USA alone (a population whose diet contained a lot of white flour), deficiencies of B vitamins became highly prevalent and caused thousands of deaths.[33] To fix this health crisis, the federal government ordered white flour to be fortified with at least eight essential vitamins and minerals (the same ones the industrial processing removed).

Using technology in our agricultural practices brought even further nutritional deficiencies. Modern agriculture changed our farming approach into intensive monocropping. This new model of food production has been destroying the quality of our soils. While growing more crops at faster speeds, we end up depleting our soils of nutrients and consequently produce nutritionally impaired foods.[34] Even the US Senate recognized in 1936, "The alarming fact is that foods—fruits, vegetables, and grains—now being raised on millions of acres of land that no longer contains enough of certain needed nutrients, are starving us—no matter how much we eat of them."[35]

After the great world wars, things only got worse. A lot of money had been invested in the chemical industry trying to find an edge during the wars. Now, without conflict, the chemical industry had to focus elsewhere. This led us to the development of synthetic herbicides, fungicides, and insecticides. Coincidently, we also discovered that antibiotics and synthetic hormones made our livestock grow a lot faster. Since this was good for business, we started pumping our animals with both.

During this time, the pharmaceutical industry also took off. New medications were being created by the day. We no longer needed to be responsible for our health. We could forget all the knowledge from the past on how to prevent disease. Now, you could do whatever you wanted without consequences since there would be a pill to fix your dietary mistakes. Even medical school changed. Nutrition and lifestyle were no longer relevant, and all the focus shifted toward learning about these new drugs, their uses, and their side effects.

Eventually, we reached a point in our technological evolution where it was possible to genetically modify our crops (GMO). This was a game changer, because now we could program these organisms to grow faster, produce their own pesticides, and even make them more tolerant to the chemical herbicides we were using.

This was great for business. But what about our health? Let me just quote what best-selling author Dave Asprey wrote in his book *The Bulletproof Diet*: "As GMOs have become popular over the past 3 decades, there has also been a 400 percent increase in allergies, a 300 percent increase in asthma, a 400 percent increase in attention deficit/hyperactivity disorder, and a 1,500 percent increase in autism spectrum disorder."[36] Obviously we need more research to link with certainty the rise of many diseases with the consumption of GMOs, but the warning signs are scary enough to cause concern.

Neo Note: Bt Toxin

The Bt (*Bacillus thuringiensis*) delta-endotoxin has been genetically added to crops like corn, potatoes, and soybeans to work as an insecticide. This toxin creates pores in the intestines of the insect, which eventually causes their death.[37] The concerning issue is that a study has shown that Bt toxin can puncture holes through the human digestive tract as well.[38] The toxin has also been shown to be carried by pregnant women and transmitted to their fetuses, possibly predisposing the babies to food intolerances.[39] Furthermore, studies show a connection between Bt toxin and autoimmune response to foods that were previously digestible and even the development of intestinal permeability.[40,41]

GMOs also allowed for an increase in the use of herbicides, fungicides, and insecticides. Crops were now immune to these, so to get better yields, we could just spray the crap out of them.

The most common chemical used is glyphosate (Roundup).[42] Glyphosate is used not only to prevent weeds from attacking crops but also to dry them out faster before harvesting.[43]

According to author Max Lugavere, "more than thirteen billion pounds of glyphosate-based herbicides have doused the world's crops over the last decade. In the United States alone, its usage has increased nearly sixteenfold between 1992 and 2009."[44]

The heavy spraying spreads this chemical beyond the traditional crops. Not to mention that these same crops are then used to feed our animals and even to produce other foods. Because of all this, glyphosate residue has been found in grains, fish, meat, berries, vegetables, and even baby formula.[45,46]

Glyphosate has been associated with the growth of pathogenic (bad) organisms in the human digestive tract, kidney disease, and even certain cancers.[47–50]

PORNOGRAPHIC FOOD

Technology has changed not only the way we produce our food but also the ways we prepare and process it. We went beyond simple processing like fermenting, sprouting, freezing, or canning food, to "ultraprocessing" methods that include the use of dyes, flavor enhancers, and artificial preservatives.

The more we hacked our food production, the fewer nutrients and the less flavor our foods had. In order to keep selling these cheap sources of calories, food companies had to use artificial flavors to make food taste good again. Not only that, but to make food products more commercially attractive, they had to be shelf stable for the longest time possible. If you have a product that goes bad in three days, how can you transport it and have it in stores for sale? You can't. But if this food is full of preservatives, it can last months or even years without going bad.

In the same way we have access to information about our genetic programming, the food industry also has it. They understood that if they could stimulate the hedonic (pleasure) centers in your brain, they could play your biology against you. A fondness for fat, sugar, and salt was wired into our brains in prehistoric times to make us feel pleasure, since, as discussed before, these flavors signal a high concentration of calories (and minerals, with salt), which was essential for our survival. By using and abusing these flavors, food producers knew they could sell their products.

In his book *Wired to Eat*, Paleo expert Robb Wolf explains how the food industry is following in the footsteps of the porn industry.[51] Similarly to food, sex also stimulates certain pleasure centers in your brain. There are many neurotransmitters that can give you this pleasurable sensation, but probably the most important one is dopamine. Stimulating the brain's dopamine centers creates a positive feedback loop in which a person desires more of the substance or activity that originated the initial "feel-good" chemicals. The problem with this positive feedback loop is that with time, for you to have the same level of pleasure, you need more quantity or diversity of stimuli. This is also the typical porn addiction situation. An addict might have started with a very soft five-minute clip, but now, to get the same pleasure response, that person needs to watch five or six clips of the weirdest stuff your mind can conceive.

Hyperpalatable foods are the equivalent of the kinkier porn. These foods combine several flavors in order to stimulate your taste buds like never before. After you eat a deep-fried Oreo with ice cream, eating an apple will feel comparable to eating cardboard.

Hyperpalatable foods also have another effect on us. You can't stop eating them. Lay's potato chips even used to tell you this in their slogan "Bet you can't eat just one!" The stimuli in your brain are so powerful, they completely override any satiety signal.

If this weren't enough, you also have ads about these foods being shown to you at all times of the day. They're on your phone, they're on TV, they're on the radio, they're on highway billboards, they're everywhere. We are so brainwashed that studies show that about 15 percent of our daily thoughts are some version of "What's for dinner? Do I need food right now?"[52]

THE DANGERS OF THE MODERN DIET

Ultraprocessed food (which I'm just going to call "processed food" for simplicity) has effects beyond addiction. The more than 3,000 additives in our food may interact with our biology in ways we are still uncovering to this day.

In one systematic review, researchers concluded that exposure to compounds often found in processed foods is a risk factor for developing autoimmune disease.[53,54] They even stated that those with a family history of autoimmunity should avoid these foods at all costs.

Several studies have connected the consumption of synthetic colors and flavors in processed foods to diseases of the respiratory system (asthma and cough), skin, gastrointestinal (GI) tract, and skeletal system, as well as to allergies, headaches, and behavioral disorders like ADHD.[55-59]

The issue is not exclusive to these brand-new lab-made foods, or "frankenfoods." Foods that we used to produce through traditional methods are now being processed with all kinds of additives to lower their production cost. Deli meats, for example, are now filled with hydrogenated fats and nitrites, which are associated with a greater risk of cancer.[60]

Even something that looks as harmless as microwave popcorn can create serious health issues. Research shows that microwave popcorn contains perfluorooctanoic acid (PFOA).[61] Does the name sound familiar? Possibly you heard it in the movie *Dark Waters*. If you haven't seen the film, please do. PFOA is a synthetic chemical found in nonstick pans that's been linked to cancer and hormone disruption.[62]

One of the best-known artificial flavorings is monosodium glutamate (MSG). It was created in Japan during World War II. Due to food scarcity, it was important to sell all foods even if they were spoiled. When MSG was added, any food would taste great. This was a way to keep the population fed with cheap and easy-to-produce foods. As always, this benefit comes with a cost. MSG consumption has been associated with obesity, metabolic syndrome, liver damage, cardiovascular disease, diabetes, behavioral problems, nerve damage, and increased inflammation.[63-65]

MSG is present in processed foods (especially Asian foods); chips; commercial seasoning blends; commercial soups, dressings, and sauces; frozen meals; instant noodles; and processed meats.

Even though I've focused mostly on these examples, there are many other artificial additives that bring serious consequences for your health. For more information, I highly recommend the book *Food Forensics*, by Mike Adams.

I hope you've been able to see through this very condensed human evolution section how our diet and lifestyle have significantly impacted our health. We still have those Paleo genes, but we live in a much different world. For a period of time, we were able to find strategies to make them work in a new environment, but then with the Industrial Revolution, we lost this ancient wisdom that had been successfully followed for centuries.

What we now eat differs substantially from what we used to eat. Moreover, the way our food is now produced depletes it of nutrients and, worse, makes it toxic for us. We are getting fatter, sicker, and dumber, but we can change all this if we start using food as medicine, like our ancestors once did.

The great news is that you are about to learn how to change all this.

NEO SUMMARY

• DNA does not control your destiny. Epigenetic factors such as diet, lifestyle and environmental exposures, will almost exclusively determine your health-span and quality of life.

• You can "turn off" your bad genes.

• You are programmed for the survival of the human species, not for your individual survival. If you don't understand and follow these biological "hints", your body might turn on its self-destruction mode. Conversely, if you understand this programing, you can trick our body into keeping you strong and healthy for longer than most.

• The evolutionary shift from scavengers to hunter-gatherers marked the transition from being "more ape" into being "more human".

• The transition into the Neolithic Era was an essential move toward life as we know it, but it also created a genetic mismatch between our DNA and our lifestyle.

• Ancient civilizations had a wealth of knowledge that allowed them to thrive.

• The Industrial Revolution disconnected us with the past and lead to the development of our modern diet, depleted of nutrients and full of toxins that are making us sick.

• The food industry has been using your biology against you. The food they promote might be bad for you but great for business.

NEO ACTION

• Forgive yourself. It's not your fault. The food industry has been messing with your biology.

• Eliminate processed foods from your diet. Stay away from any food that has been created/modified in a factory. If you can't find it in nature, don't eat it.

• Cook more. That's the only way to control the quality of the ingredients you are consuming. Favor locally-grown and organic produce.

NEO RECOMMENDATIONS

SCAN ME

• *Deep Nutrition* by Dr. Catherine Shanahan
• *Dirty Genes* by Dr. Ben Lynch
• *Dr. Gundry's Diet Evolution* by Dr. Steven Gundry
• *Food Forensics* by Mike Adams
• *Paleo Principles* by Sarah Ballantyne
• *Real Food, Fake Food* By Larry Olmsted
• *Seeds of Deception* by Jeffrey Smith
• *The New Evolution Diet* by Arthur De Vany
• *The Story of the Human Body* by Daniel Lieberman
• *Undoctored* by Dr. William Davis
• *Wired to Eat* by Robb Wolf

my.neodiet.co/neorecommendations

It's Kind of a Sh*tty Story

"Take all that is given whether wealth, love or language, nothing comes by mistake and with good digestion all can be turned to health."
George Herbert

DIGESTION 101

In this chapter, we are going to talk about the digestive journey inside us. Well, technically, the journey is not inside us but outside, but I'll get to that detail later. This anatomy and physiology lesson is important because it's a lot easier to make positive changes if you understand what on earth is going on inside you.

Most of us think of our gastrointestinal (GI) tract as this long and twisted tunnel that extends from your mouth to your anus. The truth is that this "tunnel" is a lot more complex than most assume. Not only is your digestive system responsible for breaking down your food, absorbing nutrients, and removing waste products, but three-quarters of your immune system resides in your GI tract.

Similarly to your skin, your GI tract is responsible for keeping the outside environment away from your insides. It's almost like a tunnel under a river. The cars (food) enter through one side and exit through the other side. In their entire journey, even though the tunnel takes them through the river, they are not in contact with the water (the rest of your insides). Get it?

Your digestive system creates this selective barrier that chooses what should and should not go inside of you. If this barrier gets penetrated by the wrong things, inflammation and disease will result.

Let's pretend for a second that the magic bus we used in the previous chapter can now shrink to pill size and take us on another field trip.

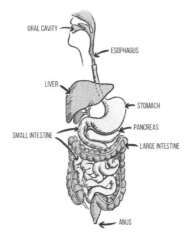

First stop is in your mouth. Just by thinking about food, you cause glands in your mouth to produce saliva. Saliva is rich in digestive enzymes that, along with the physical process of chewing, start breaking down the food. Without trying to sound like your parents . . . please chew your food, people! It's one of those things that sound so obvious, yet most of us just swallow our food in a rush to go back to whatever we were doing. By not chewing properly, you make it more likely that some food will go all the way to your intestines still undigested, which can lead to abdominal pain and gas. Not to mention that you miss out on nutrition still locked up in those undigested bits of food.

While you have all this action happening in your mouth, your stomach is already setting the mood for the next step. It releases hydrochloric acid and more enzymes to make sure you have the right chemical bomb to "melt" the food. In order to access the stomach, we need to go down the water slide called the esophagus. At the end of the slide . . . splash. We drop in the middle of all the digestive juices that were already waiting for us. While starches (carbohydrates) were already being slowly digested by your saliva, in the stomach we start breaking down protein. This occurs because of the highly acidic environment created by hydrochloric acid (the pH of the stomach should be around 2 to 2.5) and due to the action of the enzyme pepsin.

Inside this J-shaped organ, we also have muscular action from its walls to ensure that the food and all these juices are decently ground and mixed.

Possibly because of all the antacid ads on TV, many of us think stomach acid is a bad thing. As we've learned, though, this acidic environment is essential to breaking down protein. But that's not all. The acid facilitates the absorption of calcium and vitamin B_{12}, and it is crucial for destroying harmful microorganisms present in food. If you don't have enough stomach acid (a condition called hypochlorhydria), most likely food particles that would normally be broken down will now reach your lower intestines undigested. Here, they become fuel for pathogenic microorganisms and cause their overgrowth. As you will learn later, this is not a good thing. These undigested food particles might also pass through a damaged intestinal wall and trigger a full-blown immune reaction. Also a big no-no.

Hypochlorhydria (whether natural or produced by excessive consumption of antacids) is a serious problem and can contribute to various infections, anemia, osteoporosis, vitamin B_{12} deficiency, pathogenic stomach and intestinal bacteria overgrowth, and even stomach cancer.[1-6]

In his book *Why Stomach Acid Is Good for You*, Dr. Jonathan V. Wright claims that half of the American population over 50 years of age lacks the appropriate amount of stomach acid to fully digest their food.[7] This might result from taking acid-blocking medications and also from stress, poor diet, or harmful chemicals.[8]

But what about heartburn? We've been told all our lives that heartburn is produced by excess acid. Recently, many authors have been asserting the exact opposite: that most heartburn may be caused by insufficient acid. If you don't have enough acid, food will linger in your stomach longer than it should. The more time it stays there, the higher the risk of food fermentation and irritation of the stomach lining. Additionally, in a low-acid environment, pathogenic microbes such as *H. pylori* can proliferate and further inflame the stomach lining, causing heartburn.[9]

Heartburn is one of the symptoms of gastroesophageal reflux disease (GERD). According to nutrition expert Ann Louise Gittleman, heartburn might simply be a mechanical issue.[10] In people with GERD, the lower esophageal sphincter (LES), the valve that separates the end of the esophagus from the beginning of the stomach, might fail to close properly. When this happens, reflux occurs and the acid (even in people with hypochlorhydria) irritates the sensitive esophagus, creating the burning sensation. Overeating, consumption of alcohol, and the delayed emptying of the stomach (due to low acid), for example, can increase stomach pressure and make the LES malfunction.[11,12]

> **Neo Note: Are You Producing Enough Acid?**
> If you have GERD symptoms and want to assess whether you're producing enough acid but don't want to go to your doctor, here is a simple DIY test I learned from Ben Greenfield's book *Boundless*.[13]
> 1. Mix ¼ teaspoon of baking soda into ½ to ¾ cup of cold water.
> 2. Drink the baking soda solution before eating or drinking anything else, then time how long it takes for you to burp or belch.
> 3. If you don't burp within five minutes of drinking the solution, then you aren't producing enough stomach acid.

BILIARY SYSTEM DETOUR

After the stomach, our mini submersible will reach the small intestine. Before we continue our journey in search of the light at the end of the tunnel, let's pause for a minute. Even though they are not part of the "digestive tunnel," we have a couple of organs that need to be mentioned because of their role in your digestion.

We'll start our detour with the gallbladder. The gallbladder is a small, pear-shaped organ located right beneath your liver. Although the digestive substance called bile is produced in the liver, the gallbladder is essential because it works as a container where bile is concentrated and released when the time comes. Without this container, bile would continually trickle to your small intestine independently of what and how much you ate. This may not sound like something to really worry about, but it is. After the removal of the gallbladder, patients face an increased risk of obesity, metabolic syndrome, type 2 diabetes, fatty liver, and heart disease.[14-17]

Bile helps break down and absorb fats. It also has an important role in the absorption of the fat-soluble vitamins (A, D, E, and K) and the recycling of bilirubin (a waste product from the destruction of aged or abnormal red blood cells) in the body.[18] In addition, bile helps to maintain healthy bowel movements, buffer the acids from the stomach, and, because of its ability to interact with fats, facilitate the detoxification of "bad" fats and toxins by flushing them out.[19,20]

Finally, bile acids function in a manner similar to hormones, taking part in metabolic functions such as energy balance, regulation of fat metabolism, and glycemic control.[21]

Due to a poor diet and exposure to a high toxic load (more about these soon), your bile can become thick and even lead to the formation of gallstones. Thick bile will have many nasty consequences for your health. In Ann Louise Gittleman's book *Radical Metabolism*, she explains that "without healthy bile, you simply can't get those fabulous fat-blasting, immunity-boosting, cell membrane–protecting, fuel-providing benefits—no matter how good your diet is. What you will get is gas, bloating, reflux, constipation, and weight gain."[22]

As mentioned earlier, bile also works as a buffer for the stomach acids. If you're not secreting enough bile, your body, to protect your small intestine from being corroded (causing duodenal ulcers, intestinal irritation, or leaky gut, for example), will ratchet back the amount of hydrochloric acid (HCl) in your stomach. And you already know the consequences of that.

Since bile also works like a toxin magnet, helping flush out contaminants inside you, if you don't have proper bile flow, your body will accumulate them at a faster pace. Accumulation of toxins in your body can trigger many health problems, including obesity, hormone imbalance, insulin resistance, hypothyroidism, and autoimmune issues.[23-26]

> **Neo Note: Bile and Hypothyroidism**
> Did you know that people with reduced bile flow have greater rates of hypothyroidism?[27,28]
> This happens because bile triggers the release of an enzyme that converts T4 (less-active thyroid hormone) into T3 (the more active form). Besides that, the raw materials needed to produce active thyroid hormones come from the proper digestion of dietary fats. Without proper bile flow, you can't adequately digest and absorb these raw materials.
> To make things worse, hypothyroidism slows emptying of the biliary tract, which puts you in a vicious circle.

Unfortunately, most people don't realize they have a gallbladder problem or gallstones until they experience a serious crisis. Here is a list of symptoms that can be connected with poor bile flow: burping; gas; bloating; constant feeling of fullness; constipation; dry skin and hair; GERD; headache over the eyes; hemorrhoids; hypothyroidism; difficulty losing weight; light-colored or floating stools; mood changes such as irritability, depression, or anxiety; nausea after meals; pain between the shoulder blades, in the right shoulder, or up the right side of the neck; and varicose veins.

We cannot continue our journey without a quick shout-out to my OG, the liver. Besides producing bile, the liver is involved in many metabolic, hormonal, immune, and detox processes. To be fair, the liver is involved in just about everything happening in your body. We are not going into detail here, but just remember that this is one of the most important organs you have.

Finally, we can't forget about the pancreas. Usually, people only think about the pancreas as the organ that produces insulin. The truth is that the pancreas also secretes enzymes into the small intestine that are essential in the digestion of carbohydrates, fats, and protein.

THE NOT-SO-SMALL INTESTINE

Let's resume our trip, shall we? After it's been partially digested by acid in the stomach, food passes into the duodenum, the first part of the small intestine. *Small* is misleading since, in reality, if we straightened out all the twists, the small intestine would be about 20 feet (or 6 meters) long. But let's not get sidetracked here.

The duodenum is the place to be. It receives the predigested food from the stomach and mixes it with bile and pancreatic juices. These digestive fluids are added to buffer the stomach acid and to further digest the food. Ideally, at the end of this step, proteins are broken down into peptides and amino acids; fats are broken down into fatty acids and glycerol; and carbohydrates are broken down into oligosaccharides and monosaccharides (i.e., glucose). Apart from continuing to digest the food, the small intestine is also responsible for most nutrient absorption.

The mucosa that covers the walls of the small intestine is coated with finger-like projections called villi. The villi, in turn, are covered with hair-like projections called microvilli. Thanks to this design, the surface area available for nutrient absorption is roughly the size of half of a badminton court.[29] Inside each villus, there are blood capillaries and special lymphatic capillaries called lacteals. Most nutrients are absorbed by the blood capillaries, while fat and fat-soluble vitamins are absorbed by the lacteals.

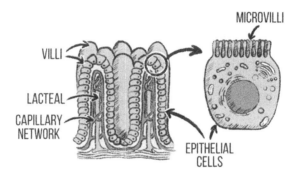

Water-soluble nutrients (proteins, carbohydrates, and some vitamins and minerals) pass into the bloodstream through the capillaries, where they are transported to your warehouse manager, the liver, to be processed and then sent to whatever organs and tissues need them.

Once the fats and fat-soluble vitamins are absorbed through the lacteals, these nutrients combine with lymphatic fluid and take a ride through your lymphatic vessels until eventually they reach your bloodstream for distribution.

Regardless of all the steps involved, your body can run this process smoothly, as long as you have a strong digestion (enough chewing, enough saliva, enough stomach acid, enough bile and pancreatic juices) and your gut lining is intact.

But if you are not breaking down food as you should and/or if you have damage to your villi or microvilli, absorption is compromised. Or worse, this can cause holes in your intestinal walls. Without the intestines' proper integrity, you will have stuff that should not be getting absorbed going inside your system and creating havoc.

Assuming all goes well, by the time the food slurry leaves the small intestine and enters the large intestine (a.k.a. the colon), around 90 percent of the nutrients have been extracted and absorbed. In the colon you will have absorption of water and other remaining vitamins, like vitamins K, B_1, and B_2.[30] Then, although you can't digest anything else in your large intestine, you have gut bacteria living there that are able to take care of the rest. These trillions of bacteria continue the digestive process by fermenting the undigested foods. This fermentation also creates short-chain fatty acids (SCFAs), which promote healthy colon cell growth and support our health in many other ways.

If everything is working as it should, this whole digestive process should take around 24 hours. When you get to this point, the human hosting our field trip will follow the *Star Wars* motto and "Use the Force." *Splash.* We reached the toilet. End of field trip.

Obviously, I've tried to simplify these concepts as much as I could. I'm sure there could have been ways to explore this in more detail, but let's not be anal about it. (Sorry. Couldn't resist.)

WE HAVE NO LOVE FOR LYMPH

Hippocrates (460–377 BC) was possibly the first person to explore the lymphatic system, calling lymph "white blood." However, proper research and documentation only commenced in the 17th century, although even then, not much importance was given to this system.[31] Luckily for us, more research has been done in the past two decades, and this has led us to better understand the importance of the lymphatic system. Not only is it crucial because of its role in our digestion, but it also plays a major role in immunity, the regulation of tissue pressure, and detoxification of the body.[32]

> **Neo Note: The Lymphatic System beyond Digestion**
> Our lymphatic system is mainly made up of a network of lymphatic vessels and lymph nodes, along with our tonsils, spleen, and thymus.
>
> Your lymph nodes are oval-shaped tanks that serve as a collection and filtration system for the lymphatic fluid, or lymph, removing damaged cells, infectious organisms, foreign particles, and toxins. Lymph nodes also contain specialized white blood cells designed to engulf and destroy these aggressors. Most lymph nodes are found in the neck, axillae (armpits), and inguinal region (groin).
>
> Your tonsils (at the sides of your throat) are an important part of your immune response since they produce antibodies and also trap bacteria and viruses entering your body through your mouth and nose.
>
> The spleen is the largest lymphatic organ. It filters and purifies your blood and produces mature immune cells that can identify and destroy pathogens.
>
> Finally, the thymus is located in front of your heart and helps your immune system by creating T cells—a specific type of white blood cell that protects the body from certain threats, including viruses and infections.

In your GI tract, the lymphatic system starts in the intestinal lining as lacteals within the villi. These lacteals absorb fat and other fatty acids from the small intestine. What I didn't mention before is that beyond these lacteals, we have a whole complex lymphatic network working closely with your intestinal epithelium (the first line of cells that make up the "you-shall-not-pass" wall) to protect you. The gut-associated lymphatic tissue (GALT) is your second line of defense. Whenever large, undigested proteins, fat-soluble toxins, or even pathogenic bacteria are able to cross your first line of defense, the GALT is there to identify these unauthorized visitors and escort them to jail (the lymph nodes), where they'll be processed and eventually eliminated.[33-35]

We cannot expect our first line of defense to always work, and some action for the GALT is actually good to keep it sharp and ready to respond. How can a soldier be prepared if there's never an opportunity to practice? The problem here is that our poor diet and toxic lifestyle are making our digestive process weaker and also increasing the permeability of our intestinal walls. This allows invaders to be a lot more frequent. And that causes your lymph to become congested.

Studies suggest that congested (full of toxins) lymph can move into the body's fat cells and intercellular spaces, causing toxicity that has been linked to the production and metastasis of tumors.[36-39] Lymphatic congestion has also been associated with inflammation, autoimmunity, depression, and mood alterations.[40-50] Other signs and symptoms connected with a congested lymphatic system are eczema, hives, arthritis, chronic fatigue, fibromyalgia, depressed immune system (frequent infections or viruses), lymph node swelling, and muscle and joint pain.[51]

As you now can understand, your digestive system and your lymphatic system are the gateway to your health. By having them operating at full force, you are guaranteed to feel amazing.

Next, we are going to break myths about healthy eating. It will shock you to learn that some of the foods you've been told to eat more of are actually making you sick. I know, it's hard to digest . . . literally!

NEO SUMMARY
• Your digestion starts in your mouth with chewing and mixing your food with saliva.
• Your digestive system is your first line of defense.
• Most of your digestive issues are not the result of excessive stomach acid, but the contrary, lack of it.
• A fully functional gallbladder is essential not only for your digestive system but also for your detox and metabolic processes.
• Your small intestine is where most of the digestion and absorption occurs.
• The "neglected" lymphatic system is essential for your digestion and immune response.

NEO ACTION
• Chew your food thoroughly.
• Eat in a relaxed state of mind. Don't rush.
• Avoid overeating.
• Antacids should be the last approach, not the first.

NEO RECOMMENDATIONS
• *Biohacker's Handbook* by Olli Sovijärvi, Teemu Arina, Jaakko Halmetoja
• *Eat Wheat* by Dr. John Douillard
• *Lymph & Longevity* by Dr. Gerald Lemole
• *Radical Metabolism* by Ann Louise Gittleman
• *Why Stomach Acid Is Good for You* by Dr. Jonathan V. Wright
• *Wired to Eat* by Robb Wolf

SCAN ME

my.neodiet.co/neorecommendations

LET'S TALK ABOUT ANTINUTRIENTS

These "Healthy" Foods Are Making You Sick

"You shall know the truth, and the truth shall make you mad."
Aldous Huxley

THINK TWICE

One thing we've all grown to know is that plant foods are the healthiest foods available to us. If it comes from a plant, it cannot cause any harm. It's a fact!

But is it, though?

I'm not exactly sure how this myth started, but somehow we have all been brainwashed to believe that plants are these benign beings happy to feed us.

No question that plants have plenty of nutrients that are imperative for our health, but research has also shown us that many plants contain compounds that might block the absorption of these nutrients. And, worse, some plants contain substances capable of attacking our bodies and making us sick. Why is this research not mainstream? I don't know, but in this chapter we're going to unveil the truth so you learn the entire story.

In chapter 1, we learned that all living things have engraved in their DNA the instructions to ensure the survival of the species. That is always priority number one. Plants also want to stay alive as long as possible. It's not like they are there hoping to be "chosen" by the "gods" (us) who will deliver them to "the great beyond" (like in the *Sausage Party* movie). No way. They are just creative in the ways they attack their predators, you included.

It's said that plants appeared about 450 million years ago, while insects only got here about 90 million years later.[1] During the time before insects came on the scene, plants had a blast. They could grow and reproduce with no one trying to kill them. When insects and, later, other animals were added to the equation, the story changed. Suddenly they were being eaten left and right, and they had no way of fighting it.

With time, plants adapted to this new reality and began learning how to protect themselves. Some developed colors to improve their camouflage game, others evolved to have hard or pointy outer coatings, and some even started producing sticky substances like resin to trap their predators. Most of them, though, became chemical experts and created compounds that, when ingested, would taste bad, make the predator sick, or even kill it. These compounds are called antinutrients.

As the name suggests, antinutrients' key feature is the obstruction of the absorption of nutrients. They bind to them and block your ability to absorb them, which consequently leads to nutritional deficiencies. Some also function as enzyme inhibitors that will affect your digestive process and cause GI distress or disease. There are even antinutrients so toxic they can disrupt the functions of cells and tissues.[2-7]

One thing we have to keep in mind is that these chemical defenses were initially built to fight off plants' main predators, insects. Obviously, a larger animal has a better ability to tolerate these compounds. But does this mean they're harmless for larger animals, including humans? Of course not. Some antinutrients are strong enough to kill if consumed in sufficient quantities.

In the natural world, if an animal consumes a plant with enough antinutrients to make it feel unwell, it won't eat that plant again. Intuitively, animals also know to stay away from these plants. Years of evolution and information being passed down created this innate intelligence. This "intuition," though, is not just seen in animals. Have you ever wondered why most children hate vegetables? Dr. Steven Gundry justifies this as part of our genetic programming, our inner intelligence. Since many vegetables are full of antinutrients, your body tries to keep you away from them while you are still fragile and in development. It does this by making your taste buds perceive these flavors as bad and even nauseating. As you grow and your body is stronger to tolerate these antinutrients, suddenly they no longer taste as bad as before.[8]

Nausea in early pregnancy might be a similar defensive mechanism against antinutrients.[9] Nausea is usually present in the first trimester, which, coincidentally or not, is also the most critical period in the development of the fetus's organs. Then, like magic, for most women the nausea is gone.

As you are going to learn, there are several plants that are safe to eat, and there are even ways to prepare "harmful plants" in order to reduce their toxicity. Then we also have to consider the different parts of the plant. For example, the plants' seeds, since they are responsible for the next generation and the survival of the species, need to be protected at all costs. Therefore, many seeds are full of antinutrients, while ripe fruits, designed to be eaten to spread the seed in the soil, are mostly harmless. However, if you eat some fruits before they're ready to "go on their journey," you can develop a host of problems, from fever to encephalopathy, to death.[10]

Don't panic. You have been consuming antinutrients and you are still here. Your body has a fantastic detoxification system that is able to eliminate a lot of these toxins. The problem occurs when your consumption of these compounds is greater than your ability to get rid of them.

Back in the day, we would listen to our bodies. If we felt unwell, we would stop eating (or cut back on) the foods that were making us sick. This would give our detox systems the breather they needed to catch up.

Now, with our modern medical approach, as soon as you start feeling something, instead of paying attention to these warnings, you shut them off. If you experience a heavy stomach, you take Nexium. If you have diarrhea, you take Imodium. If you feel aches and pains, you take ibuprofen. Our current approach is like having the house on fire but deciding to just take the batteries out of the fire alarm. Yes, it shuts down the noise, but it doesn't fix the problem.

You are not doing yourself any favors by hiding these symptoms. Things might start just with digestive distress. However, eventually they will progress to nutritional deficiencies, and even full-blown autoimmune reactions attacking different systems in your body.[11]

> **Neo Note: Medicating Our Cattle**
> Cows, in their natural environment, pasture on grasses and other forage. That's what they like and are designed to eat. Unfortunately, in industrial farms –(concentrated animal feeding operations, or CAFOs) they are fed corn and soybeans. These foods are cheap to produce and make them grow and fatten up faster. The faster the animal reaches market weight, the sooner it can be sold, and the farmer paid.
>
> The problem is that corn and soy are full of lectins (a type of antinutrient). These compounds cause such severe heartburn and pain that the cows eventually stop eating. To solve this issue, farmers add antacids to their food to ensure that they continue to eat and get fat quickly. [12]

Besides our erroneous medical approach, we cannot forget that we also live in a much more toxic world than before. Our detox systems are constantly overwhelmed and cannot tolerate the same amounts of antinutrients. This makes it essential to know more about these substances so we can be more thoughtful about our diets. Some of the most known antinutrients are chaconine, flavonoids, gluten, isoflavones, lectins, oxalates, phytic acid (also called phytate), polyphenols, saponins, solanine, tannins, and trypsin inhibitors.[13]

But aren't polyphenols and tannins good for us? Some antinutrients, in certain doses, have many health benefits, as we'll discuss later in this chapter. For now, we're going to focus on the ones my research led me to believe are the most dangerous and the ones to be avoided as much as possible.

LECTINS

Among all the antinutrients I just mentioned, lectins are probably the best known. Many articles have been written about their effects on our health, and many authors have made them "Internet famous."

Lectins were described for the first time by Peter Hermann Stillmark in his doctoral thesis in 1888 about the toxic effects of ricin, the lectin in castor beans.[14] Ricin is so toxic that a dose the size of a few grains of salt is enough to kill an adult. Fortunately, most lectins are not this strong. Nonetheless, they still have a significant impact on our health.

It's easy to find hundreds of recorded lectin-related food poisoning outbreaks. In the UK, between 1976 and 1989, there were 50 incidents of food poisoning from red kidney beans. Similar outbreaks have also been reported in Canada and Australia.[15]

But lectins can cause more than just your typical food-poisoning sweaty diarrhea. Several studies have linked them to weight gain, arthritis, brain fog, leaky gut syndrome, and other inflammatory conditions.[16–18]

So, what are lectins anyway? They are mostly large, "sticky" proteins that permanently attach themselves to the sugars in your body. By sticking to these sugars, lectins compromise cell communication and cause inflammatory reactions in several bodily systems.[19] According to Dr. Gundry, lectins also facilitate the binding of viruses and bacteria to their intended targets.[20]

Not all lectins are created equal, nor do all of us react to them the same way. Some of us are more sensitive than others to specific types of lectins. You might be allergic to peanuts (full of the lectin peanut agglutinin—PNA) and die, while I just get the runs. Quantity also matters. The more peanuts I eat, the more digestive distress I get, eventually having problems beyond my GI tract like brain fog, sore joints, skin issues, or migraines.

How Lectins Interact with Our Bodies

Our first line of defense against these bad boys is to spit on them. Well, kind of. The mucus in our noses and the saliva in our mouths are full of mucopolysaccharides (complex sugars).[21] As you know, lectins are suckers for sugar, so, when in contact with these fluids, they bind to the mucopolysaccharides, and your body is able to neutralize a good percentage of these lectins.

The human body is so clever that it will even produce more mucus when it feels that you are eating high-lectin foods. Remember what happened the last time you ate something super spicy? Your body produced plenty of mucus to fight off the lectins in those spices. That's why you cried like a baby. *No more diablo enchiladas for you, Kevin!*

The second line of defense is your stomach acid. As we learned, if working properly, your stomach can be an incredibly acidic environment. Acidic enough even to digest some of these lectins.

The ones that survive these chemical defenses now have to face our gut soldiers. Bacteria that live in your gut can learn how to break down some of these lectins. The longer you've been eating a particular plant lectin, the longer you've been producing gut bacteria specifically designed to defuse it.

The fourth and final line of defense is . . . drumroll, please . . . more mucus. I know, it's disappointing, but it is important. The same way you produce mucus in your nose, mouth, and throat, your gut also creates mucus. This mucus not only will work as a physical barrier so the lectins don't invade you, but will also trap and absorb these lectins, escorting them to your toilet.

It seems like we have a pretty strong anti-lectin game, right? Technically, yes. Unfortunately, our digestion is not at its best nowadays. At the same time, we are eating a lot more of these foods, so there are a lot more invaders to take care of.

Mechanisms Lectins Use to Harm Us
1. Intestinal Permeability

In chapter 2, we talked about the mucosal wall that lines your intestines. What I did not mention is that this "mighty barrier" is made up of only a single layer of cells. Say *whaaaat*?! With a strong digestion and proper diet and lifestyle, this is actually a good thing because the lining is strong enough to protect you, but simultaneously it facilitates the absorption of vitamins, minerals, fats, sugars, and simple proteins.

When our defenses can't take care of lectins, these large proteins will do all they can to squeeze through the mucosal wall and invade you.[22] As they destroy your mucous barrier, they move closer and closer to the cell walls. Once they get there, receptors in the cell walls bind to lectins and produce a compound called zonulin. Zonulin instructs the tight junctions of your intestinal wall (the gates that keep the space between these cells closed) to open.[23] Supposedly this is done as a defense mechanism to allow immune cells to move into the gut to fight off invaders and restore the mucous layer. Unfortunately, when you have a lot of lectins in your gut, the immune response is insufficient. Many lectins will go through the tight junctions and access your lymphatic system and eventually your bloodstream. From here, they can travel to cause issues anywhere.

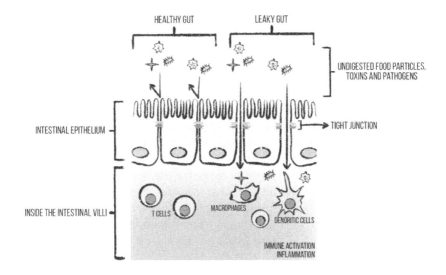

2. Molecular Mimicry

In the science world, molecular mimicry is defined as the "theoretical possibility that sequence similarities between foreign and self-peptides are sufficient to result in the cross-activation of autoreactive T or B cells by pathogen-derived peptides."[24] I know that is a mouthful. Let me give you an example to explain this in *waaaaay* easier manner.

Let's say there's a biker bar in town that is going to host a completely free all-you-can-eat steak dinner. Tony, who never rode a bike in his life, totally wants to go because he loves steak. On the day of the event, he dresses up and goes to the bar. At the entrance, because he looks like (mimics) a biker, the bouncer lets him in. Success!

Eventually, this goes sideways when the biker sitting next to Tony asks him questions about motorcycles. Tony is giving nonsense answers, since he doesn't know a thing about bikes. He is caught as the impostor he is. The biker curses him and tells him to leave immediately. Tony only has time to kick the guy in the balls and run out of the bar. This triggers an old-school bar brawl that causes so much destruction the party has to be shut down. Okay, I feel like I got carried away there, but let me explain this analogy.

Lectins are like Tony. They look like certain proteins in your body (molecular mimicry) and confuse your immune system (the bouncer). Eventually, your body is able to figure out that there is an impostor inside you. Some of your immune cells have toll-like receptors (TLRs) that act sort of like barcode scanners (like the guy asking questions about bikes) to identify proteins as friends or enemies. When these TLRs pick up the information about a certain barcode being compromised, they instruct our immune system to attack all proteins that have a similar barcode, even if those proteins (like the innocent bikers caught up in the brawl) are not the impostor lectins. This is what we call autoimmunity. Your body is attacking itself. In order to destroy one lectin, it attacks thousands of your own proteins just because their barcodes are similar. The more you eat that specific lectin, the more exacerbated this autoimmune response becomes.

The good news is that we can avert this by avoiding the consumption of these lectins. In fact, avoiding lectins has been reported in some scientific literature as a possible cure for autoimmune diseases.[25]

3. Cellular Communication Disruption

As if autoimmunity weren't bad enough, some lectins will also disrupt transmissions between your cells by mimicking or blocking hormonal signals. Lectins that look like some of your hormones might bind to the receptors designed for these hormones and mess up the entire system.

For example, the hormone insulin tells your cells to allow glucose in. When you have too much glucose circulating in your bloodstream, insulin attaches to fat cells and signals them to store glucose as fat, to be used later. Whenever the glucose levels stabilize, insulin detaches from the fat cells, so conversion of glucose into fat shuts down.

Now, there is a lectin called wheat germ agglutinin (WGA) that looks a lot like insulin.[26] If you have WGA circulating in your bloodstream, it might attach to the fat cell receptors like insulin would and stay there forever, which might cause your muscles, organs, and brain not to get enough glucose (to be converted into energy) because all is being used to create more fat. And presto, you become sick, weaker, dumber, and fat. Not the best attribute combo.

Why Are We Having More Issues with Lectins Now?

As you know, our digestive health has been declining, affecting our ability to eliminate these lectins. We also discussed how our constant intake of medication is compromising our innate intuition, so we end up eating more of these antinutrients.

Along with these changes, we also have disconnected from our ancient traditional knowledge of how to prepare these foods. Our ancestors who consumed these foods would go through several steps to prepare them, ensuring that they eliminated as many toxins as possible. Nowadays, with our industrial food production methods, we are eating these foods with the lectins in full force.

Our modern diet of processed food is also boosting our consumption of lectin-rich foods like corn, soy, and tomatoes. Look at any boxed food in the supermarket and I guarantee you it will have one of these three ingredients, or at least some variation of them. But it's not just processed foods. Even whole foods that are touted as superfoods, like goji berries, chia, or quinoa, are filled with these toxins. For reference, the plants with the most lectins include the nightshade family (eggplants, goji berries, ground-cherries, most peppers, tobacco, tomatoes, and white or red potatoes), most of the legume family (most beans and legumes like peanuts and cashews), most of the grain family (and even pseudograins such as amaranth and quinoa), the squash family (acorn squash, pumpkins, zucchini), and most seeds.[27,28]

Coincidentally or not, many of these foods originally came from the Americas after the 1500s. They were foods that Africans, Asians, and Europeans had never eaten before—so their bodies had never learned how to tolerate and process them. Natives of the Americas had several traditions for preparing these foods, like soaking, sprouting, deseeding, peeling, fermenting, and other elaborate ways to cook them. The rest of the world had to slowly come up with their own ways to make these foods less toxic. About the time everything was looking good, boom, we entered the Industrial Revolution and kicked all that knowledge to the curb.

In many European countries, in the 1800s and even the early 1900s, corn was seen as unfit for human consumption. In his book *The Plant Paradox*, Dr. Gundry recounts that the adoption of corn as a main grain in Northern Italy in the late 1800s prompted an outbreak of congenital mental retardation (cretinism).[29] Corn was mostly used to feed and fatten pigs. Now, corn (and even worse, GMO corn) is in most of the processed foods humans eat.

Did you know that in the late 1700s, a large percentage of Europeans feared tomatoes (at the time nicknamed "poison apples")?[30] Even Italians took almost two centuries to use them in their cuisine. This raises another question: Why aren't Italians sick all the time from all the tomato sauces? The likely answer: Italians haven't lost touch with their ancient traditions. They peel and deseed tomatoes before making tomato sauce, because it's in the peels and seeds that you find the great majority of the lectins. Italians also hybridized the Roma tomato to maximize the ratio of pulp to skin and seeds. Their famous red peppers? Also no peels, nor seeds.

What about the so-called superfood quinoa? Yes, quinoa is indeed nutritionally rich, but it is also filled with lectins. Without the proper preparation, it will do you more harm than good. Preparation is, once again, the keyword here. The truth is that if I asked my grandmother or even my great-grandmother what were the best ways to cook quinoa, do you know what would be their answer? Their answer would be *What in God's name is quinoa?!* My point is, most people outside of the Americas do not know how to prepare this food. The Incas had three detoxification processes to remove the lectins from quinoa. They would soak it, let it rot (ferment), and then cook it. When was the last time you followed these steps? Thought so!

Neo Note: Brown Rice

We are told that brown rice is healthier for us than white rice. The logic behind this is that the hull of rice contains fiber, vitamins, and mineral. But if this is true, why do Asian cultures, who have been consuming rice for thousands of years, go through the extra step of removing the hull? There must be a justification for this.

Through experimentation, Asian cultures realized the hull would cause them digestive issues, but when they removed it, these issues would not develop. At the time, they didn't know why; they just knew how they felt, and that was enough. Now we know the why. Even though the hull has nutrients, it is also full of digestion-destroying lectins.

Yes, white rice has less fiber and is often demonized as a cause of obesity. But is it, though? If we look at Asian cultures that eat white rice daily, they show better overall health outcomes, with less obesity, heart disease, and diabetes compared with Western cultures.[31]

Legumes are dietary staples of many people around the world, especially in developing countries, where they help compensate for the lack of other proteins. But once again, if not properly prepared, legumes can cause several issues. One lectin present in beans is phytohemagglutinin (PHA). PHA has been found to damage the surface of the intestine and to cause inflammation.[32,33] The soybean lectin (SBA) and peanut lectin (PNA) have also been shown to permeate the intestinal wall and may even contribute to atherosclerosis.[34,35] PNA has also been shown to modify the growth of rectal mucosa in a manner consistent with the development of colorectal cancer.[36]

Neo Note: Lectins and Parkinson's

Animal studies in which the worm *C. elegans* was fed PHA detected lectins being transported from the gut to the brain. Here, they then accumulated on dopamine-secreting neurons. PHA appeared to be toxic to these neurons, reducing their number and function. The study authors concluded that dietary plant lectins might be a potential dietary cause of Parkinson's disease.[37]

Dealing with Lectins

The best way to deal with lectins, at least during the initial healing stage, is to reduce your consumption of the foods rich in these antinutrients. Eliminating lectins as much as possible will be essential to letting your digestive system recover and become stronger. Later, you can slowly reintroduce some of these foods, but you should always prepare them in a way that will reduce their lectin content. For example, fermentation eliminates 98 percent of the lectins in lentils.[38]

Also, remember to deseed and peel lectin-rich foods, since the seeds and skins or hulls are the parts of the plant with the most antinutrient content.

Traditionally, although there is some controversy about these methods, we have also been soaking and sprouting these foods to reduce their toxic content.[39,40] Dr. Gundry also recommends using a pressure cooker, since, according to him, this cooking method will substantially eliminate the lectin content in most of these foods.[41] Please note that many bean lectins, particularly PHA, are not completely destroyed even after soaking and cooking, so it's essential to be cautious.[42]

One strategy to consider when you are "forced" to eat these foods is to take a lectin-binding supplement. These supplements contain particular substances that will bind to lectins, making them less likely to invade you. But please don't look at this as the solution. Easy fixes are never the solution. As I said, this is just a way to minimize the damage whenever you need to eat these foods in a social setting. You can find some recommendations in the book's resources (last pages) or by going directly to my.neodiet.co/resources.

GLUTEN

Gluten, the Al Capone of the diet world. Loved by some, feared by most. Although gluten is part of the lectin family, because of its notoriety I decided to do a separate section just for this antinutrient.

When we think about gluten, I'm sure most of us think of bread. I don't want to go into conspiracy theories here, but . . . did you know that the French word for bread is *pain*? I wonder, is it called *pain* because it's so good that it hurts or because it literally harms you from the inside out? That's what we are going to find out.

We associate the consumption of wheat and grains with the Neolithic era, but as we learned earlier in the book, there is evidence suggesting that we've been consuming grains since Paleolithic times. According to research findings, our Paleo ancestors might have started grinding them into flour about 30,000 years ago.[43–45] Nonetheless, it was during the Neolithic era that bread and cereals became seasonal dietary staples.[46–48]

Gluten is a complex mixture of hundreds of related but distinct proteins found in wheat, barley, bulgur, durum, einkorn, emmer, farro, Kamut, rye, semolina, spelt, and triticale.[49] Some also add oats to this list, not only because of contamination in the processing facilities but also due to its (less problematic) protein avenin.[50] Gluten acts like a glue (it's also a "sticky protein"), helping foods bind and preserve their shape, which is why it was added to many culinary traditions.

The problem with this protein nowadays is that "modern gluten" differs greatly from the gluten our ancestors consumed. In the last few decades, with advances in agricultural technology such as the hybridization and genetic manipulation of our grains and the use of synthetic pesticides and herbicides, we completely changed this old dietary staple. The grains that we have access to today are nothing like the grains we had before. As a result, in recent years we're seeing consequences like growing incidence of celiac disease, gluten-related sensitivities, and many other serious health conditions. In his book *Grain Brain*, Dr. David Perlmutter asserts that the excessive consumption of our "modern" gluten-containing grains is associated with autonomic dysregulation, cerebellar ataxia, hypotonia, developmental delay, learning disorders, depression, migraines, headaches, and even autism, schizophrenia, and hallucinations.[51]

How Gluten Interacts with Our Bodies

Since most of the population doesn't suffer from celiac disease, I am going to focus on nonceliac gluten sensitivities (a.k.a. "celiac light"), which are a lot more prevalent. The best place to start is by learning more about gliadin, since it is one of the main proteins said to be responsible for these gluten sensitivities. Gliadin sensitivity was initially considered to be more prevalent in people with European ancestry. Now, with new serological tests, this perception has changed. Gliadin sensitivity has also been found in developing countries where the major dietary staple is wheat, such as Southern Asia, the Middle East, Northwest and East Africa, and South America.[52] Considering these findings, it's pretty fair to say that several of us have pretty good chances of exhibiting some kind of nonceliac gluten sensitivity.

Having gliadin sensitivity is not like having a full-blown allergic reaction where you go into anaphylactic shock, but it still has substantial effects in your body, especially long term. What many authors claim is that when you consume foods with gliadin and you are sensitive to it, your body will produce an inflammatory response. Intestinal walls swell, the blood vessels in the gut enlarge, and a bunch of immune cells go into your small intestine to fight off these invaders (gliadin proteins). It is a fierce battle, but your body can take care of the situation. In his book *Boundless*, Ben Greenfield states that it takes between 12 and 15 hours for this inflammatory response in your gut to subside. Only then is the gut able to begin to slowly heal.[53] End of story, right?

Unfortunately, if you keep eating these gliadin-rich foods, this inflammatory response will continue to occur and your gut will never be able to recover. Considering this, Greenfield advises against the "weekly cheat meal" of pizza and other bread-heavy foods. As he puts it, "you literally never give your gut a chance to fully heal, which generally takes around two weeks after removal of gliadin from the diet. So be patient if you do begin to moderate or remove gliadin."[54]

Please keep in mind that the healing process may take around two weeks to start, not to be completed. By consuming these gut-wrecking foods all these years, you've had an ongoing war inside your gut that has left a lot of damage to be fixed. During this time, the mucous layer that lines your intestinal walls has probably been severely damaged. The less mucus you have, the less protection you have against toxins and other foreign particles trying to harm you.

Besides messing up your mucus, the inflammation in your gut can even destroy your villi and lacteals. As discussed in chapter 2, the villi and microvilli are essential to increasing the intestinal transit area and facilitating the absorption of nutrients from your food. If your lacteals are damaged or destroyed, you can no longer absorb fats and fat-soluble vitamins, which are essential for stabilizing your metabolism, repairing your nervous system, balancing hormone production, and optimizing your antioxidant levels.

After this damage is done, you can eat the best diet in the world and buy the most expensive supplements, but without functional villi and lacteals, this fancy diet and supplements will not work (or at least not at 100 percent), since you'll barely be absorbing them.

In gliadin-sensitive individuals, long-term consumption of gliadin is also said to cause digestive distress symptoms like bloating, hyperactive bowel, and uncomfortable bowel movements. Beyond digestive issues, some people may experience allergies, brain fog, memory loss, ADHD, headaches, chronic fatigue, insomnia, asthma, rashes, joint pain, anxiety, depression, food cravings, and weight gain.[55] Feel like you're having a déjà vu moment? Yes, many of these symptoms are similar to the symptoms I described when we were talking about lectins. Let's not forget that gluten is part of the lectin family.

Gliadin is possibly the most known and surely the most studied gluten protein. Other proteins like secalin in rye, hordein in barley, or even avenin in oats are believed to trigger similar responses. Each individual might be more reactive to one or the other, but the physiological mechanisms in your body seem not to differ that much.[56]

Why Are We Having More Issues with Gluten Now?

While introducing gluten, I briefly mentioned some of the reasons we are encountering more issues with this lectin lately. Now, let's dig in and really look at these in detail.

First, we have to consider our overconsumption of gluten-rich foods. In his book *Eat Wheat*, Dr. John Douillard describes our interaction with wheat and other grains throughout history. He explains that wheat is a cool-climate grain that used to be harvested only once a year, in the fall. The grain would then be prepared so it would sustain us during the winter. Eating wheat was seasonal or even just left for special ceremonies.[57] For the past 50 years, this seasonal staple has become a three-times-a-day, everyday food. Logically, this exponential increase in consumption is potentially overloading our ability to digest it and even to recover from any alleged damage caused by its proteins.

Now, let's make this a bit more interesting. Studies suggest that ancient wild wheat had more gluten than our current wheat. What?! That's right, these studies compared the gliadin content of two ancient wheat varieties, Kamut and Graziella Ra, with modern varieties. They concluded that the ancient wheats had almost twice the total gliadin levels of the modern wheat varieties.[58,59]

In another study, 22 subjects were divided and assigned to eat either Kamut (ancient wheat) or a modern wheat strain for eight weeks. The group that ate the Kamut (with almost twice the amount of gliadin) showed more than a two-times-greater reduction in common inflammatory markers associated with gluten sensitivity compared with the group that ate the modern wheat. In that same study, the Kamut lowered total cholesterol and fasting blood sugar and increased magnesium and potassium levels in the blood compared with the modern wheat.[60]

How is it possible that a grain with more gliadin is presenting better health outcomes? Wasn't gliadin one of the main triggers of gluten sensitivities?

Some justify this by considering studies that found that ancient wheat had more antioxidants than modern wheat.[61,62] I agree that the increased antioxidant content could potentially offset the inflammation caused by the higher gluten levels, but I continue to believe there has to be more to this story.

Wheat is one of the most-consumed cereal grains worldwide.[63] Apart from containing gliadin and other proteins, whole wheat also contains WGA, the lectin I mentioned earlier when explaining cellular communication disruption. As you probably noticed, many of the symptoms associated with gliadin sensitivity are not that different from symptoms caused by other lectins. Is it possible that some symptoms we are experiencing might come from WGA instead of from gliadin sensitivity?

We know how WGA can mimic insulin in your body and how that can mess with your endocrine (hormonal) function and metabolism. But that's not all that it does. WGA, like most lectins, triggers an inflammatory response in your gut that will produce similar damage to what gliadin would. Also, since it is a particularly small protein, it's especially sneaky and good at going past your intestinal wall. Once it reaches your lymphatic system and then your bloodstream, it can invade many other organs and systems, causing autoimmune responses there. This can trigger serious health issues throughout your body.

Right after college, I became more interested in learning about nutrition and diet. I started my health journey following mainstream health advice. Part of that advice was to eat a ton of whole grains. Immediately, I stopped eating anything white. Instead, I was eating whole grain breads, brown rice, and whole grain pasta every day. At the time, I couldn't understand why, but instead of feeling better, I was actually feeling worse than when I was on my "white grain" diet. It's embarrassing to admit, but I was always filled with gas. I had to interrupt several appointments with my clients just to go outside and let one (or six) fly. This was the only way to minimize all the abdominal pressure and pain I would experience.

That was when I learned about WGA. This lectin is found only in the bran of the grain. Processed grains (what I called white grains a moment ago) don't have the bran, so they don't have WGA (or if they do, it's a very small percentage). When I transitioned to the "healthy" whole grains, without knowing it, I started taking in a bunch of WGA that I hadn't been consuming before. I definitely felt the difference—just not the difference I was hoping for.

By the way, I chose to discuss only WGA because of our significant consumption of wheat compared with other grains. Please keep in mind that there are other lectins with similar effects (called chitin-binding lectins— CBLs) in grains like barley, rye, and rice, so this is not just a whole wheat issue.[64,65]

1. Preparation

If we look back in time, we see we used to prepare our grains completely differently relative to our modern techniques. Grains used to be soaked, sprouted, and fermented before being baked and consumed. Here is another piece of the puzzle. These extra steps made grains easier to digest by breaking down gluten and other antinutrients, and would even boost their nutritional content (by increasing minerals and amino acids).[66–68]

So why do we skip these steps now? Simple. It's better for business. Consider this example. A traditionally made bread (following all those extra steps) will take a couple of days to prepare. Skipping or substantially shortening the time spent on these steps allows us to produce a lot more bread.

The soaking and sprouting methods still have the scientific community divided, but fermentation has been shown to be extremely effective in making these foods better. During the fermentation process, the microbes naturally present in wheat (lactobacilli) eat the sugars and gluten in the wheat. This not only lowers the wheat's glycemic index but also reduces the gluten content significantly.[69,70] The same research even shows that sourdough bread produced with a particular strain of lactobacilli presented gluten levels of only 12 parts per million (ppm). And we consider anything less than 20 ppm to be gluten-free.[71] This slower fermentation required to make sourdough bread also makes iron, zinc, magnesium, B vitamins, and antioxidants more available for our bodies to absorb.[72]

Finally, in one small study, celiac patients ate sourdough bread for 60 days and did not present any clinical complaints. They even underwent biopsies, which detected no changes in the intestinal lining.[73]

2. Artificial Selection

Over time, in our process of domesticating wheat, we gave preference to and selected seeds that were larger and easier to remove when threshing. The larger the wheat seed, the more starch (sugar) and less protein (and gluten) the grain had. We've already learned about our current wheat having less gluten. What I didn't mention is that it also gained a lot more sugar. This hybridization process made the glycemic index (how quickly a food leads to a rise in blood sugar) of our wheat higher than before.[74] For example, a slice of white bread is about a 70 on the glycemic scale of 1 to 100, while a slice of 100 percent stone-ground whole wheat bread rates only a 55.

In chapter 7, we have an entire section on the effects of excess sugar in your body. As you might guess, they are not very positive.

The outcome of wheat's domestication and hybridization is that the increase in sugar content of our wheat made it less healthy.

3. Transglutaminase

The food industry started using transglutaminase (TG)—a baking enzyme—instead of the traditional yeasts.[75] Using this enzyme was more cost-efficient than traditional leavening methods. The problem with using TG instead of yeast is that without yeast, we no longer have fermentation and the consequent decrease in gluten and sugar. With TG, you get the full dose.

TG has been approved for use in many countries worldwide and is quite common in industrial baking. TG is also used in most "gluten-free" baked products. It makes them fluffier and more appealing.

In his book *Plant Paradox*, Dr. Gundry reveals that TG can pass the blood-brain barrier and act as a neurotransmitter disrupter, making it extremely harmful. He says TG is often responsible for the condition known as gluten ataxia, which is similar to Parkinson's.[76]

4. Preservatives and Other Additives

Food is supposed to spoil. Microbes in foods and in the environment end up decomposing the food as they use it for their own fuel. Same thing happens to us when we die. That is the cycle of life.

In order to make our food last longer, we have come up with several methods, such as salting, putting it in fat or sugar, dehydrating, fermenting, smoking, canning, sealing it in vacuum packaging, putting it in fridges, and even freezing it.

Traditional artisan breads had a brief shelf life. One day they would be nurturing and delicious; the following day they would become bricks. Then we came up with synthetic preservatives and changed the game. In an oversimplified explanation, one way preservatives work is by functioning as antimicrobials, inhibiting the growth of the microbes in food.[77] When we keep microbes at a minimum, it takes a lot more time for them to decompose food.

Preservatives made it possible for foods like bread that would spoil in one day to last weeks or even months.

Another way to preserve food, especially processed foods made with whole grains, is by using synthetic chemicals like *butylated* hydroxytoluene (BHT). BHT works by blocking the oxidation of the oils (fat) in those whole grains. Unfortunately, BHT is suspected of being an endocrine disruptor.[78] By mimicking estrogen, overconsumption of BHT can promote, among many things, weight gain, early puberty in girls, and male gynecomastia (aka "man boobs").

On top of preservatives, we've also added all kinds of additives, like artificial food dyes, artificial flavors, and artificial sweeteners. One of the most famous sweeteners used in processed foods is high-fructose corn syrup (HFCS). HFCS is used to replace sugar in (or even add more sugar to) baked goods and cereals. In a nutshell, this makes bread more addictive, harder to digest, and toxic. A real "cereal killer," I tell you. And these are just a few examples of the many food additives that are changing the way our foods interact with our bodies.

5. Poison in Our Grains

In our evolution, we have hybridized and crossbred grains with other species to increase yields. We also started using massive amounts of chemical fertilizers, pesticides, and herbicides, again to bump up our yields. The US Department of Agriculture (USDA) completed a study in 2004 that found traces of 16 pesticides in wheat flour.[79] Imagine how many of these chemicals we are consuming with our grains.

To make matters worse, glyphosate (one of the most-used herbicides in grains) also bonds with gluten, making it more inflammatory even to people who don't experience gluten sensitivities.[80] Glyphosate also paralyzes key liver enzymes (cytochrome P450 enzymes). These enzymes are essential in our detoxification process. Without them, we have a harder time getting glyphosate and other toxins out of our system.[81] Not only does the glyphosate in grains poison you, but it also ensures you stay poisoned. What a double whammy.

As a final note, studies show that these toxins can change the proteins in wheat and also impair our digestive enzymes (those that break down gluten and other hard-to-digest proteins).[82,83] It's no wonder that gluten now is becoming more inflammatory. By using these chemicals, we altered gluten's structure (making it more difficult to digest) and also destroyed the enzymes that would help us digest it.

6. Mold

In order to protect grains from mold, after the harvest they have to be thoroughly dried and sealed off from moisture before being stored. That is a lot of work and not business friendly. So, it rarely happens. We often store grains in less-than-ideal conditions, which consequently allow mold to grow and propagate. A 2001 study found that at least 25 percent of the world's grain crops are contaminated with OTA, a type of mold toxin.[84] In 2020, a survey conducted by Biomin on more than 21,000 samples from 79 countries, found that 87 percent contained at least 10 types of mold toxins and metabolites.[85] As biohacker Dave Asprey mentions in his book *Head Strong*, "this is such a big issue that animal ranchers track the global incidents of different mold toxins in grains because moldy grains make animals sick and reduce profits."[86]

How is it possible that ranchers are more aware of this issue than the companies feeding us grain products?!

As you can see, there is a lot more to this gluten story than gluten itself. All the different factors mentioned here made our grains much different (and more toxic) than they were before. I'm not saying that gluten is completely innocent, but we have to recognize that it might play a much smaller role in our health issues than we initially assumed.

Dealing with Gluten

In this section of the book, I've taken you on a journey from "gluten is the devil" to "gluten might not be that bad after all." This was the same journey I went through during my research. As I said in my introduction, we should always be open to questioning our beliefs and looking at the data from different angles. That's what I tried to do here, but of course, this is my take on the available data.

The truth is, you can find studies supporting both sides of this argument. Even though I read several studies portraying gluten as terrible, I also had to consider that these studies were often using isolated compounds and not considering how the *whole* grain could potentially have a different interaction with our bodies. On the other hand, I found dozens of studies saying that grains are the best thing in the world, studies I decided not to present here. Most of them were observational studies and were sponsored by the cereal industry. Probably not the best scientific information out there.

Now that this is out of the way . . . how should we deal with gluten?

If you suffer from celiac disease, you know what you have to do. For all others, the question needs to be addressed in a more personalized manner. Going gluten-free has consequences you should be aware of so you can make an informed decision.

During my two-year gluten hiatus, I had a couple of incidents in which, by accident, I ate something without realizing it had gluten, and I experienced immediate digestive discomfort. This was very frustrating. After all, I had stopped eating gluten long enough to allow my gut to heal. Not long enough yet, I guessed.

I knew my gut was much better, not only because I felt 90 percent better but also because I was checking my progress through different tests and exams. But I was not healed enough. Eating a bit of gluten and running to the bathroom is not the antifragile image I had of myself.

Concerned about the possibility of atrophying my gluten-digesting ability to a point of no return, I decided to slowly reintroduce some properly prepared organic grains. In the beginning I experienced some symptoms, but then, *poof*, I could eat larger quantities of grains without those crazy symptoms. More surprising than that, my gut tests were finally showing improvements after I had plateaued for months. Did those grains make me healthier?

More Research on the Benefits of Gluten

Gluten has been shown to increase certain enzymes (glutenases) in the large intestine, which fully digest the gliadins found in gluten. In that same study, gluten also acted as a fuel for beneficial gut microbes.[87] Research has shown that even a temporary gluten-reduced diet decreased the populations of good gut microbes and increased the pathogenic (bad) microbe populations.[88,89]

A low-gluten diet has also been shown to cause the loss of the genes responsible for carbohydrate metabolism.[90] By eating less gluten, we become less efficient at digesting complex carbs. Because of this, when you try to reintroduce complex carbs in the future, you will feel it right away. This was exactly what was happening to me.

In another study, whole wheat even improved intestinal integrity and reduced intestinal permeability.[91] How is that possible?

When researchers tested humans, they couldn't find any evidence of inflammation, immune activation, or increased intestinal permeability connected to the consumption of gluten in this study. But when testing this in a test tube, they could indeed find differences in immune reactivity.[92] As I mentioned before, testing isolated compounds in a lab setting doesn't always translate to the same real-life results in humans eating the whole food.

With all this information, the plot thickens. Not only are grains not the poison we thought, but they might actually be good for us. Now, it's time to learn about how to choose and prepare the right grains in order to minimize any potential side effects.

Traditional Preparation

As you know, traditionally, grains used to be sprouted and/or fermented, and cooked. These steps were used to reduce the content of several antinutrients. We already saw some of the research around fermentation and how beneficial it is. It reduces gliadin and other antinutrients, decreases glycemic index, and improves the nutritional profile of the food.

More and more we can find artisan bakeries popping up all over the place, so it's becoming easier to find good-quality sourdough bread. It is essential to get to know your baker. Sometimes, just because a bakery says that it is artisanal, it doesn't exactly mean they are using good-quality grains and preparing bread in a traditional way.

It's also a fun project to bake sourdough bread yourself at home. That is the ultimate way to control all ingredients and fermentation times. There are hundreds of blogs with sourdough recipes online, but I also share one I like in this book's resource section.

Sprouting still generates some controversy in the research community. No clear evidence has shown that sprouting affects gluten levels. Despite that, it has been shown to decrease the content of other antinutrients and improve nutrient absorption.[93,94]

Furthermore, for the seed to germinate and sprout requires energy. This energy is retrieved from starch in the grain. This can lower the sugar content in sprouted grains and consequently lower the grains' glycemic index.[95]

Finally, we should also consider better grains. Not only should you stay away from all non-organic grains, but you should also consider other varieties that might not have been hybridized as much.

Whenever possible, choose grains like einkorn, emmer, and Kamut (khorasan wheat). These more ancient grains have a better antioxidant and nutritional profile and don't score as high on the glycemic scale. Ancient wheats like einkorn and emmer might even turn off genes that increase the risk of type 2 diabetes.[96]

Other grains to consider are barley, rye, and spelt. Barley and rye have a lower glycemic index, while spelt has fewer antinutrients (phytates) and higher mineral content.[97]

Consuming Grains

Remember, if your digestive system is not healed, it doesn't matter if you are eating the best organic grains in the world, you will have issues. For now, I don't want to overwhelm you with information, but when we reach chapter 16, I'll show you how to fix your digestion and when to reintroduce grains. When that time comes and you are ready to eat more freely, prioritize sprouted and/or fermented organic grains (especially the varieties mentioned before). Please avoid all store-shelf grain products, since they are ultraprocessed and filled with all the toxic things we've covered.

As we've seen, some grains may be good, but you should not consume 7 to 11 servings of them a day, per the traditional food pyramid. No way. We are not supposed to be eating them three times a day, every day. Grains were originally a seasonal food eaten during the winter. Besides that, in chapters 6 and 7, you'll also learn more about your metabolism and the reasons why it's wise not to overindulge in grains.

Neo Note: Grains as Drugs

The gluten proteins in wheat might break down into molecules called gluteomorphins (gliadorphins).[98] A gluteomorphin is a morphine analogue that can trigger the opioid receptors in your brain. Why should you care? Because this basically means that bread can have an addictive effect, like a drug. I don't know about you, but when I see a breadbasket in a restaurant, I feel like eating the whole thing. The more bread you eat, the more you desire.

I am sharing this with you so you understand any potential urges you might have, and to enable you to control them better through knowledge.

Finally, I just want to talk about supplements. The most important supplements here would be the ones that can help you fix your gut, and that I'll describe later in this book. The only supplement I can recommend for now would be digestive enzymes (especially designed for gluten). But you are not supposed to use them and feel that now you can eat pasta every day. These are to be used on special occasions. Let's say that you are still in your healing journey but have a social event to attend. You will not binge on spaghetti-stuffed calzones, but you do want to, let's say, try a slice of the homemade pizza your best friend made. This would be the occasion to take a gluten digestive enzyme supplement. You can find my suggestions in the book's resources.

Neo Note: Gluten-Free Grains

Amaranth

Amaranth, in reality, is not a grain, and the part usually eaten is the seed. However, it is a good grain replacement. Since we consume the seeds, amaranth does have some antinutrients, like tannins, oxalates, and phytates. But their content is low and can be substantially reduced by soaking, sprouting, and cooking. This pseudograin has several important minerals and has been shown to lower inflammation.[99] Amaranth could be a gluten-free alternative to explore occasionally when a grain craving hits. Just remember to prepare it properly.

Millet

Millet has been getting a lot of attention lately, since it is growing as a gluten-free alternative for people suffering from celiac disease. Besides being low in lectins, millet is rich in fiber and other health-promoting compounds. This grain has been recognized for many health benefits, such as antioxidant, antimicrobial, antidiabetic, anti-tumorigenic, and anti-atherosclerotic effects.[100]

Sorghum

Sorghum has been used as a staple food in many developing countries, in particular semiarid regions of Africa and Asia due to its ability to resist droughts.[101] The introduction of improved food-processing techniques has made this grain easier to trade and export to other countries, gaining it a lot of popularity lately. Sorghum is gluten-free and contains organic compounds linked to health benefits similar to the ones associated with millet.[102] I personally use sorghum not as a substitute for traditional grains but as a replacement for corn. Popped sorghum is the perfect popcorn alternative. You should try it!

OXALATES

Oxalate (oxalic acid) is produced in our bodies as a normal waste product of the breakdown of certain amino acids. Normal accumulation of oxalic acid is perfectly manageable by our bodies, since we're able to safely excrete it.

One exception to this is a rare genetic disorder known as primary hyperoxaluria (PH). Individuals with this disorder produce a lot more oxalates than normal. This leads to excessive accumulation of oxalate crystals in their bones, joints, bone marrow, and even kidneys.[103]

Oxalates are considered antinutrients because they are also produced by plants, which use them not only as part of their cellular metabolism like we do, but also as a defense mechanism against predators.[104,105]

Oxalates can combine with minerals and crystalize into a needle-like shapes called raphides. Some parts of the plant are covered with these microscopic needles, which keep off insects and deter other animals from biting into the plants. Because we are much larger than these predators, we don't see or feel these needles, but consuming plants is a major way to increase the levels of oxalates in our bodies. While inside us, oxalates bind to calcium (and other minerals) in our blood and become sharp crystals that can be deposited anywhere in the body and cause numerous issues.

In healthy individuals, both small and large oxalate crystals have been observed pathologically (that is, they're causing trouble) in the thymus, thyroid, brain, blood vessels, kidneys, eyes, testicles, and breasts.[106-111]

High levels of oxalates can also result from an overgrowth of yeast and mold. This is a little more complex and discussed later in the book when we learn how to solve these issues.

How Oxalates Interact with Our Bodies

The first and probably best-known example of how oxalates affect us is the occurrence of kidney stones. You might have heard that too much calcium in the body causes kidney stones, but in reality, we are blaming calcium for what oxalates are doing. About 75 percent of kidney stones are made of calcium oxalate.[112] This means that around three-fourths of all kidney stones are being caused by excess oxalates in the body. Oxalates also induce renal (kidney) inflammation.[113]

Oxalate buildup can interfere with gallbladder function and digestion.[114] As soon as the gallbladder starts malfunctioning, this problem only gets worse. When oxalates find calcium in your small intestine, they bind to it, and your body cannot absorb this new calcium-oxalate compound.[115] Since it is not absorbed, you end up ejecting all these harmful oxalates in stool.

But if your gallbladder is not working properly, your body won't be able to absorb fat and fatty acids in your small intestine. The thing here is that calcium loves fat more than it loves oxalates. Thus, all the calcium circulating in your intestines will bind to these unabsorbed fats. Since now oxalates do not have calcium available, they remain "free," and your body absorbs them. As you can see, this then becomes a vicious circle that keeps exacerbating this issue.

You probably never heard about sulfate before. Despite being unknown by most of us, it is one of the most common molecules circulating in your blood.[116] In his book *Your Genius Body*, Dr. Andrew Rostenberg explains that sulfate helps us with many metabolic processes, including maintaining the integrity of our intestinal tract and strengthening bones, ligaments, and tendons. It is also required for the detoxification of all kinds of toxins, hormones, and heavy metals.[117]

Since sulfate uses the same transporters to move through our bodies as oxalates do, this creates a problem.[118] Whenever these transporters see oxalates, they no longer care about sulfate and prioritize the "sexier" oxalates, which then decrease the uptake of sulfate by our cells.[119]

If your cells don't get enough sulfate, then it cannot be used in the methylation cycle, and you start activating all your "bad genes." That's definitely not what you want.

Oxalates may also be involved in neurological diseases like autism.[120] More research is needed to understand the "how," but children with autism have displayed three-times-greater levels of oxalates in their blood and two-and-a-half-times-greater levels in their urine. There are also several anecdotical reports from functional-medicine doctors referring to the improvement of symptoms with oxalate-reduced diets. Something to consider, for sure.

High level of oxalates in the body have also been associated with conditions such as breast cancer, cataracts, joint pain, fibromyalgia, mitochondrial dysfunction, interstitial cystitis, sarcoidosis, thyroid dysfunction, uterine fibroids, and vulvodynia (chronic pain in the female outer genital area).[121-138]

Why Are We Having More Issues with Oxalates Now?

Oxalate toxicity is not a new issue. There have been several reports from medical literature stating these issues for about 200 years now. We can go all the way back to 1823 and find experiments done with dogs to whom they fed oxalates, which caused painful deaths.[139] In 1919, for example, Dr. H. F. Robb reported a case of death related to high oxalate consumption from rhubarb leaves and roots.[140] Oxalates are not the new kid on the block as we sometimes hear.

So why are we suddenly having more issues? It's a combination of forgetting the knowledge transmitted by our elders about which foods we should eat in moderation (or at least prepare in ways that minimize the antinutrient content) and being brainwashed into binge-eating so-called healthy foods.

There are different lists with different oxalate counts (depending on where and how the foods were tested), but it is generally accepted that oxalates can be found in bigger concentrations in raw vegetables such as spinach, rhubarb, sorrel, and Swiss chard, as well as almonds, cashews, hazelnuts, poppy seeds, sesame seeds, caraway seeds, rice bran, cinnamon, and turmeric. Some lists also include beer, beets, chocolate, coffee, macadamia nuts, peanuts, plantains, soy, and tea, which have smaller oxalate concentrations.

Some of these foods are indeed healthy if prepared correctly and eaten in moderation. But when you decide to eat them every single day, you overwhelm your digestion and detox systems and start accumulating oxalates at health-damaging levels.

A couple of years ago, during the time I adopted a vegan diet, I used to drink a green smoothie every day. In my smoothie I would add almond milk, spinach, Swiss chard, kale, avocado, cashews, peanut butter, sesame seeds, blueberries, and rice protein. Coincidentally, around this time (after being on this diet for a couple of months), I had to undergo a couple of ultrasounds. Everything came up clear, except that I had kidney stones in both kidneys. How was this possible? I was eating super healthy—I thought. While looking for answers, I found out about oxalates and that my "healthy" green smoothie was packing more than 1,500 milligrams of oxalates. That is a lot. Just for reference, there have been documented deaths related to consumption of as little as 5,000 milligrams of oxalates in a day.[141-143]

Unfortunately, stories like mine are becoming more and more common. In his book *The Carnivore Code*, Dr. Paul Saladino shares that he was committing the same mistake. He also describes other cases of people who developed severe health issues after oxalate-rich green smoothie and juice cleanses. But it's not just a green smoothie issue. Children with genitourinary problems, from bloody urine to kidney stones, were able to get these problems resolved just with the removal of almond milk.[144]

Once again, I want to reinforce that some of these foods are good for you, but they should be prepared properly and eaten in moderation. Overdosing on them every day will definitely make you sick.

Dealing with Oxalates

The most obvious way to deal with oxalates is to reduce the number of oxalate-rich foods you consume. If you don't take in these foods in high quantities every single day, most likely you can process and excrete them.

Please note that I am saying to reduce and not to eliminate. Unless you have primary hyperoxaluria, you should not completely eliminate these foods, since some of them are nutritious and can even be health promoting.

One strategy we learned from dealing with lectins also applies here. Soaking and cooking foods high in oxalates will reduce the oxalate content by leaching oxalates into the water.[145] Since there is no water involved, baking does not seem to produce significant results. In one study, boiling reduced oxalate content by 30 to 87 percent and was more effective than steaming (5 to 53 percent).[146] The key seems to be the leaching, so please discard the water.

And finally, please remember not to eat your spinach raw. Soak it and boil it. That's an order, soldier!

Another strategy is to take advantage of the crush oxalates have on calcium. Research has shown that consuming more calcium will actually prevent the development of calcium-oxalate crystals inside you.[147] This happens because oxalate will bind to calcium while in your gut, and this bound form won't be able to go past your intestinal wall.[148]

When eating oxalate-rich foods, also eat calcium-rich foods like dairy, fish, and broccoli. Another option is to take a calcium citrate supplement before your "oxalate meal." Calcium citrate has been shown to bind to oxalates in the gut and also to prevent oxalates already inside the body from binding to calcium in the kidneys.[149,150]

Neo Note: Vitamin B6

Vitamin B6 might be important in the physiological process of detoxification from oxalates. A study done in 1988 concluded that taking B6 in high therapeutic dosages of five milligrams per kilogram per day was effective at reducing high levels of urinary oxalates.[151]

More recently, in 2011, another study showed that even individuals with the genetic disease primary hyperoxaluria could improve with vitamin B6. About 30 percent of participants experienced a reversal of their condition.[152] More research is needed, but these two studies seem encouraging.

Obviously, this is something to only consider under direct supervision by a physician.

There is research suggesting that a species of bacteria called *Oxalobacter formigenes* might use oxalates in your gut as fuel, thus reducing the number of oxalates you absorb and lowering your risk of kidney stones.[153,154] The problem is that not everyone is colonized with this bacteria, and it's not clear how one can introduce it. Labs are working on putting it in supplement form, and the research seems promising.[155] I am sure that soon we will see an *Oxalobacter formigenes* probiotic being sold to the public.

At the time of this writing, the best supplements to fight oxalate accumulation are calcium citrate and vitamin B_6, as we just discussed. Additionally, chondroitin sulfate seems to prevent the formation of calcium oxalate crystals.[156] Research also shows that L-arginine and vitamin E reduce oxalate damage.[157,158]

PHYTATES

Phytate (or phytic acid) is another antinutrient produced by plants in order to deter animals and insects from eating them. They do this in a more subtle way than lectins or oxalates, for example.

Phytates block or limit the absorption of vitamins, minerals, and other nutrients. The more phytate-rich plants the animal eats, the less nourishment it receives. The animal is able to realize that it's not gaining weight and is feeling weak and rapidly learns to stay away from these plants.

Foods containing phytates include beans and other legumes, seeds, nuts, and whole grains. Phytate content varies, but it's particularly high in raw, unsprouted seeds.

How Phytates Interact with Our Bodies

Phytates interact with us in the same way they do with insects and animals. They make food less nourishing by binding to several minerals and blocking (or substantially limiting) our ability to absorb them.[159]

Unfortunately, we cannot digest phytic acid because we lack the enzyme (phytase) that breaks it down. Thus, undigested, it binds to the minerals copper, iron, magnesium, manganese, and zinc, contributing to nutritional deficiencies.[160]

Despite these negative consequences, phytates are also antioxidants and might even help us detox because of their ability to bind to heavy metals.[161,162] So we shouldn't completely eliminate them but should carefully monitor the amount and timing of their consumption.

Why Are We Having More Issues with Phytates Now?

Without trying to repeat myself, once again the issue has to do with the move away from traditional methods of preparing these foods and with mainstream health advice. We are no longer using ancient techniques to minimize the phytate content of the foods that contain them. To make matters worse, every day we are pushed into eating whole grains, legumes, and seeds without realizing the consequences of this overconsumption.

We are overwhelming our bodies with antinutrients, and they are screaming for help.

Dealing with Phytates

Ruminant animals like cows, goats, and sheep have bacteria that produce phytase and are able to digest phytates.[163] Unfortunately, that is not the case with us. Phytate content may be decreased by soaking, sprouting, and roasting, but it's unclear whether these reductions are enough to be significant.[164] Fermentation, once again, seems to be the best of the traditional techniques for decreasing phytic acid content.[165]

Beyond minimizing your consumption and making sure you properly prepare these foods, there aren't many more evidence-based approaches to dealing with phytates. I think the important thing here is to understand that these antinutrients rob you of nutrients, so you need to be careful not to over consume them.

As a final note, I just want to leave some food for thought. Next time you read about how nutritious legumes are, for example, please remember that they are full of phytates. Even though they might have a lot of nutrients, you can absorb only a tiny percentage of them thanks to these antinutrients.

"LESS-CONCERNING" ANTINUTRIENTS

Lectins, gluten, oxalates, and phytates are probably the most problematic antinutrients, which is why we've explored them in a little more depth. But before we close this section, I just want to briefly touch on some of the "less-concerning" antinutrients you should know.

Cyanogenic Glycosides

Cyanogenic glycosides are phytotoxins that function as part of a plant's defense system.

These antinutrients interfere with iodine absorption and thus might cause or promote goiter and hypothyroidism.[166] Fortunately, this problem seems to occur only in a setting of iodine deficiency or with massive overconsumption of cyanogenic glycosides.

Cyanogenic glycosides can also degrade and release potentially lethal hydrogen cyanide.[167] This sounds scary, but your liver can detoxify these compounds. This would become a serious issue only if you consumed a massive amount of these antinutrients in a short period of time.

Considering the above, you should not be concerned about acute toxic effects, but the consequences of chronic, low-level exposure are still unknown.

Plants that contain significant amounts of these compounds include almonds, bamboo shoots, cassava, sorghum, and the seeds of apricots, cherries, peaches, and plums.[168]

Saponins

Saponins (or triterpene glycosides) are bitter-tasting plant antinutrients named for their ability to form soap-like foamy structures in water. They are an essential part of the defense systems of plants that contain them.

Saponins may disrupt cholesterol absorption in the gut, induce intestinal permeability, and have toxic effects in our cells (especially red blood cells).[169–171] On the other hand, their cell-disrupting effect might also be beneficial in fighting some cancers.[172]

Humans rarely suffer severe poisoning from saponins, but the rule of quantity also applies here.

Saponins are found in asparagus, beans, ginseng, licorice root, oats, peas, quinoa, soybeans, and sunflower seeds.

Glycoalkaloids

Glycoalkaloids are naturally occurring antinutrients contained in certain plants. The most notorious such plants are the ones belonging to the nightshade family. Nightshades again? That's right. It's not just lectins. It appears Tom Brady was onto something when he eliminated them from his diet.[173]

Solanine, the glycoalkaloid found in potatoes, is incredibly poisonous if eaten raw in large quantities. It has been shown to affect cellular metabolism, break down cell membranes, and cause GI distress such as nausea, vomiting, diarrhea, and severe abdominal pain.[174–176]

Potato skins may cause intestinal damage, especially when fried and consumed often.[177]

Glycoalkaloids in eggplant (alpha-solamargine and alpha-solasonine) have been shown to cause GI disorders and even mental confusion.[178] I guess there's a reason Europeans, when they first discovered eggplants, used to call them "mad apples."

Lastly, excessive consumption of tomatine, the glycoalkaloid in tomatoes, has been said to cause swelling, skin redness, coughing, nausea, vomiting, and diarrhea.[179]

Peeling and cooking of these plant foods might decrease glycoalkaloid content, but there is plenty of contradictory research, so I can't say for sure. On the other hand, long-term storage and exposure to light might increase the antinutrient content.

Plants that contain significant amounts of these compounds include bell peppers, cayenne, chili peppers, eggplants, goji berries, ground-cherries, paprika, pimientos, potatoes, tobacco leaf, tomatillos, and tomatoes.

Goitrogens

Goitrogens are antinutrients that interfere with the normal function of the thyroid. For individuals with thyroid problems, high intake of goitrogens can worsen thyroid function, since the substance seems to block iodine absorption and interfere with thyroid hormone production.[180]

A poorly functioning thyroid has been associated with bone fractures, weight gain, heart disease, developmental delays in children, and mental decline in older adults.[181–188]

In order to minimize the effects of these antinutrients, variety is key. This applies not only to goitrogens but to most antinutrients. Consuming only a limited number of plants will increase your changes of overdosing on a particular antinutrient.

Cooking seems to be effective in decreasing some goitrogens.[189,190] So remember, no more raw kale in your smoothies or even raw broccoli with your dips.

Goitrogens are found in cruciferous vegetables like broccoli, brussels sprouts, cauliflower, Chinese cabbage, kale, and radishes, as well as horseradish, linseeds, peaches, peanuts, pine nuts, rapeseeds, soybeans, spinach, and strawberries.

Phytoestrogens

Phytoestrogens are plant-derived compounds that mimic the hormone estrogen in our bodies. The body recognizes them as human estrogen and lets them bind to estrogen receptors, which may interfere with processes regulated by this hormone.

For the longest time, it was believed that phytoestrogens had a problematic effect on male fertility and testosterone levels. More recent studies have shown that this notion might be incorrect after all.[191]

To be honest, the science here is not 100 percent clear, and in order to be cautious, it's recommended that pregnant women and those trying to become pregnant avoid phytoestrogens. Using soy-based infant formula (high in phytoestrogens) is also not recommended.[192]

The foods that contain the highest amounts of these compounds are soybeans and soy-based products. Other sources include alfalfa, cereal products, legumes, processed meat products, and vegetable oils (canola and sunflower).

NEO SUMMARY

• Plants do not want to be eaten. So, they produce antinutrients as chemical defenses against insects and animals.

• We can detoxify these compounds if we do not overconsume them.

• Mainstream health advice has been promoting the overconsumption of antinutrients and the health consequences of this poor advice are visible.

• Traditional preparation methods such as soaking, sprouting and fermenting may help to decrease the antinutrient content in several foods.

• Lectins, oxalates and phytates are probably the most well-studied antinutrients because of their vast deleterious effects in the human health.

• Most antinutrients are concentrated in the seeds and peels of plants.

• Grains should not be the main staple of our diet like in the food pyramid. But, they also aren't the terrifying food some health authors claim them to be.

• Soaking, sprouting and fermenting organic whole grains is your best option in terms of increasing their digestibility and nutrient content.

• Foods rich in phytates are not as nutritious as experts claim, since you cannot absorb most of the minerals in them.

• Cooking can significantly decrease the antinutrient content of foods.

NEO ACTION

• Peel and deseed plants.
• Soak, spout, ferment, and cook grains.
• Make your own sourdough bread at home.
• Use a pressure cooker to eliminate most of the antinutrients.
• Soak and boil (and then discard the water) of oxalate rich-plants.
• Take calcium citrate with unavoidable oxalate-heavy meals.
• Cook your cruciferous vegetables.

NEO RECOMMENDATIONS

• *Biohacker's Handbook* by Olli Sovijärvi, Teemu Arina, Jaakko Halmetoja
• *Boundless* by Ben Greenfield
• *Eat Smarter* by Shawn Stevenson
• *Eat Wheat* by Dr. John Douillard
• *Fiber Fueled* by Dr. Will Bulsiewicz
• *Grain Brain* by Dr. David Perlmutter
• *The Bulletproof Diet* by Dave Asprey
• *The Carnivore Code* by Dr. Paul Saladino
• *The Paleo Diet* by Dr. Loren Cordain
• *The Plant Paradox* by Dr. Steven Gundry
• *Wheat Belly* by Dr. William Davis
• *Your Genius Body* by Dr. Andrew Rostenberg

SCAN ME

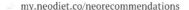
my.neodiet.co/neorecommendations

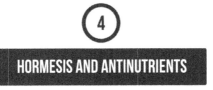

HORMESIS AND ANTINUTRIENTS

Becoming Stronger Than Super(wo)man by Microdosing on Kryptonite

"That which does not kill us makes us stronger."
Friedrich Nietzsche

HORMESIS

Legend has it that in 120 BC, King Mithridates V (King of Pontus) died in the middle of a banquet, after being poisoned by his wife. His eldest son, Mithridates VI Eupator, convinced his mother was going to do the same to him, decided to escape. During this time, he began ingesting small, nonlethal doses of known poisons, believing that he would train his body to become immune to them. Eventually, he returned and claimed his throne. It's said that during his 60 years of rule, he carried with him a potion containing 54 known poisonous compounds mixed in small doses, which he consumed daily as an elixir of health.[1]

Eventually, when people rebelled against his rule, he attempted suicide by poison. Ironically, the attempt failed because he had developed immunity to the poison.[2]

This idea of ingesting small amounts of poison (or exposing your body to stressors) with the goal of getting stronger is called hormesis. Hormesis is the concept behind inoculation and vaccination—being exposed to diseases so you can develop antibodies to them—eating small portions of certain foods so you slowly develop the enzymes to digest them, or even, as many do in college, drinking alcohol every day to improve one's skill at not passing out. Mithridates VI would have been proud!

Some damage is good for us. As they say in toxicology, *the dose makes the poison*. The key here is to control how much damage you expose yourself to. For example, you can build more muscle or completely tear one apart, depending on the amount and intensity of exercise you do.

Hormesis, in a way, is the process your body uses to prepare for harder times. As it experiences these small aggressions, your body thinks this will become the new normal and believes it needs to get stronger to survive.

In his book *Lifespan*, Dr. David Sinclair explains that we have always pushed our biology against the perceived boundaries in order to become healthier. We do this by challenging our bodies' survival mechanisms to the point right before actual damage. In this state of perceived adversity, your body is forced to adapt and grow stronger.[3]

AUTOPHAGY

In group sports, when one player is injured, the coach will remove that player so the team has a better chance of winning. If the player is not removed, the team will have a noncontributing member making it weaker.

Same happens in your body. If you have cells that are not performing, they need to be removed from the game so the others can do their job without being disturbed. This cell "housekeeping" process is called autophagy. The word *autophagy* (from *auto*, "self," plus *phage*, "eat") was coined by the Nobel Prize–winning biochemist Christian de Duve in 1963 and refers to the mechanism by which the body collects and destroys damaged cells and proteins. I know how this sounds, but remember that just like in sports, these cells are doing more harm than good by staying in play. By removing them, we make room for new, healthy cells to take over. This "survival of the fittest" process is absolutely essential for optimal health.[4] Hormetic stressors make cells step up DNA repair, and boost antioxidant enzymes and neurotrophic factors (compounds that guide tissue to grow).[5-7]

A decrease in autophagy has been linked to health issues such as accelerated aging, infections, heart disease, neurodegeneration, and even cancer.[8]

In this book, we are going to discuss different external hormetic factors (xenohormesis), but our main one will obviously be your diet. To use xenohormetic components of the diet, a person consumes "less-harmful" antinutrients that can have beneficial effects when eaten in moderation.[9]

GOOD ANTINUTRIENTS

Certainly, you've heard on TV or have even read online articles about phytochemicals (chemicals from plants) or phytonutrients like curcumin, flavonoids, polyphenols, quercetin, resveratrol, and sulforaphane, just to name a few. As you know, they are recognized as tools for optimizing your health. They're said to boost immunity, reduce inflammation, and have anticarcinogenic and antiaging effects.[10]

What you might not know is that most of these compounds are actually antinutrients.

Wait, aren't antinutrients bad? Yes, they are! But these are not as bad as lectins, oxalates, or phytates. And, if consumed in controlled doses, they can trigger hormetic processes in our body. Thus, they are good for you because they are (slightly) bad for you.

These phytochemicals become beneficial because they create a small amount of stress in our cells. In his book *Genius Foods*, Max Lugavere suggests that "eating polyphenol-rich foods is like giving our cells a workout, challenging them to detoxify, adapt, and grow more resilient to stress."[11]

When we consume these compounds, our cells, trying to defend themselves, respond by ramping up the production of antioxidants (substances that fight the harmful compounds). In fact, research has even shown that these internally made antioxidants produced after consuming polyphenols, for example, are more powerful than the antioxidants (like vitamin C and vitamin E) that we would obtain through food.[12] What this means is that you might have better (or at worst, the same) long-term immune system improvement by occasionally subjecting your body to some of these "good" antinutrients than by eating antioxidant-rich foods every day.

THE BEST-KNOWN PHYTOCHEMICALS

Some researchers estimate that there are over 25,000 phytochemicals in existence.[13] In the next few pages, we are going to discuss them one by one. Just kidding. As the viral YouTube video says, "Ain't nobody got time for that!" Instead, I am briefly going to present the phytochemicals with the most evidence-based benefits and the foods where you can find them.

• **Ajoene**—found in garlic. Research shows that this compound has strong antibacterial properties against the growth of *E. coli*.[14] Ajoene has also been concluded to have antioxidant, neuroprotective, and tumor-fighting properties.[15]

• **Allicin**—found in chives, garlic, leeks, onions, and shallots. It has similar properties to those of ajoene.[16] In addition, research also shows cardioprotective and detoxification properties.[17,18]

• **Allyl isothiocyanate**—found in bok choy, broccoli, brussels sprouts, cabbage, cauliflower, horseradish, kale, kohlrabi, mustard greens, radishes, rutabagas, turnips, and watercress. Research shows anti-inflammatory effects and even protective action against brain, bladder, colorectal, liver, and prostate cancers.[19-31]

• **Anthocyanins**—found in berries, red grapes, and red onions. Research shows that their anti-inflammatory, antimicrobial, and antioxidant properties may provide protective effects against cancer, cardiovascular disease, metabolic disease, neurological disease, type 2 diabetes, and weight gain.[32-36] Anthocyanins have also been shown to be beneficial for gut health.[37]

• **Apigenin**—found in parsley, rosemary, sage, and thyme. Research shows that this compound seems to have strong neuroprotective properties, especially in the brain.[38–41] It also may promote the health of the urinary system and have an effective anticarcinogenic action.[42–44]

• **Carvacrol**—found in oregano oil, thyme oil, wild bergamot—and tequila. Research has shown that this compound, similar to allyl isothiocyanate, is a strong anticarcinogenic agent.[45–48] Carvacrol also has antimicrobial, anti-inflammatory, antioxidant, and cardioprotective effects.[49–52] Shot of tequila, anyone?

• **Catechins and epicatechins**—found in apples, avocados, blackberries, black grapes, cherries, cocoa, dark chocolate, fava beans, guavas, peaches, pears, purple potatoes, raspberries, red wine, sweet potatoes, and especially in green tea. Research shows that these compounds are neuroprotective. They seem to protect the brain from cognitive decline and even improve memory, cognition, and spatial awareness.[53,54] They may even lower the risk of developing Parkinson's and Alzheimer's diseases.[55–57] If that weren't enough, catechins have been shown to have cardioprotective, antiobesity, antiviral, antimicrobial, anti-inflammatory, and anticarcinogenic properties.[58–67] Whew . . . Green tea for the win!

• **Curcumin**—found in turmeric. Possibly one of the most famous phytonutrients on this list. Research has shown that it has anti-inflammatory, antioxidant, antimicrobial, antiviral, antimutagenic (combating gene mutations), hepato-protective (liver protective), and immune-system-stimulating properties.[68,69]

• **Eugenol**—found in basil, cinnamon, cloves, and nutmeg. Research shows that it has strong antioxidant properties (five times stronger than those of vitamin E).[70] Besides that, it seems to promote bone and liver health, and even protect against cancer.[71–75]

• **Fisetin**—found in apples, cucumbers, grapes, kiwis, onions, persimmons, and strawberries. Research shows powerful antioxidant effects as well as possible cardioprotective, antiaging, antimicrobial, anticarcinogenic, and cognitive and mood-boosting properties.[76–96]

• **Oleocanthal**—found in extra-virgin olive oil (EVOO). Research supports oleocanthal as a strong anti-inflammatory compound. It seems to be even stronger than ibuprofen.[97–99] Oleocanthal also appears to support cardiovascular health and healthy cell and brain function.[100–106]

• **Punicalagin**—found in pomegranates. Research, once again, points to strong antioxidant properties (three times stronger than the phytonutrients in wine and green tea).[107] Punicalagin may also be associated with lowering blood glucose, reducing inflammation, and improving memory.[108–113]

• **Quercetin**—found in apples, broccoli, capers, grapes, leafy greens, peppers, and red onions. Research shows quercetin's ability to reduce allergy symptoms, risk of degenerative brain disorders, cardiovascular disease, inflammation in the body, and even cancer.[114–123] Quercetin has also been deemed an age-fighting compound.[124,125]

• **Resveratrol**—found in blueberries, cranberries, dark chocolate, grapes, lingonberries, mulberries, peanuts, pistachios, red currants, strawberries, and probably most famously, red wine. Research has found that resveratrol may lower blood pressure, balance cholesterol levels, protect the brain, increase insulin sensitivity, reduce joint pain, fight cancer, and increase our life span.[126–143]

• **Sulforaphane**—found in cruciferous vegetables, especially broccoli sprouts, but also arugula, bok choy, broccoli, brussels sprouts, cabbage, cauliflower, collard greens, kale, mustard greens, turnips, and watercress. Research shows that this compound may help with blood glucose control, support cardiovascular health, protect against brain damage, and even ease some symptoms associated with autism spectrum disorder.[144–151] But sulforaphane seems to shine brightest as a cancer-fighting agent. Several studies indicate that it has anticarcinogenic properties and may help prevent cancer.[152–157]

• **Ursolic acid**—found in apple and cranberry skins, as well as in basil, blueberries, cherries, marjoram, oregano, plums, pomegranates, rosemary, sage, and thyme. Research suggests ursolic acid may fight inflammation, function as an antimicrobial agent, lower anxiety and depression, and help us lose weight and build muscle.[158–166] More human studies are needed to confirm some of these properties, though.

THE DANGERS OF OVERCONSUMPTION

I recognize that we, as human beings, have a tendency to take things to extremes. Many authors, forgetting that these substances are still antinutrients, recommend that you eat tons of these compounds every day. Please note, just because some phytochemicals have beneficial effects, this does not imply that we should overconsume them. Dosage is still key here.

Imagine the example of a man who hires a dominatrix once a week to slightly rough him up. That dose (one dominatrix once a week) makes him happy about life. But if he suddenly decides to hire 10 dominatrices every day for a week, instead of this experience taking him to his "happy place," it will take him to the hospital. The same goes for these antinutrients. A little works like a potion; too much works like a poison. In fact, research has demonstrated that excessive consumption of these phytochemicals can cause hormonal dysfunction, liver and thyroid damage, digestive problems, and damage to DNA.[167]

Let me give you some concrete examples here. If you go to a supplement store, you will see curcumin supplements everywhere. Even though there is research supporting the many benefits of this phytonutrient, as we saw earlier, there is also plenty of research warning us about its overconsumption. For starters, turmeric (what curcumin comes from) is one of the plants with the highest concentration of oxalates, and I don't need to remind you the consequences of too much oxalate consumption. Curcumin has been shown to cause chromosome aberrations and DNA damage.[168–171] It is also a potent iron chelator (it binds to iron and makes it unusable), which can lead to iron deficiencies.[172]

Please don't get me wrong, I still recommend taking curcumin whenever you're under higher inflammation or oxidative stress (like after sleep deprivation or exposure to toxins), but I do not recommend taking a curcumin/turmeric supplement daily.

Eugenol, which we also discussed before, has also been found to be toxic in high amounts. In a case study, a two-year-old boy suffered serious liver damage caused by consumption of clove oil (rich in eugenol).[173]

Finally, we also have the example of sulforaphane. As we learned, this is one of the phytonutrients with the most potential in terms of health benefits. On the other hand, excessive amounts of this compound have been associated with genetic dysfunction and autoimmunity.[174] In mice, sulforaphane increased susceptibility to seizures.[175] To be fair, the amounts studied here are difficult to reach by just eating broccoli or other vegetables. Even so, it's wise not to overconsume sulforaphane and especially to stay away from high-concentration supplements.

If you've read this far, I'm sure we can agree on one thing: The way our bodies operate is not as linear as many experts present it to you. Our bodies work in complex ways, and even the best science might not give us all the answers. While I was doing my research on antinutrients, I noticed this pattern of discrepancies between test-tube studies with isolated compounds and similar studies with whole foods, as well as discrepancies between animal and human studies.

The interaction between the various substances in the whole food seems to add up to completely different results than when these substances are isolated. Moreover, I also noticed that the impact in the animals or humans also depended on the digestive health of the subjects, more specifically, the gut health. As it seems, the bacteria in our gut interact with phytonutrients. Depending on the specific bacteria that populate you, you might have better or worse outcomes after consuming antinutrients and other phytonutrients. This might explain why in some test-tube studies, certain phytonutrients produce serious damage to human tissue, while, in whole-food-consumption experiences, the same substances actually prove beneficial.

Is it possible that these benefits are coming from the interaction between our gut microbes with these compounds? That's what we are going to find out in the next chapter.

NEO SUMMARY
• Hormesis is the concept of exposing our bodies to small doses of stressors in order for them to grow stronger.
• Autophagy is the mechanism in which the body collects and destroys damaged cells and proteins, so new ones can take their place.
• Hormesis induced through food is a form of xenohormesis.
• There are several "less harmful" antinutrients and other phytonutrients (plant compounds) that appear to have health-promoting properties.
• Overconsumption of these same substances may make you sick depending on your intestinal health status.

NEO ACTION
• Explore the list of phytonutrients and start testing how you feel with some of those foods. Remember, do not overconsume them.

NEO RECOMMENDATIONS
• *Genius Foods* by Max Lugavere
• *Lifespan* by Dr. David A. Sinclair
• *Regenerate* by Sayer Ji
• *Stronger by Stress* by Siim Land
• *The Longevity Solution* by Dr. James DiNicolantonio & Dr. Jason Fung
• *Total Gut Balance* by Dr. Mahmoud Ghannoum

SCAN ME

my.neodiet.co/neorecommendations

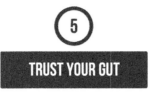

TRUST YOUR GUT

The Fascinating World Inside You

"The gut is the seat of all feeling. Polluting the gut not only cripples your immune system, but also destroys your sense of empathy, the ability to identify with other humans."
Suzy Kassem

YOU HAVE COMPANY

In 2014, while I was battling depression, no matter what I did, I felt that there was always something bringing me down. Later, as I was trying to find a path to heal myself, I learned that our mental health is deeply connected to the health of our gut. After learning this, somehow I knew the solution to my problem would be here. *I don't know. Call it a gut feeling.* Luckily for me, I was right. Things have changed a lot since then, and this chapter results from my in-depth research. I am really excited to share it with you.

First major breakthrough was realizing that I wasn't alone. I'm not saying this in the sense of the hundreds of anecdotal reports I read about people going through the same issues I was. I am being a little more literal. Within our bodies (in our skin, mouth, nose, intestines, and genitals), and even in a cloud around us, we have hundreds of trillions of different microorganisms. Not only do we have communities of bacteria living with us, but we also have fungi, parasites (yes, like worms . . . yuck!), protozoa, amoebas, archaea, viruses, and bacteriophages.

If we really think about this, at first it can seem gross, I know. But the reality is that we have to coexist to live. They depend on us for food, and we depend on them in order to be healthy. We are so deeply connected that these microbes even create chemical messengers that will control our mood and behavior. They are a big part of us. As Dr. Gundry says, "one of our biggest health misconceptions comes from our collective lack of awareness of who we really are. The real you—or the whole you—is actually what you think of as 'you,' plus those multitudinous microbes."[1]

We could get into a discussion about consciousness and the role these microorganisms may play in the perception of the different facets of our living experience. Sure, we might just be meat robots being controlled by these guys living inside us, just like in *The Matrix*. Certainly, the exploration of this topic would be interesting and hilarious. But I'll leave it to someone else. What's important here is that you know that at the most basic level, you are not alone. And the interactions you have with your "roommates" will dictate how you feel and perform.

YOUR BUGS MAKE YOU COMPLEX

Genetically speaking, the human being is not that complex. There are other animals and even plants with more genetic information than you have. I kid you not. Corn has around 32,000 genes, while you have a little more than 20,000.[2]

How did we become so complex, then? As we learned when we discussed the human genome project, looking just at our genetic information is not the answer. After all, genetically speaking, humans are not that different from our chimp "cousins." The big difference, as you are certainly guessing, comes from the bugs living inside of you. Researchers with the National Institutes of Health (NIH) concluded that the microbiome contributes 8 million unique genes to our human bodies.[3] An extra 8 million genes is a lot of processing power. And since we can borrow some of that juice, it's easy to understand how we became this complex.

NO LONGER FOES

In the late 1800s, medicine was struggling to find a solution to all the infectious diseases affecting us. The turning point in this situation was when a French chemist named Louis Pasteur came up with the germ theory. The germ theory maintains that certain diseases are caused by the body's invasion by pathogenic microorganisms (germs). And, even though this is true, the scientific community took this concept to the extreme and deemed microbes to be the only cause behind diseases. This conditioning made us perceive the microscopic world as these devilish agents that should be eliminated at all costs. As they say in the Marines, "Kill 'em all. Let God sort 'em out."

This was the leading thought for many, many years, until we discovered the microbiome. These newer findings spurred a paradigm shift in how we see the microscopic world. Yes, there are plenty of pathogenic microbes, but there are also tons of good microbes that help you stay alive, every day.

If we look the "bugs" in our microbiome, we can find a mix of mutualists (good), pathogens (bad), and commensals (neutral).[4] What determines your health is the ratio between them. In his book *Eat Dirt*, Dr. Josh Axe suggests that the average healthy mix of microbes should be about 85 percent mutualists and commensals, and 15 percent pathogens.[5] Yes, it is good to have some bad guys. Like elsewhere in nature, if you remove the top predator, you can destroy the entire ecosystem. Your gut is no different.

If we can keep these numbers, we are in a state of homeostasis (equilibrium), and we have a symbiotic (mutually positive) relationship with our bugs. On the other hand, if the pathogen population increase their presence, you enter a state of dysbiosis (negative imbalance in the microbiome), which can cause health issues, of course. Shortly, we'll look into some consequences of dysbiosis, but for now, what you need to know is that you have control over this balance. The microbiome feeds on what you eat. So, by carefully selecting what you eat, you can make the bad guys grow or starve. The goal is to starve them so they don't last long enough to make us ill. The Neo Diet is designed to support the good bugs and simultaneously create an internal environment that's inhospitable to disease-causing bacteria, fungi, and viruses.

Diversity is also important. You might have the proper 85:15 ratio, but if you don't have a variety of different species of mutualists, you won't be as healthy as someone who does.

Let me explain this. Imagine your gut as a city. Your city has active, "ethical" workers (mutualists), mobsters (pathogens), and retired people (commensals). When you have a good ratio, you have enough active workers (assuming they have the right to perform a citizen's arrest) to keep the mobsters under control. The perps end up doing only some smaller crimes, and violence is kept in check.

However, it's not just about quantity of mutualists but also their diversity. Let's say that among your active workers, you have a very limited diversity of professions. Suddenly, the streets need paving and we have to have the barbers doing it because you don't have engineers or construction workers. Either the work won't be done at all or it will be done poorly. This also happens in your microbiome. Different species are good at different tasks, and for you to have the most help possible, you should have a diverse microbiome.

SYMBIOTIC RELATIONSHIP

In a perfect scenario, we have a rich and diverse microbiome living in harmony in our large intestine (that's where the big majority should be). Here, they can munch on what we could not digest in our small intestine. They work in teams to break down these hard-to-digest foods and allow you to absorb the nutrients you need. We rely on our bugs to digest a lot of our food because they are much better at it than we are. For example, the digestive enzymes we produce have a hard time digesting the rigid outer cell walls of raw leaves and vegetables. For your microbiome, that's peanuts. In the process, they also help us out by synthesizing micronutrients like vitamin K.[6]

They even let you know whether you're doing a good job providing for them. If they are well fed, they stimulate the production of feel-good hormones like serotonin. In fact, 95 percent of the serotonin in your body is manufactured and stored in your gut.[7,8] To sum things up, if your microbiome is well fed, you will be happy.[9]

In his book *Fiber Fueled*, Dr. Will Bulsiewicz points out, "If I were to boldly define the entirety of human health, there would be five essential elements: immunity, metabolism, hormonal balance, cognition, and gene expression. That would cover our bases for everything we need to thrive as humans, and what's amazing is that the microbiota is intertwined with all five axes of human health."[10]

Directly or indirectly, your microbiome influences your metabolism, digestion, detoxification, skin health, kidney function, liver function, longevity, and emotional and cognitive states (including the risk of development of diseases like depression, Parkinson's disease, Alzheimer's disease, autism spectrum disorder, and attention-deficit/hyperactivity disorder).[11-19] Your microbiome is so important for your health that some researchers have said we should consider it an organ.[20]

Even though I won't go into an in-depth explanation of how the microbiome is involved in all the processes mentioned above, I think it is important to briefly explain some of them. In chapter 2, we understood how crucial it is to have a healthy digestive system not only for your ability to absorb the nutrients from food but also to have a strong immune system. What I did not mention at the time was that the microbiome is an essential part of those two functions.

Your microbiome will help you unpack the hard-to-digest foods and in the process will produce brand-new nutrients or unlock nutrients hidden inside these foods, like amino acids, conjugated linoleic acid (CLA), B vitamins, and vitamins C and K.[21-24] All these are building blocks for all the systems mentioned above. Beyond that, your microbiome will also help you maintain the integrity of your intestinal wall and is deeply connected with your immune response.[25]

Since they live inside you, your bugs have a vital interest in keeping their house clean and safe. They are in constant communication with your immune system to make sure things stay this way.[26] Although our immune system gets along with our microbiome, your bugs are still foreign to you, having their own DNA.[27] So communication between your microbiome and immune system is essential to toning the immune response. Your microbiome helps your immune system by signaling when pathogens are invading[28]—almost like alerting the immune system that this new invading nasty bug is not part of the community and should be removed. Like the public transportation slogan, if you see something, say something. This helps your immune system stay sharp.

Recently, it has also been discovered that there may be links between the microbiome and longevity. In a study with 1,000 participants ages three to over 100, it was discovered that the participants who were over 100 possessed very similar microbiomes to those of the 30-year-olds. The researchers concluded that a healthy gut was the key indicator for individuals who live into their 100s.[29] In another study, researchers actually identified the specific types of bacteria (Ruminococcaceae, Lachnospiraceae, and Bacteroidaceae families) allegedly responsible for this greater longevity.[30] These specific families of bacteria tend to be lost as we age. People who live to be 105 years old or beyond, however, seem to hold on to them. These microbial populations seem to be a determining factor in this longevity.

Our microbiome is so connected to us that it is a major part of what creates our bio-individuality (biological uniqueness) and how we respond to our environment and the food we eat. Researchers, using solely information on the individual's gut microbial profile, were able to accurately predict which foods would cause more or less of a blood sugar spike. And this measure was different for every person.[31]

These unique microbial profiles might even control your love life. Have you ever noticed feeling attracted or turned off by someone's smell? It's been demonstrated in animal studies that bacteria control the release of compounds called pheromones that are deeply connected with sexual attraction and mating behavior.[32–34] Furthermore, this phenomenon might also apply to kissing. Even though anthropologists don't seem to concur with this, some theorize that kissing may have evolved as a way of sampling a potential lover's microbiome for compatibility.[35-37]

OMG, I just had a million-dollar idea! I am going to create a dating service in which you spit in a vial and send it to a lab. We will identify your microbial profile and find the perfect match for you. Do you know someone interested in investing?

IT ALL STARTED WITH YOUR MOTHER

You start developing your bug collection through your mother. In her womb, you received your first microbes via her placenta.[38] Then, at birth, as you went through the birth canal, you were bathed in your mother's vaginal biome. Interestingly enough, a mother's vaginal biome changes. Before you were born, your mom had a microbiome rich in *Lactobacilli*.[39] Yes, the famous bacteria you hear about in all yogurt commercials (*Lactobacilli* love to feed on dairy). Among other functions, this rich community was there to be part of your initial microbiome and help you digest your mother's milk (while they also expanded their presence in your gut). Research shows that children born via the vaginal canal have much more robust and diverse microbiomes than their counterparts born via C-section.[40] In another study, it was shown that children delivered vaginally have a gut biome that is like the mother's gut biome. In contrast, children delivered by C-section have a gut biome that is more similar to the mother's skin biome.[41]

These differences in the microbiome will have significant consequences for a child's immunity. It's believed that Csection babies' microbiome populations can only catch up around the six-month mark and that this delay might even have long-term consequences.[42] As the authors of this 2012 study say, "infants born by Cesarean section and initially colonized by bacterial species of epidermal, rather than vaginal, origin are predisposed to development of allergies and asthma later in life."[43] Other studies found that C-section babies present an increased risk of developing asthma, lower respiratory tract infections, juvenile arthritis, celiac disease, ulcerative colitis, type 1 diabetes, and obesity.[44,45]

Obviously, I understand that not every woman can deliver vaginally. A possible solution might be to swab the newborn C-section baby with microbes from the mother's vagina. Yes, I'm suggesting to expose the baby to the vaginal juices. Of course, there is a discussion on how effective this practice might be, but it's low risk and definitely worth a try.

The next big microbiome builder is the mother's milk. Breast milk contains up to 600 different species of bacteria, which will be a great a contributing factor in the child's microbiome diversity.[46] Breast milk also contains several nondigestible molecules that become fuel for the microbiome[47]—increasing not only the diversity but also the quantity of the baby's microbiome populations.

Unfortunately, baby formula does not confer all these benefits. Research shows that formula-fed children have less-diverse microbiomes as well as an increase in the potentially harmful bacteria *C. difficile*.[48] Babies with an underdeveloped microbiome have been shown to be at an increased risk of autoimmunity, allergies, asthma, allergic rhinitis, coronary artery disease, diabetes, obesity, and late-onset sepsis.[49–52] A poor early microbiome, in particular the absence of *bifidobacteria*, has been shown to lead to systemic inflammation and a greater likelihood that vaccines will cause adverse effects on the infant.[53]

For all these reasons, the World Health Organization (WHO) has recommended that babies should be exclusively breastfed for the first six months of life and should continue to nurse at the breast until the child's second birthday.[54]

If you were not breastfed, you are not alone. Many infants, including yours truly, were not breastfed. Sometimes this decision was forced because of physiological or emotional reasons, but many times it was, and it still is, significantly influenced by marketing propaganda from the baby formula industry. In my particular case, I suffered the consequences of my mother's inability to breastfeed, as I already shared. Even now, after all these years, I know I need to take good care of myself so I don't go back to my fragile former self.

EARLY-LIFE EXPOSURES AND THE HYGIENE HYPOTHESIS

As you continue to develop, your environment becomes the major source of exposure to microorganisms. Early-life exposure to animals, dirt, germs, and bugs aids in the development of your microbiome and consequently of your immune system. This is probably why industrialized countries have higher rates of inflammatory and autoimmune diseases than less-developed countries (where children typically play outside in the dirt).[55]

This phenomenon is justified by the hygiene hypothesis. The hygiene hypothesis proposes that early-life exposures to certain microorganisms protect children from allergic diseases through training the immune system.[56] In other words, human beings were designed to have these exposures to microbes when we're growing up. We were not supposed to live in a sterile bubble. Our exposures to good and bad microorganisms teach our immune system how to operate.[57] It's like having an army. If the soldiers don't practice, they won't be prepared when the actual war arrives. Growing up, being exposed to the natural world is the equivalent of practicing. Your immune system starts to identify the good and bad microorganisms, and becomes stronger and better equipped to deal with more serious threats.

Due to the influence of our dear Louis Pasteur, most developed societies bathe their kids in antibacterial lotions constantly. If the kid touches a bit of dirt, parents have a heart attack. To make matters worse, at the earliest sneeze, they get prescribed antibiotics immediately. This microbiome nuclear bomb extinguishes the few defenses these poor younglings had.

These kids become so poorly prepared to deal with pathogens that at the slightest exposure to them in the future, their immune system attacks in full force. It's almost like a fly entering your house and you deciding to use a machine gun to kill it. You might kill the fly, but in the process, you will also destroy your entire house. In your body, this is the equivalent of allergies and autoimmunity. Your immune system reacts to things that aren't threats, things like pollens, foods, or animal hair, and creates a full-blown war that will also attack your body's healthy tissue.

I'm not saying we should throw the concepts of hygiene and sanitation out the window. Please continue to shower, for God's sake. Some hygienic measures have greatly reduced infectious diseases and infant mortality. But being germophobic is causing more harm than good.

Neo Note: COVID-19 and the Hygiene Hypothesis

As I am writing this chapter (summer of 2021), we are noticing through anecdotal reports how the sanitation measures imposed by the health authorities might be making our kids sicker. Please note that I am not questioning their efficacy or importance. But the reality is that social isolation and constant disinfection are decimating the environmental microbial exposure of these kids. The full long-term consequences are yet to be studied, but all indicators point toward worse health outcomes for these oversanitized and isolated children.[58–60]

Early-life (before six years old) exposures to pets seem to be important to train our immune system. This is further supported by the fact that if the first exposure occurs later in life (after age six), it may be detrimental.[61] At this stage, since there haven't been any previous exposures, the immune system will overreact to this first contact. Early exposure is the key here. How early? Probably even before birth. Researchers found that if, while pregnant, the mother had exposure to farm animals, the child demonstrated protection from the development of immune disorders later in life. Additionally, the researchers also noticed that the more animals the mom was exposed to, the better health outcomes the child presented. This prebirth exposure even presented better outcomes than if the child was just 12 months old when he or she first encountered animals.[62]

Exposure to plants is also connected to better health outcomes. People with plants around their homes have more diverse skin microbiota.[63] In fact, teenagers with a variety of plant life surrounding their homes presented a lower level of skin allergies, such as rashes and eczema.[64]

Finally, even exposure to other humans will influence your microbiome. Have you ever heard the expression *you are the average of the five people you spend the most time with*? This might be more literal than you think. Researchers have found out that people share a more similar microbiome profile with the people they spend the most time with (even if not related) than with their biological parents or siblings.[65] Like my grandfather used to say, choose wisely who you spend your time with!

THE "BIOTICS"

For the past 15 to 20 years, we have been bombarded by ads about probiotics. It all started with yogurt and being able to poop, then eventually moved on to kombucha and taking advantage of probiotics to lose weight. More recently, the craze migrated to prebiotics and even postbiotics. But what exactly are all these "biotics"?

In this section I am going to briefly introduce these concepts so you know what they mean when they recur throughout the book. Later, as we discuss different foods (filled with these "miraculous" substances) and even the strategies to heal your gut, we will uncover more research about these microbes' uses and benefits. For now, let's keep it light and simple.

Probiotics are nothing more than living bacteria—the same families of bacteria that become the mutualist microbes of your microbiota. They've been named *probiotics* because *pro-* means "positive" and *biotic* means "pertaining to life or caused by living organisms." Basically, probiotics are living organisms that benefit the host. *Pre-*, of course, denotes "what comes before." In this instance, prebiotics are the food that allows the probiotics to grow. Finally, postbiotics are the compounds that probiotics produce after eating lots of prebiotics. In other words, prebiotics + probiotics = postbiotics.

Probiotics

There are several claims about probiotic supplements being superb for you. But we are left to wonder: Is this assumption backed by science, or are these supplements just marketing and hippie-dippy medicine?

The truth is that good probiotics do work. I say "good" because, as with many other supplements, you have excellent companies that produce wonderful products and bad companies that sell you "encapsulated fillers" (with barely no active substance). Quality is key. Here is a recap of some studies and their conclusions about probiotics.

• Probiotics can increase the production of proteins that are responsible for the integrity of the intestinal wall. They also enhance your gut's protective mucous membrane and stimulate the immune system.[66,67]
• Probiotics can help clear infections from the gut and resolve dysbiosis.[68,69]
• Probiotics help the body detoxify and reduce its levels of toxic free radicals.[70]
• Probiotics can enhance the effectiveness of antibiotics. They also help return the gut microbiota to normal after a course of antibiotics.[71-75]
• Probiotics have been shown to improve anger, anxiety, depression, hostility, and stress-hormone levels.[76] They help make you happier, with fewer negative thoughts and less sadness.[77-79]

These are some of the benefits backed by the most significant research, but there are many more studies referring to other potential benefits. Either way, we can clearly conclude that probiotics are beneficial and can be a powerful tool for improving our health.

Since they are beneficial, should we take them every day? You know me well enough by now to guess my answer. Supplements are intended to supplement a treatment plan, not to be taken indefinitely. Taking probiotics every day without solving the underlying issues is just creating dependence. As soon as you stop taking them, the symptoms will return. The key is to take them while you are healing, but then stop.

Prebiotics and Postbiotics

Prebiotics are the food that fuels the beneficial bacteria and other microorganisms in our gut. They are composed mostly of nondigestible carbohydrates and dietary fiber. When your microbiome critters ferment and metabolize these prebiotics, they originate by-products such as butyrate and other short-chain fatty acids (SCFAs). These postbiotic compounds have numerous health benefits, like helping to stimulate the integrity of your intestinal wall, soothing inflammation, and boosting cellular health.[80–82] As I said, I'm keeping this brief for now, but in chapter 10 we'll run down the best sources of prebiotics, and we'll also take a look at further research.

To end this section, let me just answer the usual question. If prebiotics are good at feeding our probiotics so as to create beneficial postbiotics, should we eat tons of prebiotic-rich foods? The answer is: It depends. Let's say that you are not used to eating a lot of prebiotics and suddenly you go nuts on them. This might cause bloating, gas, cramping, constipation, or diarrhea. Another example is the case of people that have an overgrowth of bacteria, as with small intestinal bacterial overgrowth (SIBO). They already have more bugs than they're supposed to. Providing them a ton of food will just make the matter worse. On the other hand, if you are healthy and don't have any dysbiosis going on, slowly building up your tolerance and increasing your consumption of prebiotics can be an incredibly healthy move. But even that strategy has a ceiling, as we will see later on.

> **Neo Note: Modbiotics**
> The new "biotics" term on the streets is *modbiotics*. These are compounds that "modify" your microbiome through their antibacterial, antifungal, and antiparasitic properties. They are not live organisms and they are not indiscriminate killers like antibiotics. They are antinutrients or phytochemicals like polyphenols that balance your microbiome by thinning the herd of harmful microorganisms as well as increasing the beneficial species that have anti-inflammatory properties.

THE GUT AS A CENTRAL PILLAR OF HEALTH

As a kid, while spending time with my father during the holidays, I always noticed that when the plants in his garden looked sick, he would dig around the plant to look at the roots. Any experienced gardener will tell you that even if the problem seems to be in the leaves, most likely it's coming from the roots. The roots are essential because they are the part of the plant that absorbs water and nutrients from the soil. If the roots are healthy, you will have a healthy plant.

The gut is our equivalent to a plant's roots. The gut is where you absorb water and nutrients. And if your gut is not healthy, you might develop symptoms that will show up in other parts of your body.

This modern lifestyle we've adopted has been taking a toll on our gut and consequently is making us sick. As you know, the immune, nervous, and endocrine systems are deeply connected with your digestive system, and they all communicate with each other. The digestive system is your engine. It allows all other physiological processes to have the raw materials and building blocks to work.

When your gut is healthy, you are resilient, sharp, and full of energy. You are in superhuman mode. But when your gut has issues like dysbiosis, increased permeability, and inflammation, you are in wimpy-human mode. Not only do you have uncomfortable and embarrassing digestive symptoms, but you also experience brain fog and lack of energy. You may even start developing chronic and serious diseases.

WHEN THINGS START TO GO SOUTH

The balance among the different microorganisms living inside your gut is an essential part of your health equation. Good, neutral, and bad, they all coexist in a complex ecosystem. The mutualists, when in the majority, keep things neat and supervise the pathogens. If needed, the mutualists go full Fight Club on them and make sure their real estate is in great condition. The commensals are like that weird cousin who comes to the family gatherings but just stays in the corner the whole time. He's harmless, just let him be.

If you, as the landlord, can provide favorable living conditions for your good guys, they make sure to keep you healthy. On the other hand, if you create a toxic environment, they will start dying and losing their diversity. When this happens, they lose their influence on the "streets," and the pathogens gang up and start wreaking havoc inside your gut.

As modern humans, we have become poor landlords. It's not like we do it on purpose, but the lifestyles we have are not gut friendly. Every day, we expose ourselves to things that will have a direct impact on our digestive health. We take antibiotics and other strong medications like they were candy; we eat fast food full of inflammatory substances; we barely get prebiotics in our diets; we live in a toxic world full of dangerous chemicals; we are completely disconnected from nature; we are always rushing and under stress; we don't sleep enough; and some of us top things off with high consumption of alcohol to numb the emotional pain we feel inside. All these things will have consequences. One of them is dysbiosis. Trust me, it's no joke.

Clostridium difficile (*C. diff*) is a pathogenic bacteria that can live in the colon. Even healthy people can have some *C. diff* on board but have no issues because the good guys keep it in check. The problem with *C. diff* is when the number of good guys starts to fall and *C. diff* doesn't have enough mutualists to stop it. All hell breaks loose. *C. diff* will cause severe inflammation of the colon that only gets worse as the pathogen grows and multiplies. This will cause abdominal pain, fever, and explosive and bloody diarrhea. It can get so bad that some people end up losing parts of their colon or, worse, their lives. As scary as this sounds, this issue is becoming more and more frequent.[83] According to the Mayo Clinic, each year in the United States alone, about half a million people get sick from *C. diff*, and in recent years, *C. diff* infections have become more severe and difficult to treat.[84]

The standard medical treatment for this infection is antibiotics. The irony is that *C. diff* infections often start because of the prior use of antibiotics, which kill off the good bugs.[85] Unfortunately, the use of antibiotics as treatment is becoming less efficient, and doctors have to keep trying new antibiotics as *C. diff* develops resistance to them.[86,87]

Desperate times require desperate measures. Medical experts decided to look at ancient treatments in an attempt to solve this growing issue. Do you know what approach they tried that has been producing very promising results? Fecal microbiota transplantation (a.k.a. fecal bacteriotherapy), or fecal transplants for short.[88,89] Yes, it's exactly what it sounds like. You take some poop from a healthy person and transfer it to the colon of the sick person. The "healthy poop" is full of good bacteria that can go full Chuck Norris on *C. diff*. In case you didn't understand the martial-arts-hero reference, by adding healthy poop, you repopulate the gut with good bacteria and restore the balance of the microbiome.

It's kind of disgusting, but it works. I hope this never happens to you (if you follow the Neo Diet, it won't . . . *cough, cough*), but if it does, just pretend the poop is coming from Dwayne Johnson or Beyoncé—depending on your preference. Still nasty, but it sure is some powerful poop!

What is the moral of the story here? Most issues don't arise from the increase of the bad bugs but because of the loss of the good ones. It's not a matter of trying to get rid of all the bad guys, like many experts preach. That will never happen! That type of ideology is the same one that created the hygiene hypothesis. The goal here is to have a diverse and thriving community of good guys. And then just let them do their job.

Neo Note: Firmicutes and Bacteroidetes

Let me tell you about Firmicutes and Bacteroidetes. These two large groups of bacteria are present in the gut, and some experts say that Firmicutes are bad and Bacteroidetes are good. People make this claim because folks with obesity have high levels of Firmicutes compared with Bacteroidetes, meaning they have a high Firmicutes/Bacteroidetes ratio.[90] Does this mean Firmicutes are "bad"? Not really.[91] Firmicutes are important for the production of the postbiotic butyrate (which is fantastic for cellular energy) and they may even be involved in the absorption of calcium.[92,93] Firmicutes are good. But if they grow too much in relationship to Bacteroidetes, it creates a disarrangement in your intestinal ecosystem. The key is to keep everything in balance and not let one particular strain dominate your gut.

In conclusion, our westernization is causing us to lose biome diversity.[94] This loss in diversity is at the root of many Western diseases.[95] But fear not! The Neo Diet will help you empower the good guys, increasing their diversity and restoring the balance in your gut. Easy peasy!

DYSBIOSIS

Similarly to plants, you might have an issue in your "roots," but the symptoms only appear in your "leaves." Dysbiosis can go undiagnosed for years, because many of the clinical symptoms might show up far away from the gut.

Believe it or not, researchers report that dysbiosis might cause the following symptoms and conditions: acne, ADHD, allergies, anxiety, asthma, atopic dermatitis, autism, candidiasis (yeast infection), *C. diff* infection, celiac disease, chronic fatigue syndrome, chronic skin rashes, depression, gastroesophageal reflux disease (GERD), *H. pylori* infection, inflammatory bowel diseases (IBS, Crohn's disease, and ulcerative colitis), joint pain, metabolic syndrome and prediabetes, migraines, multiple sclerosis (MS), obesity, premenstrual syndrome (PMS), rheumatoid arthritis, schizophrenia, small intestinal bacterial/fungal overgrowth (SIBO or SIFO), and systemic lupus erythematosus.[96-124]

This is an impressive list, and my goal in sharing it is to show how important your microbiome balance is. If you have one of the above-mentioned diseases or symptoms, your microbiome and gut may need some attention. Later, I'll provide you with strategies to correct these imbalances. For now, let's explore how your gut is impacting some of these issues.

SMALL INTESTINAL MICROBIAL OVERGROWTHS

SIBO, once thought to be rare, is now one of the conditions experts in functional medicine talk about the most. Contrary to before, with our modern technology, it has become easy to diagnose. Because of this, we now know that it's way more common than once believed.[125] SIBO and its counterpart SIFO are serious problems and deserve their section in this book.

> **Neo Note: The Mycobiome**
> When talking about the microbiome, many experts focus mostly on the bacteria (bacteriome) but completely neglect all the other organisms that make up this gut community. No question that bacteria is the most representative faction in your intestinal population, but other residents—fungi, in particular—also affect your health. Fungi usually have a bad rep, but they aren't all bad. Some are very helpful in small amounts.
> The reason we don't hear a lot about your fungi, your mycobiome, is because most research focuses on bacteria, and only bacteria. We have forgotten about the other guys, but luckily, things are changing. Your

mycobiome may not outnumber your bacteriome, but according to microbiome specialist Dr. Mahmoud Ghannoum, it can compromise your health, contributing to weight gain, digestive problems, inflammatory bowel disorders, and even mood disorders and other mental illnesses.[126]

Fungi are multicellular organisms that, similar to animals and plants, have a nucleus and other organelles. The fungus family has many members, but some of the most famous are mushrooms, yeast, and mold. To answer your question, no, you do not have mushrooms growing inside of you.

Another famous fungus celebrity is Penicillium. The name sounds familiar, right? That's because some members of this family of fungi produce penicillin, the mold derivative that has been used as an antibiotic. This was a tremendous medical discovery back in the early 20th century and has saved many lives.[127] Unfortunately, there are other types like *Candida*, *Aspergillus*, Mucorales, and *Fusarium* that have also made us incredibly sick and even caused death.[128]

While fungi represent only 0.1 percent of your microbial species, they still compete with bacteria for the spotlight, because fungi are larger.[129] Gut bacteria shift slowly with your dietary changes. Gut fungi, by contrast, can shift significantly with every meal, so we can use this in our favor to rebalance the mycobiome.

Under normal conditions, most of your gut bacteria live in your colon (large intestine), but with both SIBO and SIFO, these microorganisms decide to set up shop in your small intestine—where they are not supposed to live. When they move into the small intestine, they not only cause classic GI distress symptoms (like diarrhea, gas, bloating, nausea, burping, and indigestion) but also interfere with digestion and absorption of nutrients. They're also associated with inflammation because they damage the intestinal lining.[130]

As discussed in chapter 2, you digest and absorb most of your food in your small intestine. If you now have hungry microorganisms there, they will eat your food and you won't be able to absorb the nutrients you need. Over time, this can lead to malnutrition and deficiencies in calcium, iron, and vitamins A, B_{12}, D, and E.[131] To make matters worse, while feasting on your food, they will produce toxins. These can cause neurological and cognitive symptoms, such as depression and even autism.[132-134]

Why are these microbes invading your small intestine? Experts suggest two chief causes: dysmotility and low acid.[135]

Dysmotility is a condition in which the food is not moving through the GI tract as quickly or efficiently as it should due to compromised muscle activity. It's a reduction in peristalsis (wave-like muscle contractions that move food through the GI tract). These peristaltic waves should occur between meals, every 45 minutes to three hours. In patients with SIBO or SIFO, the timing is delayed, which allows your food and microbes to sit there a lot longer.[136] In a very basic way, they are not pushed down as fast as they can climb up.

Acid-blocking medications commonly prescribed for acid reflux are also associated with causing SIBO and SIFO.[137] Your microbes like to live in a low-acid environment, so your colon is the perfect spot. As food leaves the stomach (super acidic), it starts being exposed to alkaline fluids from your gallbladder and pancreas, which causes a dilution of the acid. Along its journey, the food becomes less and less acid—a process called acid gradient. When the mixture reaches the colon, the acid has been so diluted that it no longer causes harm to your bugs.

When you produce low stomach acid, your small intestine becomes less acidic than normal and allows your bugs to feel comfortable there. *Guys, pack your things, we're moving!*

> **Neo Note: Overgrowths Make Everything Worse**
> Research has found that individuals with celiac disease frequently have SIBO as well.[138-144] Even though not all studies agree with this, there seems to be enough evidence to suggest this correlation. The interesting part is that many times, people with celiac disease don't undergo an improvement in their symptoms when they go gluten-free.[145] But when they treat their SIBO, the symptoms finally disappear.[146] By all means, I am not saying that celiac disease is not real or that all the symptoms are being caused by SIBO. What I am trying to explain is that SIBO is surely making the symptoms more persistent. A similar relationship has been documented regarding SIFO and Crohn's disease (CD), IBS, and ulcerative colitis (UC).[147-151]

CANDIDA OVERGROWTH

With SIBO, several species of bacteria might be the culprit. With SIFO, however, *Candida* is responsible for the majority of the cases. (*Aspergillus* is the runner-up.)[152] In the US, *Candida* species are the fourth-most-common cause of hospital-acquired infections.[153] One study even showed that these *Candida*-infected patients had a 40 percent mortality rate, even when being treated for the infection.[154] It's a serious issue!

Candida is an opportunistic yeast. When the environment is right, it can quickly multiply and grow out of control. It used to be believed that this occurred only in individuals with suppressed immune systems, but now we know it also happens in people with normal immunity. Usually, it occurs more often in cases of malnutrition and after the use of corticosteroids and antibiotics.[155-157] In the case of antibiotics, this happens because of the indiscriminate killing of bacteria, which allows *Candida* to grow and flourish without competition.

Candida (and other yeast) overgrowth can cause another disorder called gut fermentation syndrome (GFS), a.k.a. auto-brewery syndrome.[158] This uncommon digestive disorder can result in feeling drunk . . . all the time. *Sounds fun!* Not really. The symptoms include asthma, sinus infections, extreme difficulty concentrating, brain fog, chronic fatigue, depression, lower immunity, bloating, and constipation.[159] There is even one case reported by CNN in which a woman was fined for drunk driving but was able to get the fine dismissed after providing evidence that she suffered from GFS.[160]

Candida might also have mental health implications. Researchers have gone as far as to suggest that preventing *Candida* overgrowth can ease symptoms of manic depression, schizophrenia, ADHD, and autism.[161]

Recent findings also show that *Candida* has the ability to interact with bacteria and other fungi to create biofilms (digestive plaque) that shield it from the immune system and even from antibiotic and antifungal treatment. These biofilms act like a bunker, and the doors only open when the residents want to eat or take out the trash. That's it! In his book *Total Gut Balance*, Dr. Ghannoum states that not even desiccation, oxidation, or radiation can readily penetrate the exterior of these biofilms, which is why it's so difficult to treat biofilm-associated infections.[162]

Fungal pathogens like *Candida* even release anti-inflammatory signals to fool the immune system, and create camouflage molecules on the surface of the biofilm that make it more difficult to locate.[163] Biofilms provide pathogenic microbes a safe haven where they can reproduce and grow, which only aggravates the already-dangerous situation. These biofilms have been linked to the disruption of the intestinal mucosal barrier, Crohn's disease, and colon cancer.[164–168]

Neo Note: *Candida* Arthritis

In some severe cases of *Candida* infection, this yeast can invade and degrade joints like hips and knees (most common), and also shoulders, ankles, elbows, wrists, toes, and vertebrae. This *Candida*-produced arthritis can erode and destroy bone, marrow, and cartilage, increasing fracture risk and causing pain and inflammation.[169]

There is still a lot we don't know about *Candida* and other fungal infections, but one thing is certain: they are proven opportunistic pathogens with the ability to cause a lot of trouble. There is no question they need to be dealt with. However, standard treatment is to take antibiotics or antifungal medications, which, as we already know, carry the risk of increasing dysbiosis. In chapters 16 to 18, you will encounter a new way of eating for gut health. We will stimulate the growth and diversity of the good bacteria and keep bad bacteria and fungi under control. It will be all good in the hood.

AUTOIMMUNITY

According to a study in the *Journal of the American Medical Association*, diseases such as obesity, asthma, and neurobehavioral disorders like autism have been on the rise. Between 1994 and 2006, these issues increased 15 percent among US children.[170] Celiac disease used to be incredibly rare, but after the 1980s its prevalence rose. Today, it affects almost 1 percent of the global population.[171] The number of children with type 1 diabetes has been exploding. Globally, the average increase in incidence has been 3 percent to 4 percent per year over the past few decades.[172] Just between 1997 and 2011, according to the Centers for Disease Control and Prevention (CDC), food allergies among children increased by a whopping 50 percent.[173] Do you know what these have in common? They are all representations of chronic inflammation believed to have an autoimmunity basis. Yes, these "isolated" diseases increasing actually represent an epidemic of autoimmunity.

We briefly discussed autoimmunity when we spoke about molecular mimicry and lectins, but let's dig a little deeper here. In a nutshell, autoimmunity is the umbrella term for conditions in which a person's immune system gets confused and hyperactivated, attacking the body's own tissues. This is the equivalent of what the military calls friendly fire.

Depending on the trigger and the tissues involved, you can have different representations. One example is food allergies. Imagine that your immune system is hyperreactive and mistakes strawberries for an aggressive pathogen. Suddenly, each time you eat strawberries, your immune system goes into full attack mode and creates inflammation around your GI tract. In a way, this is the representation of a food allergy. It's not that the food is bad per se, but your body mistakenly identifies it as bad and creates an exaggerated response to it every time you eat it.

In the case of a food allergy, it's easy to identify the trigger, but that is not the case with many other autoimmune conditions. What we know for sure is that there is some sort of molecular mimicry involved, because most autoimmune diseases tend to attack very specific tissues in the body.

For example, when your body starts attacking intestinal tissue, you can develop celiac disease or IBD; when it targets thyroid tissue, you can develop Hashimoto's disease or Graves' disease; when it goes after joint tissue, you can end up with rheumatoid arthritis; when it wreaks havoc with nervous tissue, you can develop MS or amyotrophic lateral sclerosis (ALS); and when it attacks your skin tissue, you can develop eczema and psoriasis. You get the idea!

There are many triggers for these autoimmune responses. One of them, as we already discussed, is the consumption of lectins. Because of their molecular mimicry abilities, they get our "immune scanners" (TLRs) confused and have them order the attack on similar-looking tissues in our body. Other triggers include dysbiosis and exposure to toxins. What they all seem to share is their ability to create inflammation and alter the gut lining's permeability. This phenomenon is commonly called leaky gut syndrome.

LEAKY GUT SYNDROME

As you'll recall, our gut lining is an integral part of our digestion. The mucosal cells absorb nutrients and pass them into our circulatory system to eventually be distributed where they're needed. The gut lining is simultaneously responsible for keeping toxins and other pathogens outside of us. Some even say that about 70 percent of our immune system surrounds the gut.[174] Almost like the customs and immigration services at the airport, they decide who may enter and who needs to be barred. Every day, thousands of microorganisms and by-products of digestion come in contact with this one-cell-layer-thick wall. This wall is almost like a castle fortification, but it has thousands and thousands of gates. These microscopic gates (the tight junctions between your cells) are slightly open, just enough to let nutrients pass through into your bloodstream, but not open enough to allow larger and potentially dangerous microorganisms in. If all this works well, your gut lining is efficiently triaging who enters and who needs to be stopped, and the rest of your innate immune system regulates your interaction with the microbiome, keeping things quiet.

But when you suffer from dysbiosis or consume excessive quantities of antinutrients and other toxins, the mucus that coats the walls gets thinner, and the gates start losing their ability to stay closed enough to block these pathogenic microorganisms or toxins. As the intestinal lining loses its integrity, it becomes the entry point for unwanted particles, or pathogens. When they then enter the bloodstream, an immune response is triggered.

To make matters worse, either dysbiosis or the consumption of some lectins (or both) can trigger the release of zonulin.[175] As we learned in chapter 3, zonulin has the ability to tell the tight junctions to open. What used to be a helpful immune response now becomes a constant event that keeps the gates wide open, day and night. When this happens, your gut "leaks" and cannot block the passage of these pathogens.

Leaky gut (a.k.a. intestinal hyperpermeability) was considered a myth for many years. I'm not sure if it was treated that way because of the silly name it was given, but recent studies have proved its existence. Research has even suggested the possibility of its being the "gateway disease" to many other, more complex health problems.[176] Once bacteria or toxins are able to sneak past the intestinal lining of someone suffering from leaky gut, these aggressors go to different parts of the body and trigger an autoimmune response.[177] In other words, leaky gut might be the first stage of development of many known diseases.

To support this theory, studies have linked leaky gut to conditions such as:

- ADHD[178]
- Allergies and food sensitivities[179]
- ALS[180]
- Alzheimer's disease[181]
- Anxiety and depression[182]
- Autism[183]
- Celiac disease and nonceliac gluten sensitivity[184]
- Chronic fatigue syndrome[185]
- Crohn's disease[186]
- Fibromyalgia[187]
- Hashimoto's disease[188]
- IBS[189]
- Metabolic syndrome[190]
- MS[191]
- Nonalcoholic fatty liver disease[192]
- Parkinson's disease[193]
- Polycystic ovary syndrome[194]
- Restless leg syndrome[195]
- Rheumatoid arthritis[196]
- Skin disorders such as acne, dermatitis, eczema, psoriasis, and rosacea[197]
- Systemic lupus erythematosus[198]
- Type 1 and type 2 diabetes[199–201]
- Ulcerative colitis[202]

Trust me. This list is only scratching the surface. As more research is done, more conditions will continually be added.

After analyzing this information, some will look at this and feel like it's the end of the world. Leaky gut can cause so many serious conditions. On the other hand, some (myself included) will look at this and think, *I can heal most of these conditions just by healing leaky gut. With one therapeutic approach, I can heal multiple problems.* Makes sense, right? That was exactly what Dr. Gundry and his team tried to prove in a study they did with 102 patients with biomarker-proven autoimmune diseases. After following a leaky-gut healing program (similar to what we are going to present later in the book) for six months, 94 percent of them were disease-free, were off their medications, and presented negative biomarkers.[203] Yes, this is just a small study, but it definitely shows that our theory about healing autoimmunity by fixing leaky gut has tremendous potential.

IRRITABLE BOWEL SYNDROME

Irritable bowel syndrome (IBS) is one of the most common intestinal disorders.[204] Although I won't go into detail, I feel it is important to write a short section about this disease since it affects many people. This condition is characterized by abdominal pain, bloating, gas, and constipation or diarrhea. According to a 2009 study, individuals with IBS go to the doctor more frequently, undergo more diagnostic tests, are prescribed more medications, are less productive, miss more workdays, and are hospitalized more often than other patients.[205] Other studies suggest that individuals being treated for IBS have lower measures of physical, social, and emotional well-being compared with healthy people and even those with other chronic illnesses.[206,207]

A clear structural cause has not been found, but we have learned that one of the key elements of this disease is visceral hypersensitivity.[208] What this means is that people with IBS have increased sensitivity of all the nerves that surround the gut (that is, the enteric nervous system). This causes an exacerbated perception of triggers that most people would not feel at all. For example, IBS sufferers think they produce more gas, but in reality they produce the same amount; they just feel it more due to the hyperactivation of these nerves. This altered response from the nerves around the gut produces not only sensitivity issues but also mechanical issues that alter the normal motility (transit control) of the gut.[209] What causes the nerve dysfunction? Again, no definite answers here, but it's thought to be caused by inflammation produced by dysbiosis and leaky gut.[210] If IBS goes untreated, it can lead to severe digestive issues that can contribute to malabsorption of nutrients, toxin buildup, and mental health problems.[211]

IRRITABLE BOWEL DISEASE

Irritable bowel disease (IBD) is an umbrella term that includes both ulcerative colitis (UC) and Crohn's disease (CD). Granted that IBD is different from IBS, but in my way of seeing things, IBD is the 2.0 version of IBS. It's IBS with a kick of autoimmunity. UC and CD involve relatively similar symptoms but affect different locations and layers within the lower digestive system. UC tends to affect only the colon, while CD can affect the upper GI tract as well. In terms of symptoms, IBD can start with issues similar to IBS but then develop into more complicated ones like bloody stools, anemia, weight loss, bowel obstruction, intestinal perforation, and colorectal cancer.[212,213]

During the past few decades, the incidence of IBD has been increasing with the industrialization of our diet and lifestyle.[214,215] *Can you see the pattern once again?* Scientists believe IBD may have a genetic component, but that needs to be taken with a grain of salt because of epigenetics, as you know.[216] That being said, a clear etiology (cause) is not recognized by the medical community, but IBD's pathogenesis (development) is undoubtably associated with autoimmunity.[217] After what you just read about autoimmunity, do I need to tell you what might be causing IBD? Thought so! Just in case you are a bit insecure . . . yes, you were right . . . it's leaky gut.

I hope that by now you can see all the patterns and understand that at the most basic level, most of these diseases are the product of our consumption of toxins (antinutrients included), states of dysbiosis, and leaky gut. In the Neo Diet, we are going to skip the traditional medical approach of addressing these different diseases by looking at the symptoms. Instead, we will be laser focused on fixing the cause, and healing several problems at once.

THE MICROBIOME-GUT-BRAIN AXIS

Have you ever met a special someone and felt "butterflies" in your stomach? What about having GI distress before an exam or a big meeting? These are some of the very basic day-to-day things that show the deep connection between your gut and your brain. This deep-rooted connection is known as the microbiome-gut-brain axis (MGB axis). This sounds like a recent discovery, but if we look at ancient medical approaches like Ayurveda, we can see that the large intestine has been considered the "seat of the entire nervous system"—meaning that the brain and the rest of the nervous system are governed by what happens in the gut.[218-222]

Please note that your gut talks to your brain, but your brain also talks to your gut—this is a bidirectional conversation.[223] Studies show that negative changes in the microbiome and digestive system can affect the function and structure of the brain, causing depression and anxiety. Likewise, changes in cognitive function affect the microbiome and the GI system.[224]

Initially, the MGB axis was called simply the gut-brain axis. Most recently, researchers decided to emphasize the importance of the microbiome. Studies have shown the tremendous influence it has on your brain and behavior.[225] Your microbiome has even been shown to have a direct correlation with your personality traits.[226] All the recent research done in this area has led to a concept called psychobiotics.[227] In his book *The Psychobiotic Revolution*, science journalist Scott C. Anderson explains, "this field focuses on the treatment of mental health issues by changing the gut microbiome through probiotics and prebiotics."[228]

How are these distinct regions of our body connected? Early in your development as a fetus, a group of cells called the neural crest appears and divides into two parts. One part turns into the central nervous system, and the other becomes the enteric nervous system (the nerves around your gut, also called "the second brain"). Later in your development, these two systems connect through the longest of all cranial nerves, the vagus nerve. *Vagus* means "wanderer," and the nerve was given this name because on its way from the brain to the gut, it makes minor detours to connect (and innervate) most of the body's major organs. The vagus nerve is the major component of the parasympathetic nervous system and regulates involuntary bodily processes like breathing, your heartbeat, and peristalsis.[229] For this chapter, the most important thing you need to know is that the vagus nerve works as the physical bridge between gut and brain. Recent studies even have suggested that "gut invader" lectins use the vagus nerve to go from the gut into the brain.[230]

Your gut and brain not only communicate via landline but also use Wi-Fi. The equivalent of Wi-Fi in your body is the use of chemical messengers. Let's look at some of these messengers.

• **Serotonin:** As you know, this is a "feel-good hormone" produced mostly in the gut, but also in your brain. This compound acts as a hormone and a neurotransmitter, regulating your emotional state. An imbalance in serotonin levels can be associated with anxiety, depression, and autism.[231] Similarly, it also regulates gastric acid secretion, GI blood flow, and peristalsis.[232]

• **Dopamine:** This is a neurotransmitter that is associated with feelings of euphoria, motivation, and concentration. Dopamine is released by your brain when you experience pleasure, but it's said that about half of this neurotransmitter is produced in your gut.[233] Dopamine influences movement control, sleep, learning, mood, memory, and libido, and is even associated with mental health conditions such as anxiety, depression, schizophrenia, and Parkinson's disease.[234-239] It is also involved in gastric secretion, intestinal motility, and mucosal blood flow.[240-242]

• **GABA:** The neurotransmitter gamma-aminobutyric acid (GABA) is produced and consumed by multiple species of intestinal bacteria.[243] It promotes relaxation, reduces stress, balances mood, eases pain, and facilitates better sleep.[244-246] GABA also helps with intestinal motility, reduces inflammation, and improves immune function.[247,248]

• **Postbiotics:** Short-chain fatty acids (SCFAs) such as butyrate, propionate, and acetate, known for their role in fueling the cells of your gut and regulating your immune response, also seem to exert physiological effects on several organs, including the brain.[249-253] As we already discussed, gut dysbiosis has been connected to behavioral and neurologic diseases, such as depression, Alzheimer's and Parkinson's diseases, and autism spectrum disorder. Likewise, the field of psychobiotics has been successfully manipulating the microbiome and, consequently, the production of SCFAs to treat these and other mental health diseases.[254]

In conclusion, the MGB axis is a network of biochemical signals between the digestive system and the central nervous system (the brain and spinal cord). Physically through the vagus nerve, and chemically through neurotransmitters, hormones, and postbiotics, the MGB axis also connects the endocrine system, the immune system, the autonomic nervous system, and the gut microbiome.

LEAKY BRAIN SYNDROME

In your brain, you have a tight junction system similar to the one in your intestinal barrier, called the blood-brain barrier (BBB). Its main role is to choose which particles are allowed into the brain and to block the ones that should not have access to it. The walls in your gut and the ones in your brain are so alike that they are susceptible to the same type of assault from dietary and environmental aggressors. Thus, a dysfunctional or "leaky" BBB can cause a brain invasion by inflammatory toxins and pathogens.[255] When these bad boys enter the brain, they can cause inflammation, neuronal oxidative stress, sepsis, neuronal death, and brain damage.[256]

This hyperpermeability of the BBB walks hand in hand with leaky gut. If a person didn't have a leaky gut, the toxins and pathogens would not have access to the brain. Of course, there are exceptions, like a wound infection, for example. But the majority of our exposure to these inflammatory molecules and organisms occurs through the GI tract. With leaky gut sufferers, once these troublemakers pass through the gut walls, they have two main highways to the brain: the bloodstream and the vagus nerve. The culprits can even cause damage at a distance. These invaders can lead to an increase in cytokines (proteins that signal your immune system to intervene).[257] Cytokines can then cause brain inflammation and damage.[258,259] The rest of the story, you already know.

The same way a leaky gut can lead to a leaky brain, a healthy microbiome and strong gut can keep you happy, relaxed, sharp, and full of energy. I start to feel bad about constantly repeating myself, but once again, to heal many of the cognitive and behavioral issues we experience, one should heal the gut first.

Neo Note: "Leaky Balls"

You already know how leaky gut can cause leaky brain. Now, it's time to learn how it can also cause "leaky balls." I know, it sounds goofy and not very scientific, but it's true. In a leaky gut situation, you can have pathogenic bacteria in your bloodstream. The same way they can go up north to your brain, they can also go down under. I'm not talking about Australia, mate. I'm talking about testicles! This theory even has a fancy name. It's the GELDING theory (gut endotoxin leading to a decline in gonadal function).

Yes, studies have shown gut bacterial endotoxin in the testes. Here they cause loss of testosterone and decreased sperm production.[260] Men become less ballsy, one might say.

Joking aside, this is a serious situation that should be addressed by healing the gut. One study done with mice suggests that the consumption of probiotics to regulate the microbiome can improve testicular performance and prevent "shrinkage."[261] Considering this and all we've discussed up to this point, we can theorize that healing the gut might reverse this issue.

COGNITIVE AND BEHAVIORAL DISEASES

Throughout the different sections of this chapter, we've discussed several studies connecting gut health with cognitive and behavioral diseases. That being said, I don't feel the necessity to go into detail about the mechanisms behind the development of each of these diseases. If that's something you're interested in, I got you. At the end of this section, I recommend some fantastic books about this matter. In this section, I'll briefly discuss some of the major issues.

Let's start with Alzheimer's disease. This disease was the reason I saw my grandfather "dying"—not his body but his mind—years before his actual death. I understand the pain this disease has caused to many people, so that is why I'm sharing my findings.

Alzheimer's is the most common form of age-related dementia, and its prevalence among seniors has been booming for the past few years.[262] For decades, it has been known for causing the accumulation of amyloid plaques in the brain (almost like the equivalent of kidney stones but in the brain).[263] In his book *The End of Alzheimer's*, Dr. Dale Bredesen shares that amyloid plaques behind this disease can be produced by the microbiome and then make their way to the brain.[264] Here they stimulate even more amyloid production.[265]

A 2021 study theorized that not all amyloid is bad, though. According to the findings, cognitive impairment (associated with Alzheimer's) could actually be caused by a *decline* in soluble amyloid-beta peptide (Aβ42) instead of the corresponding accumulation of amyloid plaques.[266] Apparently, regardless of the amount of plaque in the brain, in this study the individuals with high levels of the Aβ42 peptide were cognitively normal. More studies need to be done to explore this further, but either way, these findings are making us question the way we've been looking at this disease. Independently of that, I still believe that there is a strong gut-Alzheimer's connection, since Aβ42 is heavily influenced by the microbiome.[267-269]

The next on the list is Parkinson's disease (PD). This disease affects, on average, 1 or 2 people in every 1,000. Unfortunately, PD's prevalence is increasing, and it's believed to affect 1 percent of the population above age 60.[270] The most common trait of PD is the loss of dopaminergic neurons (producers of dopamine) in the substantia nigra (a region of your brain), which translates into tremors and impairment of voluntary movements.[271]

Once again, the medical community doesn't yet recognize a clear etiology, but there are many theories out there. One of them has been described by an author I have mentioned several times already (and strongly admire), Dr. Steven Gundry. In *The Plant Paradox*, he shares a study showing that lectins climb the vagus nerve and can then "hide" in the substantia nigra.[272] Knowing this, we can now understand a large Chinese study in which patients who have had a vagotomy (a procedure that cuts the vagus nerve in an attempt to solve digestive issues) many years before, had a 40 percent lower incidence of PD compared with age-matched control subjects.[273] Quoting Dr. Gundry: "Lectins weren't reaching the brain as readily, and therefore weren't able to cause as much harm. It also explains why Parkinson's is more prevalent among vegetarians, as they consume more plants (and therefore more lectins)."[274]

Your brain has specialized cells, in particular microglia and astrocytes (both are glial cells), that handle maintenance and security in your central nervous system.[275] Inside your skull, these two help your brain by nourishing and supporting the neurons and cleaning up waste and dead cells. Similarly to a gardener working with trees and other plants, these glial cells prune away weak dendrites (branches of the neurons) so stronger ones can grow in their place. This is a perfectly normal and healthy process. The problem starts when the glial cells detect that bad guys (lectins and bacteria, for example) or cytokines are coming. When this happens, they prune more intensively in order to contain a possible spread of these aggressors.[276]

While this physiological response is essential during an acute emergency like an infection, for example, it has catastrophic results when it happens all the time as the consequence of a gut dysfunction. Microglial hyperactivation ("hyperpruning") has been associated with the feeling of poor mental performance that you experience when stressed and sleep deprived.[277,278] Unfortunately, that's just a "light" example. Prolonged microglial hyperactivation is responsible for neural inflammation, which has been considered to be the potential mechanism for the occurrence or worsening of neurodegenerative diseases.[279]

I would go even further and add behavioral diseases into the mix. Depression, for example, has been associated with brain inflammation. Depressed individuals who were prescribed anti-inflammatory drugs for pain (unrelated to their depression) saw improvements in their depression symptoms.[280] This after they had demonstrated a poor response to traditional antidepressant drugs. These findings were discovered by accident, but they show that when inflammation in the brain was reduced, the symptoms of depression got better. Imagine how many more cognitive and behavioral diseases might share this.

One of these diseases might be autism spectrum disorder (ASD). Research shows that the pathogenesis of ASD is linked to maternal immune responses that induce inflammation in the brain of the offspring.[281] The inflammation can then lead to brain malformation and alterations that can cause the development of ASD and other neurodevelopmental disorders like ADHD and schizophrenia.[282–284]

As we already discussed before, dysbiosis is linked to ASD (especially to late-onset ASD).[285] What I did not mention was that this was not only applicable to the children. Dysbiosis in the pregnant mother might be one cause creating the inflammation in the fetus's developing brain.[286]

HEALING BRAIN DISEASE THROUGH THE GUT

I don't want to beat a dead horse here. I believe I've shared enough data to support how the gut and brain are deeply connected. Like in a marriage, they are together *in sickness and in health*. If the gut is healthy, the brain is healthy. If the gut is sick, the brain will become sick. The good news is that, contrary to what you've been told before, you are in complete control over your health. Each time you eat, you are deciding between eating something that will make you sick or something that will empower you to be strong and healthy.

If you avoid "toxic" foods, fuel yourself with the right nutrients, and properly feed your microbiome, you will heal your gut. By healing your gut, you not only prevent toxins and pathogens from reaching your brain and causing further damage, but you can also reverse that same damage. The postbiotics produced by your bugs can cross your BBB, nourish your brain, and bring down the inflammation.[287,288] Butyrate, for example, has been shown to stimulate the formation of new brain cells, calm the microglial hyperactivation, slow down age-related memory decline, and reverse anxiety and depression.[289-291] If you have kids, butyrate might even help make them more well behaved.[292] To me, that's a really nice side effect.

Let's use the power of your second brain to heal the first one!

THE GUT IS SICKER THAN EVER

What is the principal cause of this gut disease epidemic we are witnessing? In my humble opinion, the answer lies in our modern lifestyle. Just in the US alone, there are more than 80,000 chemicals on the market. Many of them are in products we come into contact with every day. But incredibly, only about 1 percent have been studied for safety.[293] Imagine what these untested chemicals might be doing to you.

We consume genetically modified crops and eat processed foods filled with additives and preservatives. Not to mention the residue of the harsh pesticides and herbicides still present in these foods. Our obsession with hygiene has led us to use incredibly toxic personal and home cleaning products that have been overloading our detox systems, annihilating our microbiomes, and making our immune systems confused and hyperactivated. If this weren't enough, we then try to heal ourselves by overmedicating our bodies with synthetic chemicals that are only hiding symptoms while making us worse with their huge lists of side effects.

While it would be almost impossible to list and discuss every single agent destroying our guts, in this section, I'll present what I consider the top five offenders.

1. Glyphosate

The first offender is the infamous glyphosate. As mentioned in chapter 1, this is the world's most widely used herbicide, and unfortunately, it has been associated with several serious health problems.

A study done in California tracked urine levels of glyphosate in 100 individuals between 1993 and 2016. Levels of the chemical increased by about 1,200 percent over the 23-year period.[294] In another study done in Germany, city workers, journalists, and lawyers who had no direct contact with glyphosate (or agriculture) were tested for glyphosate contamination. The study found glyphosate in all urine samples at values ranging from 0.5 to 2 nanograms of glyphosate per milliliter of urine. These values are 2 to 20 times greater than the "safe" drinking-water limit of 0.1 nanograms per milliliter.[295]

Despite the evidence that levels are rising, potentially putting us at greater risk of harm, some still continue to say that glyphosate is perfectly safe for humans. A study from the University of Wyoming even stated that glyphosate is less toxic than the other 94 percent of herbicides they tested.[296] The most interesting part of this study was the footnotes, where the researchers noted that this university receives funding from several chemical companies, including Monsanto, the company behind Roundup (a commercial name for a glyphosate-based herbicide). I'm not making any accusations here, just sharing this publicly available info so you can make your own conclusions— *cough, cough.*

How does glyphosate work, anyway? It kills plants by disrupting a metabolic process called the shikimate pathway. This physiologic mechanism is present in plants, fungi, and bacteria but not in animals.[297] The shikimate pathway is an essential process for these living organisms since it is part of the mechanism that will ultimately produce important amino acids (L-phenylalanine, L-tyrosine, and L-tryptophan), vitamins B_9, E, and K, and other metabolites (alkaloids, quinones, etc.).[298]

In reality, as humans, we do not use this pathway, but our friendly gut bacteria and fungi do. So, when we ingest glyphosate by eating GMO crops or non-organic foods that have been sprayed with it, we can observe a reduction in good bacteria and an overgrowth of harmful strains of bacteria in the gut.[299] In other words, it leads to dysbiosis and all its consequences.

Glyphosate is also known for inhibiting cytochrome P450 enzymes, which are essential to detoxifying the body.[300] The more toxins you have, the more health problems you develop, including inflammation of your bowels. Glyphosate also appears to make the tight junctions of the intestinal wall and the BBB more permeable.[301-303] Yes, this means it might cause leaky gut and leaky brain. If all this weren't enough, glyphosate can also cause deficiencies in important minerals (cobalt, iron, and molybdenum), as well as inadequate vitamin D_3 activation, which is essential for several physiological processes in the body, including cellular metabolism and immunity.[304,305] In a nutshell, long-term exposure to glyphosate can lead to chronic intestinal and systemic inflammation of the body, which can then develop into incredibly serious diseases.

2. Ultraprocessed Foods

In chapter 1, we already discussed how the consumption of synthetic colors and flavors in processed foods can cause several health concerns. We also looked at the case of MSG and all its negative physiological consequences. I also shared with you resources on how to further explore the effects of most of the artificial additives being used today. So, I'll keep this section brief and just mention a couple of findings about some of the ones with greater impact on your gut.

First on the list is sodium nitrate. This chemical is commonly used to add color and flavor to preserved meats. Unfortunately, this compound can interact with heat and your stomach acid to produce nitrosamines, which are linked to an increased risk of colon cancer.[306]

Then we have the case of sulfites. Research found that sulfites commonly used in food preservatives killed or inhibited the growth of good bacteria, even when tested at levels regarded as safe.[307]

Finally, we have the worst of them all, emulsifiers (a.k.a. surfactants). Emulsifiers are used to add texture to food products and increase their shelf life. Unfortunately, they also destroy your intestinal mucous layer, which is essential in preventing leaky gut, infection, and inflammation. Studies have shown that even trace amounts of emulsifiers can cause bacteria to leak through your gut into your bloodstream.[308]

More research also uncovered that polysorbate 80 (one type of emulsifier), over time, decreases beneficial bacteria in the gut and increases pathogenic bacteria, which leads to inflammation.[309] Another emulsifier called carboxymethylcellulose has also been associated with altering gene expression in your bugs, which caused an overproduction of flagellin, a gut-irritating protein that can cause inflammation.[310]

Emulsifiers are found in most processed foods, such as salad dressings, ice creams, nut milks, coffee creamers, and pastries. Sadly, their use in the food industry has been increasing over the years.[311]

3. Mold and Mycotoxins

The next offender on our list is mold, in particular mold toxins, also called mycotoxins. We associate mold with our homes, but, as Ben Greenfield shares in *Boundless*, the primary source of our exposure to mycotoxins actually comes from our diet. Why should you be concerned? Quoting a 2020 study, "mycotoxins are considered the most frequently occurring natural contaminants in the diet of humans and animals."[312] And, as we are about to find out, mycotoxins have been connected with several health issues.

Grains have always been the major source of mycotoxins in the diet of man and his animals, but it's now commonly found in other foods, like grain-derived products, coffee, chocolate, raisins, wine, and beer.[313,314] I know, I also shed a tear.

Eating the organic versions of these foods may not make much difference in terms of mycotoxin content.[315,316] Production methods seem to be irrelevant, since the mold toxins are believed to develop with improper conditions of processing and storage of these foods.

How do mycotoxins affect our health? Mycotoxins produce an inflammatory response in our digestive system that can manifest as abdominal pain, heartburn, and constipation or diarrhea.[317] Mold toxins are also said to promote leaky gut by weakening the tight intestinal junctions.[318] This, as you know, can lead to food allergies and autoimmune diseases. Mycotoxins are also sneaky because they target some of the organs important in your detoxification processes, like the liver and kidneys.[319] Indirectly, mycotoxins undermine your effectiveness in getting rid of them, which can cause a cumulative effect that will only worsen your condition.

Research shows that mold toxins are connected with leaky brain syndrome as well.[320] This may explain why mold has been associated with cognitive and behavioral symptoms such as brain fog, anxiety, and depression.[321]

At low levels, mold toxins can produce "light" symptoms like low energy or just feeling off, since the toxins cause mitochondrial dysfunction.[322] At higher levels, they can cause all the issues noted earlier, and as stated by Dave Asprey in his book *Head Strong*, mold toxins can cause serious illnesses such as cardiomyopathy, cancer, hypertension, kidney disease, and brain damage.[323]

4. Medications

I'm not a medical doctor, and I do not provide any medical advice. Throughout this book, I'm only sharing my research and some of my personal conclusions. What you do with that information is up to you. With that being said, my fourth disrupter is medication. While many meds save lives and we should definitively take them, there are also many times when their side effects might outweigh any good the drugs do. Not to mention that we are clearly overmedicated in general, but let's not even go there.[324] In this section, I'm going to present some of the most commonly taken meds that can disrupt your gut and overall health.

Broad-Spectrum Antibiotics

This is the perfect example of a lifesaving medicine that, used incorrectly, can also cause much harm. Like that quote from the late Bob Proctor, "you can cook a man's dinner with electricity; and you can also cook the man."

Broad-spectrum antibiotics were developed in the late 1960s, and they were (and still are) miraculous, saving people from diseases like pneumonia and septicemia. Unfortunately, this new drug made doctors lazy. Instead of trying to assess the proper cause of an infection, doctors started to simply prescribe these antibiotics all the time. Most likely, they were going to get the job done.

This overprescription of antibiotics is still present today, and, sadly, doctors even inappropriately prescribe them in situations of infections caused by viruses and not bacteria.[325] Antibiotics are great killers of bacteria but do nothing against viruses.

Why am I criticizing the overprescription of antibiotics? Well, broad-spectrum antibiotics work by killing almost all strains of bacteria, good and bad. This is necessary in some extreme situations, but taking these antibiotics and destroying your entire microbiome every other month because of a cough makes no sense whatsoever. No wonder kids are sick all the time. At the slightest thing, they get prescribed antibiotics. Their guts are like those western-movie towns with nothing but tumbleweeds rolling through. Research has found that early antibiotic use in children (and even exposure through the mother during pregnancy) is associated with issues later in life including allergies, autoimmunity, asthma, behavioral challenges, Crohn's disease, diabetes, and obesity.[326–328] In adults, broad-spectrum antibiotics also wreak havoc in our microbiomes, which can cause dysbiosis and leaky gut.[329] I'm sure I don't need to remind you of the devastating consequences of these two.

Studies also show that commonly prescribed antibiotics promote mitochondrial dysfunction by inducing high oxidative stress.[330] Certain classes of antibiotics have also been associated with neuronal damage.[331,332]

Yes, the antibiotics are helping fight a sore throat and a runny nose. In exchange, they just steal your energy, create brain fog, and make you anxious and depressed.

You know, Kevin, I am not concerned since I never take antibiotics. Good for you! Unfortunately, you might still be exposed to them indirectly. Antibiotics commonly go into animal feed, to prophylactically protect the livestock against infections or to fatten them up in record time. Even if you only eat organic (and don't use antibiotics) or if you don't eat meat at all, you might still get these meds through your vegetables, since antibiotic residues can leach out of the feedlot into the fields.[333] Even drinking water might have some.[334]

I just want to end this section by mentioning the issue we are facing with superbugs (antibiotic-resistant bacteria). The WHO has recognized that the inappropriate, indiscriminate, and irrational use of antibiotics is creating the global problem of antibiotic resistance.[335] In 2019, in the US alone, the CDC reported 2.8 million cases of infections and 35,000 deaths from 18 antibiotic-resistant bacteria. These are serious issues, folks. We need to get our shit together and stop the antibiotic craziness!

Nonsteroidal Anti-Inflammatory Drugs (NSAIDs)

NSAIDs were introduced in the pharmaceutical market in the 1970s and were only available with a prescription. Now, you can purchase them over the counter in most places. Depending on the country you live in, you can find them under different brand names, but their most common generic versions are ibuprofen, naproxen, celecoxib, diclofenac, ketorolac, and meloxicam.

For the longest time we thought they were safe "as long as you take them with some food." Now we know this is not the case. Several studies have shown that NSAIDs cause adverse effects including cardiovascular, cerebral, gastrointestinal, hepatic, pulmonary, and renal complications.[336]

The gastrointestinal adverse effects are the most common and can start with heartburn and abdominal discomfort, going all the way to more serious issues like life-threatening ulcers.[337] That's right, they don't increase the permeability of your tight junctions, they create full-size holes in your intestinal lining! Combining this with the fact that NSAIDs create dysbiosis of your microbiome, this exposes you to pathogens (and other toxins) and can lead to intestinal inflammation and autoimmunity.[338-340]

Stomach-Acid Blockers

The most common antacid drugs are proton pump inhibitors (PPIs). PPIs were introduced in the 1980s, and once again, they were prescription drugs, not over-the-counter meds like nowadays. PPIs are acid blockers that, in certain isolated situations, might be useful, but are completely unnecessary in most cases. As you already know, stomach acid is essential for your digestion and immunity, since it kills most of the pathogenic bacteria you ingest. If the stomach environment is not acidic enough, more of the interlopers survive, and that can lead to dysbiosis, leaky gut, and autoimmunity. It will also create the conditions for your stomach to be invaded by the pathogenic bacteria *H. pylori*, which can ultimately lead to gastric cancer.[341] Your small intestine also becomes more alkaline than it should be, and you substantially increase the risk of developing SIBO or SIFO and *C. diff.*[342] Beyond the adverse GI effects, PPIs are also known for crossing the BBB and poisoning your brain, contributing to brain fog, Alzheimer's, and other dementias.[343-346]

Selective Serotonin Reuptake Inhibitors (SSRIs)

SSRIs are antidepressants that work by increasing the concentration of serotonin in the brain by blocking the neurotransmitter's reabsorption. With more serotonin in your body than you're used to, you might have some GI issues like diarrhea, but the most concerning side effect is the interaction with your microbiome. Studies show that SSRIs reduce the number and diversity of the microbiome.[347] You increase serotonin's concentration in the brain but lose your major serotonin factory. Not a good trade, in my opinion.

Oral Contraceptives

Finally, a quick reference to hormonal birth control pills. As with all the previously presented medications, I am not saying you should or should not take any of them. I am just sharing the data so you can make an informed decision.

Research shows that birth control pills can significantly affect the health of the microbiome and can substantially increase the risk of developing both Crohn's disease and ulcerative colitis.[348,349] Not to mention that they completely mess up the endocrine system, but that's for another book.

5. LPSs

Lipopolysaccharides (LPSs), also known as bacterial endotoxins, are present in the outermost layer of the cell walls of gram-negative bacteria. Without going into microbiology, let's just say that most gram-negative bacteria are pathogenic and not a major part of a healthy microbiome.[350] As gram-negative bacteria die, LPSs are released into the gut. Normally, we wouldn't worry much, since a healthy microbiome can take care of these pathogenic bacteria. Unfortunately, we know dysbiosis is relatively common, and thus we may have a higher number of LPSs to process.

Having a solid microbiome is only half of the equation. The other half, which somehow seems to be the bigger half (I was never great at math), is making sure LPSs are pooped out without causing harm. To be fair, under normal circumstances, your body can take care of the issue. But you know that "normal circumstances" are long gone for most people. If we consider that most people with dysbiosis (more LPSs) also have leaky gut, you have a shit show (quite literally sometimes). To make matters worse, LPSs further increase intestinal permeability.[351]

Then we have the case of chylomicrons (a.k.a. ultra-low-density lipoproteins—ULDLs). Basically, these are particles that transport fats in food from the intestines to other locations in the body. Research has shown that LPSs can attach to chylomicrons and go past your intestinal wall.[352] Some authors then associate the consumption of fatty foods (saturated fats) with an increase in endotoxemia (LPSs causing harm in your body).

The first thing I want to point out is that chylomicrons also increase after a high-carbohydrate meal, so high fat is not the only culprit.[353] What research also shows is that chylomicrons are actually protective. They bind to LPSs not just to give them a fun ride, but to inactivate them and to assist in their excretion, preventing more serious complications.[354-358] According to another study, chylomicrons spur better health outcomes by limiting macrophage exposure to endotoxins and thereby reducing secretion of inflammatory cytokines.[359] In other words, chylomicrons take care of LPSs without causing as much inflammation as if they were not present. It appears chylomicrons may not be that bad after all.

Research shows that high levels of LPSs in the blood are associated with higher risks of ALS, Alzheimer's disease, autoimmune disease, cardiovascular disease, chronic inflammation, insulin resistance, pancreatitis, type 2 diabetes, nonalcoholic fatty liver disease, and obesity.[360-362] This is probably why Dr. Gundry calls LPSs "little pieces of shit."[363] I'm sure you won't forget about them after that one.

They are also very resourceful in finding ways to harm us. For starters, they increase intestinal permeability, which in itself it is already a gateway to body-wide inflammation and disease. Then, when they invade us, they put our immune system on red alert. Since LPSs are fragments of bacteria, the TLRs read that bacteria are inside us, and our immune system activates a response similar to the one it would use for a real bacterial infection. Each time more LPSs pass through, this intense immune response is activated, which leads to chronic inflammation and all the diseases that result from that.

LPSs don't stop here. They also interact with a protein we have in our bodies called fibrinogen. Fibrinogen is important for our health because, in the case of a wound, it creates a blood clot that stops you from bleeding to death. The problem is that LPSs change fibrinogen and create an abnormal clotting behavior that can potentially cause a heart attack or stroke.[364] LPSs also inhibit detox mechanisms in the body and increase oxidative stress, which causes even more inflammation.[365,366] Think of an LPS as a substance that makes everything worse!

THE MICROBIOME WORLD

This was a long chapter filled with a lot of information. Do not be overwhelmed if you feel this was too much to "absorb"—*ba dum tsss*. I don't expect you to memorize all this. My goal is to create a resource for you to access any time you have a doubt. The important thing here is that you know that your microbiome and your gut health are chief contributors to your ability to feel and perform like a superhuman. Later in the book, I'll give you explicit instructions on how to address these issues simultaneously and easily. Now that you are a gut expert, it's time for you to learn about the epidemic no one talks about. Curious? Follow me to the next chapter.

NEO SUMMARY
• You have trillions of microorganisms living inside your GI tract. Some good, some neutral, and some bad.
• We all have a unique microbiome configuration.
• Your microbiome will influence your mood, your weight, your energy, your memory, and your overall health.
• Imbalances in the microbiome (dysbiosis) can cause GI diseases such as SIBO, SIFO, IBS, Crohn's disease, and ulcerative colitis. Dysbiosis can also trigger issues such as autoimmunity, cognitive and behavioral diseases, and cancer.
• Your gut and your brain are physically and chemically connected. Their health is intertwined.
• Dysbiosis and toxins can cause leaky gut. This will allow pathogens and toxins to invade your body and cause inflammation and disease.
• Leaky gut and dysbiosis are the gateway issues to most chronic inflammatory diseases.
• You can heal from these chronic inflammatory diseases by fixing your gut and balancing your microbiome.
• Our modern lifestyles with processed foods, herbicide/pesticide-filled produce, mold exposure, and overconsumption of meds, are destroying our guts.
• LPSs make everything worse.

NEO ACTION
• Stay away from processed foods.
• Eliminate GMOs from your diet.
• Don't oversanitize.
• Go outdoors and expose yourself to some *bugs*.
• Be conscious of your medication consumption.
• Salute at your poop in the toilet. It's full of "about-to-retire" microbes that helped fight off disease in your gut.

NEO RECOMMENDATIONS

SCAN ME

- *A New IBS Solution* by Dr. Mark Pimentel
- *An Epidemic of Absence* by Moises Velasquez-Manoff
- *Eat Dirt* by Dr. Josh Axe
- *Eat Wheat* by Dr. John Douillard
- *Fiber Fueled* by Dr. Will Bulsiewicz
- *Genius Foods* by Max Lugavere
- *Gut and Psychology Syndrome* by Dr. Natasha Campbell-Mcbride
- *Head Strong* by Dave Asprey
- *Healthy Gut, Healthy You* by Dr. Michael Ruscio
- *Stronger by Stress* by Siim Land
- *The End of Alzheimer's* by Dr. Dale Bredesen
- *The End of Mental Illness* by Dr. Daniel Amen
- *The Energy Paradox* by Dr. Steven Gundry
- *The Good Gut* by Justin Sonnenburg & Erica Sonnenburg
- *The Gut Balance Revolution* by Dr. Gerard E. Mullin
- *The Longevity Paradox* by Dr. Steven Gundry
- *The Mind-Gut Connection* by Emeran Mayer
- *The Plant Paradox* by Dr. Steven Gundry
- *The Psychobiotic Revolution* by Scott C. Anderson
- *Total Gut Balance* by Dr. Mahmoud Ghannoum

my.neodiet.co/neorecommendations

6

INSULIN RESISTANCE, METABOLIC DISORDERS, AND INFLAMMATION

The Epidemic No One Talks About

"When diet is wrong, medicine is of no use. When diet is correct,
medicine is of no need."
Ayurvedic Proverb

BROKEN METABOLISM

During my years in college, I noticed that for the first time since before puberty, I was having difficulty managing my weight. I felt like a sponge. Everything I ate would be absorbed and turned into fat. I had to constantly control my diet to stay decently fit. At the same time, I was also experiencing more frequent injuries. The slightest awkward joint movement was enough to leave me in pain for days. Then there was the low energy issue. I woke up drained every single day. I had to drink six to 10 shots of espresso a day just to function like an average person. Why was this happening to me? I was way too young to experience these issues. Was my metabolism broken?

To answer that question, we need to start by understanding what metabolism is. Usually, we associate metabolism with the ability to "burn fat." We all have that friend who can eat whatever he/she wants because of his/her "great metabolism." *I hope you choke on that ice cream, Helder!*

The truth is that this association with burning fat is an extremely narrow definition of metabolism. The term *metabolism* comes from the Greek word for "change." So your metabolism can be understood as the physiological mechanism that changes (better yet, transforms) the food you digest into the energy that will power all your cells. Metabolic processes are happening all the time, and they control every single biological activity in your body. Your appetite, energy production, immunity, tissue repair, mood, memory, aging, and yes, fat burning, are all controlled at a cellular level.

If you have a "broken metabolism"—which is called metabolic syndrome (MetS) or syndrome X—you can experience negative effects in any bodily system, since they are all made of cells. For me, it was weight gain, low energy, and injury proneness. For you, it might be high blood pressure and high triglyceride levels, for example. MetS is not black-and-white. Technically, it's not a "real" disease by normal definition. It's more of a cluster of conditions and symptoms that increase your risk of heart disease, stroke, and type 2 diabetes.[1] These symptoms on their own are concerning, but their combination can trigger serious medical issues, since several systems become compromised simultaneously.

Metabolic dysfunction is the epidemic people don't talk about. But it's here! Researchers behind a 2018 study done in the US reached the conclusion that it was extremely hard to find people in ideal metabolic health, even in normal-weight individuals.[2] Worldwide, every day we are facing chronic diseases with a metabolic nature that used to be incredibly rare just a few decades ago. In 2019, about 17.9 million people died of cardiovascular disease around the globe (representing 32 percent of all deaths).[3] In 2020, nearly 10 million deaths were attributed to cancer.[4] A 2021 study states that around 463 million adults worldwide have diabetes.[5] According to the World Health Organization, in 2020, 39 million children under the age of five were overweight or obese. Data from 2016 also showed that 39 percent of adults ages 18 years and over were overweight, and 13 percent were obese.[6] More than half of the population is carrying extra weight and thus has a higher risk of developing metabolic disease.[7]

INSULIN RESISTANCE

The numbers are clear: we have an epidemic of metabolic disease on our hands, folks. The big question now is . . . what is causing it?

Once again, there is no clear consensus in the scientific community, but many researchers have noticed insulin resistance as the common underlying mechanism.[8]

In his book *Why We Get Sick* (which I highly recommend), researcher Benjamin Bikman states, "in fact, insulin resistance is the most common health disorder worldwide, and it affects more people—adults and children— each year than any other."[9] Historically, insulin resistance was a disease of the wealthy, but now that is no longer the case. Currently, low-income countries have a higher percentage of cases than high-income countries.[10] The worst part is that most of the people who have it have never heard about it before. They don't know the risks they're facing. That's why it's important to spread this message. The only way we can fight this issue is by sharing knowledge about it.

Well, I go to the doctor all the time, and I was never told that I had insulin resistance. Unfortunately, insulin resistance is not something doctors look for in their regular assessments. It's not because it isn't widely prevalent in their patients; it's simply not one of the commonly ordered tests. This can be due to the costs associated with these tests but may also stem from a lack of knowledge about the condition.

You cannot know for certain without a proper test, but you can "guesstimate" your risk of having insulin resistance by answering some of the following questions:

• Are you overweight?
• Do you have high blood pressure?
• Do you have high levels of triglycerides?
• Do you suffer from water retention?
• Do you have a family history of heart disease?
• Do you have a family history of type 2 diabetes?
• Do you have patches of darker-colored skin or skin tags on your neck, armpits, or other areas?
• Do you suffer from polycystic ovary syndrome (PCOS) or erectile dysfunction?

The more yes answers you gave, the higher your risk of having insulin resistance.

UNDERSTANDING INSULIN

Before we can explore the details on how insulin resistance is leading to metabolic dysfunction, we need to understand what insulin is. As a kid growing up with diabetic family members, I always thought insulin was a medication for diabetes. Later I found out that insulin is a hormone that we, in a healthy condition, produce in our bodies. I would go as far as to say that insulin is the strongest contender for MVH—most valuable hormone—this season. Insulin is one of the most important hormones in human health, since it influences every cell in every tissue of the body.

One of the main things insulin is famous for is regulating your blood sugar. When you eat, one of the end products of digestion is sugar, or glucose, to be more scientific. When these sugars go to your bloodstream, your pancreas is like your distribution manager; its goal is to get the sugar out of the bloodstream and into the cells that need it. To do this, it sends insulin to direct these sugars into the cells. Insulin does not transport the sugars into the cells (you have proteins that do that), but it connects to the cells and opens the doors so the transporters can dump the cargo.[11] Insulin also has an anabolic effect (it helps tissues grow), and it regulates how every cell in your body uses its energy.[12]

When everything works well, insulin does an amazing job at keeping you healthy and strong. The reason for this chapter is that, lately, insulin isn't working as it should. To be fair, it's not the hormone's fault. It's what we are doing to our bodies. Shortly, I'll explain everything in the proper scientific terms, but for now let me just continue with my sugar distribution example. In a normal situation, insulin goes to the warehouses (liver, muscle, and fat cells, mostly), opens the doors, and tells the trucks to dump the sugar there. Smooth process!

Unfortunately, because of our modern diet and lifestyle, we are getting a lot more sugars needing distribution. Luckily for you, your distribution manager (your pancreas) can send more insulin to help. The issue here is not insulin but the fact that the warehouses are full. When your warehouses reach max capacity, they become reluctant to accept more sugars. And so, when insulin gets there, the warehouse staff closes the door, so insulin can no longer do its job and coordinate the delivery of the sugars. When this happens, insulin calls the pancreas and asks for backup. More insulin is then sent to help open the door and proceed with the sugar delivery.

After this initial experience, the problem only gets worse because the warehouse staff build stronger and stronger doors so that insulin can't break them down in the future. This leads to more and more insulin being produced in order to bring down the stronger doors. In a nutshell, you need more and more insulin to take care of the same amount of sugar. This is what we call insulin resistance.

DIAGNOSING INSULIN RESISTANCE

It's difficult to talk about insulin resistance without talking about diabetes. Before we learn how to diagnose insulin resistance, I feel it is important to understand more about the diabetes mellitus family of diseases. *Diabetes* comes from the Greek *diabete*, meaning "to pass through," while *mellitus* is Latin for "honey-sweet." In other words, this name was used to describe the condition of passing sweet urine (glucose in the urine, a.k.a. glucosuria).[13] In the fifth century, Indian physicians determined that there were at least two types of this disease, one associated with young individuals (type 1 diabetes, also called juvenile-onset diabetes), the other with older people, commonly those who were overweight (type 2 diabetes).[14] Even though these two types seemed very different, there were limited diagnostic resources back then. So, since both presented glucose-loaded urine, excess of glucose ended up defining the disease.

Nowadays, we know that the two forms' main differentiator is insulin. Type 1 diabetes is caused by having too little (or even no) insulin (a situation that's of autoimmune origin), while type 2 results from having too much (a condition that has a metabolic origin). Type 2 is then the result of insulin resistance. However, the medical community ended up (incorrectly) wrapping up insulin resistance with hyperglycemia (excess of sugar).

The problem here is that one can have insulin resistance but not necessarily have hyperglycemia. To put it another way, you can have insulin resistance and still have completely normal blood glucose levels. This is the reason this condition often is not properly diagnosed. Most doctors focus only on the glucose levels, since, unlike insulin, these are easy and inexpensive to assess.

If the medical community used the correct test and measured insulin, they would easily see its elevated levels and quickly diagnose insulin resistance (prediabetes), even if glucose levels were normal. But, because doctors don't typically do this, they can detect insulin resistance only when it has already progressed to type 2 diabetes and its consequent hyperglycemia.

This is what is happening in the world. Most people are becoming more and more insulin resistant, while their bodies can still keep glucose levels within the normal range. This might go on for years or decades. Unfortunately, we only recognize the issue once the insulin resistance is so bad that the body can no longer keep the glucose levels in their normal range. We detect the issue when it's almost too late to fix.

INSULIN RESISTANCE AS THE CAUSE OF METABOLIC DISEASES
Type 2 Diabetes

The most obvious metabolic disease caused by insulin resistance is type 2 diabetes. Unfortunately, the traditional medical approach to this disease might not be the wisest. The medical community tends to look at this disease through the lens of "not having enough insulin" instead of considering the more effective approach of "let's decrease insulin resistance."

Although some people with advanced type 2 diabetes have significant pancreatic dysfunction (pancreatic beta cells lose their ability to produce insulin) and can have low insulin levels, this is not the case for most of the patients. Studies show that pancreatic dysfunction in these more advanced cases might even be in part reversible.[15] For most, the pancreas can still produce enough insulin, just not enough to overcome the insulin resistance. Regrettably, many doctors try to fix type 2 diabetes by giving the patient more insulin. This is like giving extra alcohol to a person with a drinking problem. Each time, you have to increase the dose of alcohol to achieve the same level of drunkenness. By giving more insulin to someone who is insulin resistant, we are simply making the resistance worse and creating a vicious circle.[16] A wiser approach is to adopt a diet and lifestyle that support insulin sensitivity, which basically means decreasing insulin resistance.

Neo Note: Blood Is Lava

Your body is a machine that likes stability. The same way your temperature and pH are kept within a controlled range, your blood glucose should also be balanced. When this balance is not kept, you suffer. At any given time, your glucose should be around 1 teaspoon of sugar diluted in 5 liters of blood. When you develop a state of insulin resistance, your body struggles to keep this average, and your glucose levels rise. High levels of glucose in the blood seem to give it "corrosive-like" abilities. It's as if your blood becomes lava.

Elevated blood glucose has been found to directly damage the gastrointestinal epithelium (external layer), the endothelium (internal layer) in the kidneys, and the BBB.[17-19] This "lava blood" appears to corrode our tissues and make them leaky. It might even corrode endothelium of our blood vessels, causing inflammation and atherosclerosis.[20,21]

Obesity

Obesity is strongly associated with the development of insulin resistance.[22] But could insulin resistance be one factor also causing obesity? Is this a two-way relationship? As you know, one of insulin's primary jobs is to regulate your blood sugar by signaling your cells to absorb it, thus removing the excess from the blood. The first warehouse to be filled with sugar is your liver, then the other main organs and your muscles, and finally your fat cells.[23] While your organs and muscles have limited capacity, your fat is more adaptable. It can expand in size and in number. Basically, it can build more warehouses to accommodate all this excess sugar.

Another part of this equation is that insulin blocks the breakdown of glycogen (stored sugar), protein, and fat to be used as fuel.[24-26] Insulin also induces the accumulation of fat (with the goal of using this fat as fuel in the future).[27,28] Finally, your fat cells have an enzyme called hormone-sensitive lipase (HSL) that helps break down body fat into fatty acids that can be used as fuel. Guess what. Insulin also suppresses the activity of HSL.[29] Considering all this, we can say that insulin turns off fuel-burning mode and keeps fuel-storage mode on.

In a case of insulin resistance, you will have chronically high levels of insulin. Since insulin is high all the time, it keeps your body in accumulation mode, thus it puts you in a position to gain more and more weight. This is not just a theory. Several studies support that high levels of insulin, as in insulin resistance, are known as a cause of obesity.[30-32]

Don't know why you can't get rid of that extra weight? Insulin resistance might be the hidden culprit.

Cardiovascular Diseases

It's no secret that insulin resistance and high blood pressure are related.[33] However, research has recently uncovered that insulin resistance is a direct cause of high blood pressure.[34] One of the ways high insulin levels increase blood pressure is through the hormone aldosterone. Your adrenal glands, right on top of your kidneys, release aldosterone to regulate the balance of sodium (salt) and water in your body. Aldosterone tells your kidneys to reabsorb sodium, which causes water retention. The more water you retain, the higher your blood volume and pressure.[35] Insulin enhances aldosterone's effects. Logically, when you have insulin resistance (and thus more insulin in your blood), your aldosterone's effect on your kidneys will be stronger. You will retain more water and increase your blood pressure.[36] To make this worse, as presented in the last Neo Note, insulin can cause inflammation of the blood vessels and hardening of the arteries.

Research shows that insulin resistance is also associated with dilated cardiomyopathy (DCM).[37] DCM is characterized by a dilation of the heart muscle (the myocardium). In theory, with this dilation, the myocardium needs more and more glucose to keep working. With insulin resistance, the heart will have a harder time accessing the needed glucose, and this can aggravate the condition.[38] Here, there is no clear evidence that insulin resistance caused the disease, but we can certainly speculate that it's making it a lot worse.

Brain Diseases

Insulin is essential for all our cells. The ones in your brain are no different. Insulin stimulates the brain to use glucose as fuel, helps brain cells grow, and plays a role in learning and memory formation.[39-41]

When insulin resistance develops, your brain functions get compromised. Insulin resistance is associated so deeply with brain disease that Alzheimer's disease (AD) has been called "insulin resistance of the brain," or type 3 diabetes.[42,43] Insulin may contribute directly to accumulation of the famous Aβ plaque between brain cells.[44,45] But as you know, there are still some questions about insulin's role in AD, so I'm not going to further explore this point.

Another important characteristic of AD is the presence of neurofibrillary tangles ("nerve knots").[46] In your brain, you have what are called tau proteins. They are part of your neurons' maintenance crew. The issue is that sometimes they get overexcited and grab the neurons and twist them, creating knots. Normal insulin levels in the brain inhibit this tau overexcitement.[47] When you have insulin resistance, less insulin is able to interact with your brain, and thus the tau proteins become overactive, potentially leading to more neurofibrillary tangles.[48] Additionally, we can't forget that with insulin resistance, your brain is not getting as much glucose as it should, and this certainly has consequences. PET scans have shown that AD patients have substantial reductions in brain-glucose uptake (absorption).[49] This suggests that AD and other dementias might just result from a starving, shrinking brain. Another consequence of starving neurons might be migraines.[50] Studies have shown that people with insulin resistance were more likely to have regular migraines compared with more insulin-sensitive individuals.[51,52]

Finally, Parkinson's disease (PD) is intrinsically connected with the loss of dopamine-producing neurons, as we discussed in the last chapter. Insulin is known for interacting with dopamine in the brain.[53] A study shows that the most insulin-resistant individuals produced the lowest quantity of dopamine in their brains.[54] PD is a complex disease with many factors involved, but these findings support that insulin resistance can at least aggravate this condition.

Bone and Joint Diseases

Insulin has an anabolic (growth) effect. This applies not only to muscles or neural tissue, but also to your bones. Insulin stimulates the activity of osteoblasts (cells that synthesize bone) and inhibits the action of osteoclasts (cells that break down bone tissue).[55,56] This means that insulin promotes bone growth while simultaneously preventing its loss. If you have insulin resistance, this signaling will not be as efficient, and that can trigger a cascade of events that can lead to osteoporosis.[57]

Osteoarthritis (OA), or joint degeneration and inflammation, has been characterized as a "wear-and-tear" disease. That's what I learned in physical therapy school, and that's what is still being taught in most medical schools around the world. But new findings are making us realize this type of arthritis might be more of a metabolic condition than just a consequence of abusing our joints.

We already learned about how oxalate crystals can accumulate in joints and trigger an inflammatory response. Lectins can also end up there and cause a similar situation. Now, we're going to look at how insulin resistance also has a role in OA.

In your joints you have cells called chondrocytes, which produce and maintain the cartilage in the joints.[58] This cartilage is what protects your joints from wear and tear. Try to guess, what do chondrocytes need in order to get their fuel (glucose)? That's right, the usual suspect, insulin![59] In states of insulin resistance, chondrocytes starve and do a poor job of maintaining the cartilage.

Then we have synovial fluid, the lubricant that keeps you moving without squeaking. Synoviocytes are the cells that produce synovial fluid. When synovial cells are exposed to too much insulin, as in insulin resistance, they trigger an inflammatory response that leads to significant shutdown of their fluid production.[60]

Putting these two together, we can conclude that insulin resistance can cause poor cartilage maintenance and decreased synovial fluid, which are major contributing factors to OA. Indeed, research shows that among individuals of similar weights, the ones with osteoarthritis are more likely to have the highest insulin resistance.[61]

Reproductive Diseases

Gestational diabetes is a condition that can occur during pregnancy when insulin resistance is present. Gestational diabetes is known for increasing the risk of preeclampsia—one of the most dangerous pregnancy issues. Research has found that women who develop more severe insulin resistance early in pregnancy have higher chances of developing preeclampsia during the second half.[62] Even if insulin resistance doesn't cause any issues during pregnancy, it can affect the mother's ability to nurse. And you know how important this is for the healthy development of the baby. Researchers uncovered that women with high insulin resistance were likely to have low milk supply.[63]

Now, let's talk about the fellas. Insulin resistance makes men "less manly." This is because higher levels of insulin lead to lower testosterone levels.[64] Having low testosterone is not a good thing. Low T can cause reduced bone mineral density, decreased athletic performance, weight gain, losses in muscle strength and mass, fatigue, depression, diminished libido, and erectile dysfunction (ED).[65,66] ED is actually directly connected with insulin resistance.[67] This link is so strong that researchers say ED could be one of the earliest signs of insulin resistance, especially in young adults.[68] How's that morning wood, boys?

Cancer

To end this section, we are going to talk about the Big C—cancer, that is. While cancer is commonly recognized as a condition that results from genetic mutations, increasing research questions this "fact." Is it possible that we've been approaching cancer incorrectly all this time? Authors of a 2019 study raise this question very eloquently:

> Could cancer causation be interpreted as an allegory not to the damaged hardware (damaged genetic material caused by chance mutation) but to an incorrect function of a software (a metabolic program)? Do we thence use wrong approaches to treat the cancer disease with chemotherapy and radiation therapy, which are aimed at destroying the hardware (killing cells), instead of a more sophisticated approach aimed at reprogramming the software inside the cells in order to restore the normal mitochondrial function and metabolism?[69]

Independently of the existence of genetic triggers in some cancers, recent scientific research shows that metabolic dysfunction might be what makes cancer develop and grow.[70] As you know, insulin has an anabolic effect. It would make sense that if your body has increased levels of insulin in the blood, this would trigger more cellular growth, especially of cancer cells. Let me clarify something. I said "especially" for two reasons: First, cancer cells loooove sugar.[71] They appear to have a sweet tooth, and in insulin-resistant states, it's almost like an all-you-can-eat sugar buffet. Second, cancer cells are metabolically wired differently.[72] They have a lot more insulin receptors than most cells.[73] This is like the warehouse having a lot more doors for sugar to be delivered. In other words, there are many more ways to get sugar into cancerous cells; that is, they're more insulin sensitive.[74] Because of their high sensitivity, they can grow a lot faster when insulin is in overabundant supply.

Breast cancer seems to be one of the cancers most commonly associated with insulin resistance. According to 2020 numbers, it's also the world's most commonly diagnosed cancer.[75] Average breast cancer tumors have over six times more insulin receptors than healthy breast tissue has.[76] Research also shows that women with the worst breast cancer outcomes are the ones with the highest levels of insulin resistance.[77] This relationship is so strong that some places have even started to treat breast cancer with insulin-sensitizing medications and have presented very interesting results.[78]

Studies show that insulin, but not glucose, is also associated with a higher risk of developing prostate cancer.[79] Indeed, considering men of the same age, race, and body weight, the ones with higher insulin levels have about a 250 percent greater likelihood of developing prostate cancer.[80] Insulin resistance might even make cancers more lethal. Research shows that insulin-resistant colorectal cancer patients are about three times more likely to die of the disease.[81]

> **Neo Note: Insulin Sensitivity and Longevity**
> Researchers are theorizing that metabolic health might be one of the key factors for longevity.[82,83] Studies have shown that people with a genetic variation in insulin-related genes are likely to live longer than those without the variation.[84] And a 2021 study reviewed several research papers and concluded that there is good evidence supporting the idea that insulin-sensitizing medications may indirectly extend longevity.[85] While the aging process cannot be rewired (at least for now), it can be delayed, and one strategy may be to have strong metabolic health.

IT ALL STARTS IN THE CELL

I'm sure that by now you understand how your metabolism is connected with several chronic diseases and how insulin resistance is the crucial factor behind these metabolic issues. Where we still have to spend more time is on the exact mechanism that makes us insulin resistant. I used the distribution-center-and-warehouse analogy to keep things simple, but it's time to understand why the warehouses are getting full and turning away glucose. As much as I would love to give you a single cause for this, that's not the case. This is a complex phenomenon with several triggers that will eventually change your cellular metabolism. Independently of the particular cause, insulin resistance starts with cellular dysfunction.

As we learned before, antinutrients like wheat germ agglutinin (WGA) can change the way your cells interact with insulin. Likewise, the thousands of toxins we are exposed to daily can alter our cellular behavior and create metabolic dysfunction. In this section, rather than discussing every single possible external trigger, we are going to focus on how your diet can affect your cellular processes.

At a fundamental level, insulin resistance seems to begin within your mitochondria. Mitochondria are organelles (tiny parts) inside your cells that are often referred to as the powerhouses of the cell. If this were an episode of

MTV Cribs, your cells would point to the mitochondria and say, "This is where the magic happens!"

It's inside mitochondria that the protein, fat, and carbohydrates we eat are ultimately converted into energy as adenosine triphosphate (ATP).[86] All your cells except your red blood cells have mitochondria.[87] Some cells, like the heart muscle cells, for example, actually have thousands of mitochondria inside them.[88] The more energy a tissue needs, the more mitochondria it develops. But when your mitochondria become damaged, they won't provide your cells enough energy, and this can promote every chronic disease you can imagine.

Think of your mitochondria as a more complex digestive system for your cells. Through a process called cellular respiration, a mitochondrion converts "food" (carbs, fat, and protein) plus oxygen into usable energy (ATP). One by-product of cellular respiration is the creation of free radicals called reactive oxygen species (ROS).[89] In a very simple way, ROS are chemically unstable molecules that react with other molecules and cause trouble. Trouble can mean inflammation, DNA damage, cell death, etc.[90,91]

Your body is designed to deal with ROS and clean them up. Within a certain range, they might even be positive. Remember hormesis? But things go off the rails when you produce ROS at a higher rate than your body's ability to inactivate them with antioxidant compounds. This is when trouble happens.

When you are overfed, while converting all that fuel, your mitochondria overproduce ROS. This excess of free radicals can lead to cell damage, and as a defense mechanism, the cell is signaled to ignore insulin and not to accept more fuel.[92-94] This, my friend, is insulin resistance.

Overeating is one of the most recognized mechanisms that can induce insulin resistance, but it's not as linear as we might think. Research shows that overfeeding (within reason) with a single macronutrient (either carbs, fat, or protein) does not appear to lead to insulin resistance. It's their combined overconsumption that seems to cause negative metabolic consequences.[95] To rephrase it, your mitochondria get overwhelmed when they are overfed with different fuels at the same time, and end up being less efficient and generating more ROS. If we compare ROS to exhaust fumes, in this case, you are producing more fumes because you are driving a less efficient car.

Why do mitochondria become less efficient with different fuels coming in at the same time? It's very simple. If you eat "natural foods," your digestion processes these fuels with different timings. If you consume a normal-size meal (of unprocessed foods) with all three macronutrients, your body breaks down and then transports them sequentially, and your mitochondria can move from fuel to fuel (a process called metabolic flexibility) in a specific order and not get overwhelmed. As you know, that is not the case nowadays.

First, we're eating too much. Second, we are no longer eating these foods in their wholesome forms. In his book *Fast Carbs, Slow Carbs*, Dr. David Kessler explains that our ultraprocessed diet is "predigested."[96] In other words, these foods are completely stripped of fiber during manufacturing, and their sugars, fats, and proteins no longer go through our normal digestive processes. This means they are absorbed and reach your mitochondria at about the same time.

Let's say that your cells are a factory and your mitochondria are the production line workers. In this factory, because it's a small place, your workers are well trained to do the different tasks of the product assembly process, but at different times. At 8 a.m. they put the screws in, at 11 a.m. they paint the product, and at 2 p.m. they put the product in boxes to be shipped. Even though these are three different tasks, because they are done in order, workers can switch from one task to the other as the day progresses (the equivalent of mitochondrial metabolic flexibility). But what if the manager decides to put thousands of products, in different assembly stages, in the production line at the same time? Now, the workers might paint one part, then put another in a box, then go back to painting, then put some screws in, and so on. They don't know what's coming next, and they're just trying to keep up. As you can imagine, it will get to a point where the workers are painting the screws, hammering the boxes, and throwing away the metal parts because their brains just melted with all that multitasking. Eventually, the manager notices and stops the production line before more damage is done.

In a way, this is what's happening with your mitochondria after you eat processed foods. The workers are not efficient and end up producing more ROS than normal. When ROS piles up, your cells get the instruction to ignore insulin so issues don't become even worse.

Have you ever wondered why some of the extreme elimination diets work incredibly well, at least in the short term? They essentially make your mitochondria more efficient. Let me explain what I mean by that. There are extreme diets on which you're supposed to eat only a very restricted list of foods. Some are so extreme they allow only a single major ingredient, like the rice diet, the cabbage soup diet, or the egg diet, for example. Because these diets require zero metabolic flexibility, your body becomes superb at processing the same foods over and over again. The same applies to diets like the no-oil vegan diet. Although there are several different foods on your menu, this diet is high carb, low fat, and low protein. The foods vary, but the macronutrient profile (the type of fuel) is always the same. Your mitochondria become pros at taking care of carbs and get to a point where they do it "with their eyes closed." Because they become so efficient, they produce less ROS, and cause less inflammation and metabolic disfunction.

Obviously, these diets do not work long term. It's very difficult, if not impossible, for most people to stay on a "mono diet" for long with all those limitations. Not to mention that any time you deviate from the plan, you won't feel good because your body is no longer used to processing these other foods and will create an exacerbated response to them.

Neo Note: Beyond Insulin Resistance

When mitochondria get overwhelmed by our lifestyle excesses, they have another defense mechanism beyond triggering insulin resistance. The mitochondria decide not to make ATP out of every single fuel molecule they receive. They let some pass unprocessed so they don't create more ROS and cause inflammation. This phenomenon is called mitochondrial uncoupling.[97] This is a perfectly normal and healthy response, unless it occurs all the time because of our chronically poor diet. When this happens all the time, your mitochondria just end up becoming lazy. They prefer to turn a blind eye and process only a percentage of the fuel. They eventually become so inefficient that the energy they produce is not even enough to cover their own ATP needs.[98] This is one reason most people always feel drained.

THE GUT-MITOCHONDRIA CONNECTION

Your cell mitochondria (mitobiome or mitobiota) and your gut bacteria (bacteriome) have more in common than we initially thought. Researchers believe your mitochondria evolved from ancient bacteria, similar to your gut bugs.[99] Both also seem to be "digestive machines." Your gut microbes help you digest your food while your mitochondria "digest" the processed version of that same food and turn it into cellular energy. It's also believed that these old family members communicate with each other. Studies have shown that mitochondrial DNA mutations can affect the function of the bacteriome, and mitochondrial ROS production can also impact the health of your microbiome and even the integrity and immune response of your intestinal barrier.[100,101] Similarly, research shows that SCFAs (butyrate in particular) produced by your microbiome are critical to controlling mitochondrial oxidative stress and can also induce an increase in cell mitochondria to improve your metabolism.[102–104]

Knowing about this interaction, we can understand how your gut health can also influence your metabolic health. If you follow a dietary lifestyle that promotes the health of your microbiome, your gut bugs will produce plenty of SCFAs that will neutralize the oxidative stress from ROS in your mitochondria, which can delay or even prevent defense mechanisms like insulin resistance. It will also signal your mitochondria to multiply and improve the cells' metabolic efficiency, once again delaying or preventing further defense mechanisms.

Finally, as we've been discussing throughout the book, your diet can either neutralize or promote inflammation in your body. Even in something as simple as chronic low inflammation triggered by obesity, your body produces cytokines and other inflammatory compounds. Several studies show that these compounds will alter insulin signaling and will cause insulin resistance.[105] To make matters worse, you now know that insulin resistance promotes even more inflammation, which can leave you stuck in a vicious circle.

UNDERSTANDING INFLAMMATION

Since the beginning of the book, I've been throwing the *inflammation* word around, but I haven't really explained much about what it is. Intrinsically, we all think of inflammation as a bad thing, but in reality it's just a natural defense response from your body. Let's say that you trip and sprain your ankle. Almost instantly, your ankle will become swollen, the skin will get warmer and will develop some redness, and the whole joint will be tender. This is inflammation. The occurrence of these symptoms is the start of the healing process. This inflammatory response will make you protect the joint from further damage and will allow increased blood flow to the region to promote the proper supply of nutrients for the repair process. We can say that inflammation is an important component of the immune system.

Inflammation becomes problematic when it gets out of control, appears by mistake, or simply doesn't go away. When any of these situations happen, inflammation shifts from a healing to damaging. If inflammation doesn't subside, it can trigger different symptoms and expand to other regions of the body. Chronic inflammation can then develop into different diseases depending on the tissues it affects. As we just discussed, chronic inflammation and metabolic dysfunction are deeply connected, and they can trigger each other and cause serious health issues.[106-108]

As many authors state, a healthy inflammation response should follow the Goldilocks principle. It shouldn't be too small, and it shouldn't be too big either. It should be just right to solve the issue and then leave.

There are many things in our modern lifestyle that can cause inflammation. Environmental pollutants, harsh chemicals, stress, poor sleep, and the medications we take contribute to inflammation. But probably the one thing that has the biggest impact is your diet. If our bodies' internal processes can change so much with just a couple of milligrams of the pharmaceutical compounds in meds we take, imagine the impact of the several pounds of food you eat every day.

I can see the metabolic connection, but what about diseases of genetic origin? Good question, my friend. Well, inflammation can regulate epigenetic factors that can contribute to "shutting off" these bad genes.[109] Inflammation can also lead to mutation of your genetic material and potentially cause some of these diseases.[110] At the end of the day, we can connect inflammation to all diseases imaginable.

Neo Note: Inflammaging

There are several theories regarding the processes behind what makes us old. One theory claims that aging is the accumulation of cellular damage as the result of chronic low-level inflammation. This is called inflammaging.[111] According to the theory, this "light" chronic inflammation inflicts more cellular oxidative stress than your body's antioxidant system can combat. This causes an accumulation of cellular damage, which "ages" you. I don't believe you will live forever just by changing your diet, but I am certain you can improve how you age. To me, that is the most important aspect of getting old. I do not want to live to 175 if I have to depend on people 24/7. I would prefer to live only to 110 and remain active and sharp until I go to the eternal dirt nap. What do you think?

IT'S ALL CONNECTED

During the months of research I did to write this book, the authors of some of the books I read asserted that all disease is caused by cellular dysfunction. Others theorized that all disease stems from insulin resistance. And then there was another group of authors who said that inflammation causes all disease. Do you want to know my opinion about who's right? In a way, they all are. As we saw, these three things are deeply connected, and it is impossible to dissociate one from the others. It's more of a question of which came first: the chicken or the egg? Independently of the answer, all three processes will eventually occur as diseases progress. There is no way we can separate cell health, metabolism, and inflammation. These belong in a unified theory.

You can look at this in two ways. Either you decide to feel defeated because you imagine the unavoidable doomsday path filled with all kinds of diseases. Or, you take the alternative path and actually get excited. You no longer have to worry about an infinite world of diseases. Instead, you see that there is only one disease but with different representations. And, by taking care of the cellular/metabolic/inflammatory cause, you can heal any problem. Mic drop!

Neo Note: Check Where You Stand

You answered the "insulin resistance questions" but are still curious about your insulin sensitivity status? Another quick way to see if you have insulin resistance is to look at your belly. Measure your waist and then divide it by your height (using the same measuring unit, whether inches or centimeters). If the number you get is at or above 0.5, there's a high likelihood that you have insulin resistance.

Another way that does not involve actually testing your insulin levels is by looking at your triglyceride and HDL levels in your regular blood work. Check these two results and then calculate the triglyceride/HDL ratio. There is plenty of controversy here, but several studies show that this is a good indicator of insulin resistance.[112–115] I couldn't find a definite cutoff value, but it seems that if you divide your triglycerides by your HDL value and get anything over 2, this puts you at high likelihood of having insulin resistance. Ideally, you should aim for 1 or lower.

Still not sure? Talk to your doctor and get your insulin levels tested.

What about inflammation? Inflammation can show up as so many things that it's difficult to give you any testing hacks. The best is to talk to your doctor and get some blood work done. Substances such as CRP, homocysteine, and Lp-PLA2 are good markers for inflammation.

NEO SUMMARY

• Metabolism is the process of transforming food into the energy that will power all the cells in the body.

• Modern diets are overloading our metabolic processes and compromising our cellular performance. This can cause all types of diseases, from obesity, diabetes, cardiovascular diseases, brain diseases, to even cancer.

• Researchers believe that this metabolic dysfunction has been mostly triggered by insulin resistance.

• Insulin resistance is a condition in which the body becomes less sensitive to the hormone insulin (needed to regulate the level of blood sugar).

• Besides causing metabolic dysfunction, the excess of sugar in the blood appears to corrode tissues from different systems and make them leaky. This can cause systemic inflammation and trigger autoimmunity.

• Insulin resistance appears to be triggered by cellular "overtaxation" due to overeating (in particular of processed foods), oxidative stress, and inflammation.

• Unfortunately, insulin resistance is not properly diagnosed, and it has become a "silent" epidemic.

• Cellular health, metabolic function and inflammation cannot be dissociated and are behind all diseases.

• The key prevent/revert most diseases is to present a high insulin sensitivity and healthy metabolism.

NEO ACTION

• Eat whole foods.
• Be mindful and don't overeat.
• Stay positive. All can be reversed.

NEO RECOMMENDATIONS

• *Fast Carbs, Slow Carbs* by David Kessler
• *Metabolical* by Dr. Robert H. Lustig
• *Mitochondria and the Future of Medicine* by Dr. Lee Know
• *Radical Metabolism* by Ann Louise Gittleman
• *The Genius Life* by Max Lugavere
• *The Inflammation Spectrum* by Dr. Will Cole
• *The Cancer Code* by Dr. Jason Fung
• *The Diabetes Code* by Dr. Jason Fung
• *The Obesity Code* by Dr. Jason Fung
• *The Paleo Cure* by Chris Kresser
• *Why We Get Sick* by Benjamin Bikman

my.neodiet.co/neorecommendations

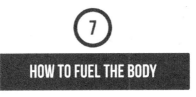

HOW TO FUEL THE BODY

Debunking Myths about Carbs, Fat, and Cholesterol

"Every truth passes through three stages before it is recognized. In the first it is ridiculed, in the second it is opposed, in the third it is regarded as self evident."
Arthur Schopenhauer

TRICKED INTO EATING MORE

We live at a time when more people are overweight than underweight.[1] You read that right! And I am not just talking about the so-called developed countries. This is a worldwide average. Why are we eating so much? The impulse is stronger than our will. People blame themselves and feel that they have no self-control, but this has nothing to do with self-control. People are physically hungry. You can be the most disciplined person in the world, but when you are hungry, food is all you can think of. Your mind will not let you do anything else until you fulfill that primitive need.

Now, this raises another question. Why are we so dang hungry? In chapter 1, we discussed how the food industry was playing with our genetics by shoving down our throats hundreds of processed, hyperpalatable foods. As you know, these foods are hypnotic. They whisper in your ear: *Hit me, baby, one more time*—sorry, Britney—and we become food junkies.

Besides hyperpalatability, processed foods also induce a phenomenon called vanishing caloric density. Steven Witherly, a food scientist and the author of *Why Humans Like Junk Food*, explains that when you eat something that almost instantly melts in your mouth (like most soft candy and salty snacks), your brain assumes there were no calories in it and ends up not sending you a signal to stop eating.[2] Therefore, one can eat a full bag of chips and still be hungry.

It's not just the bulk in foods that can trigger a satiating response. Some theorize that your body is always looking for the micronutrients it needs to thrive. If your food doesn't contain the bare minimum nutrition, your body will continue to fire off hunger signals to keep you eating until you get the missing nutrients.[3] The problem is that our modern food is depleted of nutrients. We keep eating it and getting fat, but we remain "hungry" because we can't find all the nourishment we need. We are overfed (overweight) but undernourished, what science calls the double burden of malnutrition (DBM).[4] In a developed country like the United States, data suggests that 90 percent of the population is deficient in at least one vitamin or mineral.[5] In other words, one can speculate that 90 percent of Americans have to fight their food cravings daily. I wish I had more information on other countries, but I wouldn't be surprised if the global average looked similar to that of the US.

CALORIC MISTAKE

The most scientific way to understand this overeating issue is by looking at the calories we're consuming, right? Not at all. But let me explain. The calorie was first described in 1863, as the amount of heat needed to raise the temperature of one kilogram of water from zero to one degree Celsius.[6] This concept was used in research, but it was completely unknown in the diet world. This all changed in 1918 when Dr. Lulu Hunt Peters published the best-selling book *Diet & Health: With Key to the Calories*.[7] For the first time in history, people looked at food not for what it was but for how many calories it had. This led to the development of the "calories in, calories out" (CICO) concept. This is the reigning diet theory I learned in school and that is still being taught in many medical and nutrition schools worldwide. In a simple way, this concept states that if you eat more calories than you burn, you get fat. Likewise, if you burn more calories than you eat, you lose weight.

Considering this idea, some argue that our obesity issue is not coming from overeating but from our laziness. They say we are not burning enough calories. Although there is also some truth to this statement, this entire theory is built on a flawed concept. First, a calorie only tells us how much energy is contained in a food, not how much energy your body will actually be able to "absorb" and use. For example, most foods contain indigestible components like fiber that we do not absorb but still count in our calorie intake. This, by itself, throws the equation completely off. Second, our bodies are not simple calorie reservoirs. They are complex systems that can "burn" more or fewer calories depending on how efficiently they're running. In other words, your calorie expenditure is not linear and will depend on your digestive ability and metabolic efficiency.

Obviously, if you consume 10,000 calories a day and you are not Michael Phelps, it's probably not going to work out very well for you.[8] CICO is flawed, but calories still count. You simply cannot rely on the CICO equation as an absolute truth. Focusing on calories can give us an overall idea, but it will never give us a clear understanding of how much we are eating, nor is it a solution for weight management.

> **Neo Note: Ranchers Don't Believe in CICO**
> In the ranching industry, hormone manipulation has been used to improve feed efficiency (getting animals bigger and fatter on less food).[9] The days of giving hormones like estrogens through the feed are behind us, but ranchers can still manipulate animals' metabolism by using anabolic implants with estrogen, progesterone, or trenbolone acetate (an analogue to testosterone).[10] This is just another example of how the CICO model cannot be trusted. These animals are eating the same number of calories but are growing muscle and fat a lot faster than the rest.

HUNGER REGULATION

More important than calories are hormones and neurotransmitters like insulin, leptin, ghrelin, and cortisol. These are critical elements that regulate our appetite and influence our metabolism. The key to successfully managing your weight and health is not to fight your inner voice or question your willpower; it's to understand these chemical messengers and use them in your favor. Roll up your sleeves, because I'm about to show you how to kick hunger out of your life for good.

Insulin

I'll keep this short, since we already learned about insulin in the last chapter. In a nutshell, insulin is a hormone that helps us regulate blood sugar levels by facilitating the cellular uptake of glucose or directing it to the liver, where it can be processed to become fat.

Normally, carbs release the largest amount of insulin, with protein releasing less, and fat even less.[11] In optimal metabolic health, we require only a small amount of insulin to deal with any food we eat and keep our blood sugar stable. But in cases of insulin resistance, our blood sugar rises excessively after a meal.[12] What goes up must come down. Here, blood sugars tend to then crash to abnormally low levels, which can cause blurred vision, dizziness, shakiness, sweating, irritability, and anger.[13] Interestingly, a study on married couples found that the lower the individuals' blood sugar levels, the more aggressive and angry they felt toward their partners.[14] Insulin resistance might cause your "hangriness" (hunger + anger).

For this section, what you need to consider is that the presence or absence of insulin in the blood will indirectly affect your perception of hunger or satiety. I will get to the exact mechanism shortly.

Glucagon

Glucagon is also produced in the pancreas, but it has an opposite effect to that of insulin. While insulin prompts the storage of glucose (either to be used by the cells or to be transformed into fat), glucagon sets the fuel free. When your sugar levels are low, glucagon tells the liver to engage in glycogenolysis, which is the conversion of stored glycogen into glucose.[15] When these liver reserves are depleted, glucagon can stimulate the breakdown of fat for energy and even the conversion of protein to glucose (gluconeogenesis).[16]

Glucagon can be released in states of hunger (due to low blood sugar) and with the consumption of protein. What is important to know is that glucagon and insulin are counteragents of the same feedback system, so one operates only when the levels of the other are low, and vice versa.

Leptin

Nope, not a mistake. This is leptin and not the antinutrient lectin. Memorize it this way: "Lectin causes Chaos; leptin is produced by 'Phat' (close enough) cells. Not the most grammatically correct mnemonic, but it's good enough to distinguish them. Leptin is our main "satiety" hormone, regulates our metabolism, and also intervenes in sexual development and fertility.[17] Leptin is produced by fat cells (adipocytes). When you have a lot of fat, leptin is released and your body interprets that as "I'm fat enough, I don't need to eat more." This generates a sensation of satiety and also leads to an increase of metabolic rate (you burn more calories).[18,19]

The problem here is that if you are overweight, leptin keeps being produced 24/7. Guess what this causes? You nailed it. Leptin resistance. Similarly to insulin, your body thinks all this leptin must be a mistake and starts ignoring it, no longer giving you the satiety sensation nor boosting your metabolism.[20] In broad brushstrokes, since your body no longer gets the signals from leptin, it thinks you're starving, when in reality you are far from it. In response to this, it will make you hungry and will dramatically reduce your energy expenditure.

If you are trying to lose weight by cutting calories but suffer from leptin resistance, I'm sorry to tell you it will not work long term. You can cut calories as much as you want, but you will always feel hungry, and your metabolism will be in the gutter.

Research also suggests that high leptin concentrations are directly associated with obesity and the subsequent development of insulin resistance and metabolic syndrome.[21] As you know, insulin resistance can cause further weight gain, significantly aggravating this situation.

Neo Note: *The Biggest Loser*

In a 2016 study, a team of researchers studied 14 contestants from the weight-loss reality show *The Biggest Loser*.[22] After six years, 13 out of 14 contestants had regained at least some of the weight they'd lost, and five of them regained so much that they actually weighed more than when they joined the show. On average, the participants had regained about 70 percent of their lost weight, and to make things more interesting, they also had greater appetite and slower metabolisms than other individuals at the same age and with the same body composition.

According to the study, during the time of the TV show, the contestants had drastic decreases in leptin levels that remained lower than average even after they regained the weight. The most plausible justification for this is the fact that during the show, the significant calorie restriction made their bodies assume they were going through severe starvation, which caused leptin to plummet. The less leptin in their bodies, the lower their metabolic rates became. Simultaneously, they also started to experience more and more hunger. Eventually, this uncontrollable hunger was too much to resist, and you can imagine the rest of the story.

This is the typical case of losing weight done wrong and why CICO is a recipe for failure. The good news is that if you follow the Neo Diet, you will optimize your hormones and metabolism so you'll never experience what these contestants did.

Ghrelin

The hormone ghrelin is the yin to leptin's yang. Instead of creating a sensation of satiety, it produces the feeling of hunger. Ghrelin is secreted by the stomach mostly when it's empty, and its levels decrease after meals.[23] A smaller percentage of ghrelin can also be produced by the pancreas, possibly as a response to low blood sugar.[24] Research shows that protein-rich meals keep ghrelin levels down.[25] Initially, a high-carb meal decreases ghrelin, but it sets off a high rebound effect.[26] The rebound effect causes the ghrelin levels to rise fast and consequently make you crave food. Want to avoid cravings? Eat a protein-rich meal as your first meal of the day.

Another strategy to keep ghrelin low is to eat less-frequent but larger meals. The larger (nutritionally-rich) meals and the consequent longer digestion time will lead to lower levels of ghrelin.[27] Eating small meals frequently throughout the day is terrible dietary advice. *That's right, I said it!* Several studies have shown that frequent meals do not improve metabolic rate and may increase hunger, while fewer meals produce better levels of satiety and better long-term appetite control.[28–30] In other words, eating more frequently, as most "experts" have told you to do, does not make you less hungry or cause you to burn more fat. There are even studies suggesting that increased meal frequency is a risk factor for colon cancer.[31,32]

The goal should not be to have ghrelin levels low all the time. As with insulin (and other hormones), we should aim to have high sensitivity to it so it can do what it is supposed to do. Ghrelin is much more than just a simple hunger stimulator. Ghrelin regulates blood sugar through inhibition of insulin secretion, protects your cardiovascular system, helps with muscle preservation and bone formation, regulates energy consumption, and has systemic anti-inflammatory effects.[33,34]

Cortisol

Cortisol is usually known as the stress hormone because of its part in the fight-or-flight (stress) response. However, it's involved in many other biological processes. Secreted by the adrenal glands (on top of the kidneys), cortisol is also involved in reducing inflammation, modulating the immune system, helping you learn and form memories, assisting with nutrient metabolism, increasing blood sugar, and regulating your circadian rhythms.[34-40]

Among this list of functions, the last two are the ones that interest us the most for purposes of this chapter. Let's start with the last one. Cortisol peaks in the morning, and that elevation is connected with our awakening process.[41] Cortisol has a catabolic (in this case, fat-burning) effect designed to help us get energy in the morning by breaking down our fuel reserves (fat, or even muscle as a last resort). This is a healthy mechanism, but our dietary practices have turned this against us. As Max Lugavere explains in his book *Genius Foods*, "when insulin and cortisol are both present at the same time (i.e., after a carbohydrate-rich breakfast), cortisol's fat-burning effect will be shut down, and it will only exert its catabolic effect on your muscles—clearly, not a desirable scenario."[42] Additionally, we have to consider that cortisol also ratchets up blood glucose. If you are chronically stressed, your cortisol levels will be high, and this can lead to insulin resistance and fat accumulation.[43,44]

In simple terms, eating carbs in the morning (when your cortisol is naturally high) or when you are stressed is probably not the best choice, since they will most likely be converted into fat. Even though the effects may vary between individuals, high cortisol levels are believed to increase food cravings and drive people to eat more.[45-48] This may result from cortisol's inhibitory effect on peptide YY (PYY), which acts as a satiety hormone like leptin.[49]

I know, they have lied to us. We've been manipulated into eating more than we're supposed to. Our physiology was played against us, and we were set up to fail in our emotional fight against our cravings. The sensation of hunger is not something to have willpower over; it's a warning sign that something is wrong and needs to be fixed. Throughout this chapter, we are going to uncover more lies, and I'm going to show you how you can finally be in charge of your metabolism and your health.

CARBOHYDRATES AS FUEL

Since the last chapter, I have been talking about carbohydrates as one of our primary fuel sources, but I haven't really explained much about them. At a fundamental level, carbs are macronutrients (macros). If you read about diet or fitness, you've likely read about macros. As their name suggests, macronutrients are nutrients that should make up a large part of our food intake. They are essential because they provide energy and support all functions of your physiology. Carbs can be a very useful macronutrient because they are easily converted into glucose and reach your bloodstream quickly.[50] Your body can also make glucose out of proteins using a mechanism called gluconeogenesis, but this is more out of necessity than as a preferred process.[51]

Carbs can be divided into two major categories:

• **Simple carbohydrates**, or simple sugars, are the easiest for your body to break down into glucose. Carbs are molecules that contain single, double, or multiple sugar molecules called saccharides. Simple carbs contain only one or two sugar molecules. Therefore, they can be called monosaccharides or disaccharides, respectively.[52] Examples of simple sugars are glucose, fructose, lactose, galactose, ribose, and sucrose. These can be found in candy, carbonated beverages, dairy products, desserts, fruit, honey, sports drinks, syrups, and table sugar.

• **Complex carbohydrates**, or complex sugars, require a bit more work to metabolize. Instead of containing one or two sugar molecules, they have three or more. In most cases, when they have from three to 10 sugars, we call them oligosaccharides; those with more than 10 we call polysaccharides.[53] In nutrition, you also may hear these being called starches. Even though complex carbohydrates are not sweet, they still release plenty of glucose, so make no mistake. Examples of complex sugars are cellobiose, rutinulose, amylose, cellulose, and dextrin. These can be found in whole grains, legumes, and most vegetables, although in much higher concentration in starchy vegetables like potatoes and squash.

Neo Note: Fiber as a Macronutrient

Fiber is technically considered a nondigestible complex carbohydrate. Under the traditional definition, macronutrients are energy-yielding nutrients, and since fiber does not produce energy (directly, at least), it cannot be considered a macronutrient. This can cause some discussion and confusion because since complex carbs are macronutrients, and fiber is a complex carb, some argue that fiber would also be a macronutrient. Some authors also mention that since fiber is so essential that it needs to be consumed in a "macro" scale, it should be considered a macronutrient in itself (even if it does not directly yield energy). Because of these and other arguments, the USDA extended its list of macronutrients and now recognizes fiber as an independent macronutrient.[54] Hip hooray! I have to go with USDA on this one. Even if it's scientifically controversial, in this book I am considering fiber to be a macronutrient.

Historically, our consumption of carbs has been increasing. Carbs started as a complement to our diets and slowly became dietary staples. We have been eating too much of them, and too many of the wrong kind. Nowadays, we find added sugars in most processed foods. Even if you try to avoid them and start checking the labels, you will have a hard time because the food industry disguises them. Dr. Robert Lustig, who's one of the world's leading authorities on sugar, identified 300 terms the food industry uses to hide sugar from the avid label reader.[55] Some of the most common ones are agave syrup, barley malt, beet sugar, brown rice syrup, cane juice, coconut sugar, corn syrup, date sugar, dextrose, fructose, fruit juice, glucose solids, high-fructose corn syrup, lactose, malt, maltodextrin, molasses, and sucrose.

To be fair, the issue is not just with simple sugars. Modern agriculture turned many complex carbs into less-healthy versions than in the past. Through time, we have been breeding and hybridizing grains, tubers, vegetable, and fruits for maximum content of starch and sugar. We have made our plant foods bigger and sweeter, inadvertently increasing their sugar loads to levels we were not used to.[56]

I want to make one thing clear. Carbs are not bad. Lately in the diet world, everything is taken to extremes. You either love high-carb, low-fat, or love the opposite. There is no middle ground. If you look back in history, you can find several healthy peoples that followed both spectrums of the macronutrient discussion. With high-carb, for example, indigenous groups like the Kitavans, Massas, and Tarahumara Indians all thrived on this type of diet. Obesity and chronic disease were rare in all these groups.[57-59] In Asia, until recently, we could still find entire populations following high-carb diets and living healthy lives. Okinawans, for example, are one of the longest-living populations in the world, and their traditional diet was incredibly rich in sweet potatoes.[60,61]

The issue is the type of carbs consumed in our modern (Western) diet. As soon as the individuals in those healthy populations mentioned above adopt more of a Western diet, they experience disease. A 2021 Japanese study stated, "in Japan, the number of obesity-related malignancies such as colorectal cancer, breast cancer, and prostate cancer has been increasing with the westernization of lifestyle, especially diet."[62] Other reports from China associate the expansion of Western fast-food chains with an increase in cases of diabetes and obesity.[63] Even the traditionally long-living Okinawans are now experiencing obesity and "premature death."[64]

Traditional high-carb diets were based on the consumption of complex carbs from whole foods. Western high-carb diets, on the other hand, are based on refined carbs. These refined carbs, during processing, have most of their fiber, vitamins, and minerals removed. This makes them "empty" calories that lead to rapid bursts in blood sugar and insulin levels after meals. As you know, the rebound effect that happens after these spikes from high-glycemic-index foods can be disastrous. Several studies across the world and performed with different age groups support that refined-carb consumption is causing leptin resistance, increased appetite, weight gain, inflammation, insulin resistance, diabetes, and cardiovascular disease.[65–73]

Not sure what refined carbs are? Here are some of the usual suspects: bagels, biscuits, cake, cereal, chips, cookies, crackers, doughnuts, energy bars, energy drinks, granola, ice creams, jams, juices, milk chocolate, milkshakes, muffins, pancakes, pastas, pastries, pretzels, sodas, and waffles, just to name a few.

SUGAR

We are genetically programmed to love sugar because it is an indicator of a dense source of calories. In a natural environment, that would be okay, but the food industry manipulated their products to hack our programming and destroy our palate. Never in history could we get so much sugar so quickly, without even realizing it. According to the USDA, the average American consumes 66 pounds (about 30 kilograms) of added sugar every year.[74] To give you an idea, this is like eating a full-size German shepherd made of sugar.

In chapter 1, we talked about the experiment where rats chose cocaine instead of food and water, and starved themselves to death while getting high. What's more incredible is that other studies were done with these party animals, but this time they gave them another option. This time, the researchers got a group of cocaine-addicted rats and gave them a choice between cocaine and sugar. Guess what they chose? They chose the sugar.[75] Different scientists reviewing this experiment have concluded that this happened because the reward from sugar surpassed that of cocaine.[76] In the brain, sugar acts like some of the most addictive opioids, yet it is perfectly legal and it's added everywhere.[77,78]

On top of that, research shows that consuming high doses of sugar can decrease the number of dopamine receptors in your brain (that is, create dopamine resistance).[79] What this means is that you need more and more sugar to get the same response of pleasure and energy. Just like with any other drug, those hooked on sugar can also experience withdrawal symptoms when they go too long without getting their fix.[80] They might experience difficulty in concentrating, start sweating, or even feel shakiness, jitteriness, and anxiety.[81,82]

BEYOND ADDICTION

Our problems with sugar go beyond addiction. Research suggests that excessive sugar is indirectly making us adopt a more sedentary lifestyle.[83] This means you might eat an energy bar to give you the power to go to the gym, but its sugar can convince you to go to the couch and watch Netflix instead.

Sugar intake also depresses your immune system. This is very important to consider, especially now that every four or five years we have a global viral epidemic. For example, with COVID-19, studies have shown that individuals with higher glucose levels are more prone to develop more severe forms or symptoms of the disease.[84-86] Watching videos of people being discharged from COVID units and then being given sodas by the hospital staff to celebrate created some big face-palm moments for me.

High glucose levels are associated with intestinal permeability, higher levels of inflammation, depressed response from immune cells (neutrophils and phagocytes) that protect you against infection, higher risk of developing autoimmune diseases, and an overall weak immune response.[87-94]

High blood glucose levels are associated with systemic inflammation, but in particular in the brain. As Ben Greenfield illustrates in his book *Boundless*, "high blood glucose levels increase not only astrocyte-induced neuroinflammation but also the susceptibility of your neurons to injury. This means that a diet high in sugar and starch, which spike blood glucose levels, can be damaging to the brain."[95] Consumption of high-sugar foods, including sweetened beverages like coffee and tea, has been linked with anxiety, depression, and impaired decision making and memory.[96-100]

GLYCATION

Another mechanism that can make sugar dangerous is called glycation. When was the last time you had a lollipop? Remember that after you licked the lollipop, it became sticky? Well, this is glycation. The sugar in your lollipop dissolved in the water in your saliva and then reacted to the proteins on the surface of your skin and created chemical bonds known as cross-links.[101] The stickiness is the resistance to breaking these chemical bonds. The problem with glycation is that if enough time has passed (or if heat is added, or both), oxidation occurs and the bonds become stronger and may even become permanent.[102,103] Want to see it for yourself? Go to the beach, lick some hard candy, and press it against your exposed leg. Let it "cook" for a few hours and then try to remove it. Just kidding, *please don't do this*!

As these glycated proteins continue to oxidize, they generate advanced glycation end products (AGEs).[104] If you have normal blood sugar levels, your body can clean up AGEs faster than they're produced.[105] The problem occurs when you produce AGEs faster than your body can handle. These accumulated AGEs stick to cells and alter their function. For example, in your arteries, AGEs make these semipermeable vessels become hardened and stiff.[106,107] This alters endothelial permeability (the ability for exchanges between the blood and the tissues beyond the artery or vein) and can lead to atherosclerosis.[108] AGEs can cause issues anywhere they end up. If they set up camp in your joints, they can lead to arthritis.[109-111] If they lodge in your white blood cells, they can cause immune compromise.[112] If they hang out in your eyes, they can cause cataracts.[113,114] And if they end up in your brain, they can speed up the loss of brain volume and cognitive function, impairing learning and memory, and even worsening Alzheimer's and other dementias.[115–120] I'm sure you get the point.

Chronic AGE accumulation will promote inflammation and cellular damage and will also contribute to aging of the heart, kidneys, liver, bones, and skin.[121,122]

Factors that determine the formation of AGEs in your body are how high your blood sugar is and how much oxidative stress you have going on.[123–126] In *Genius Foods*, Max Lugavere suggests that a way to determine your rate of AGE formation is by looking at your hemoglobin A1C markers (commonly tracked to manage diabetes), which reveal the amount of sugar stuck to your red blood cells.[127]

COMPLEX CARBOHYDRATES

Some authors compare simple carbs to five shots of tequila in a row, while complex carbs are more like 20 glasses of wine throughout the day. Both will get you intoxicated, but you'll experience different kinds of "drunkenness." The first will hit you like a hammer, and your alcohol levels will shoot up the roof in no time. However, in a couple of hours you'll recover, and "party's over." The second method will allow you to keep a steady buzz throughout the whole day. These authors argue that even though the rate of intoxication is different, you end up consuming a lot of harmful alcohol and endangering your health.

Although I understand this point, I can't say that I completely agree. Stepping outside of the analogy, we can see that consuming simple carbs or complex carbs will have different effects. Yes, quantity matters, but speed of absorption (glycemic index) is also important. As we saw before, several studies show that the higher a food's glycemic index, the worse the outcome. Simple sugars will cause a big rebound effect, and your body's response will be exacerbated in comparison with that of a complex carb that gets digested more slowly. That is why I can't support that the overall effects are the same.

Am I saying it's okay to binge-eat complex carbs? Of course not! A complex carb has a low glycemic index, but it also has a lot of sugars in it—*more than* you probably need. I think the main point I want to present for now is that you need to be mindful of the type and total quantity of carbs you consume. Most importantly, you need to stay away from high-glycemic refined carbs.

FRUCTOSE

Fructose is the natural sugar from fruits. It is also present in some vegetables, and in honey. Because of this, one might say that since fructose is a source of "whole" carbs, we can eat as much as we want. Well, don't put the cart before the horse. As I briefly pointed out before, fructose has been giving us our fair share of issues. Historically, we don't seem to find many issues with the consumption of fruit. Actually, it was considered an excellent source of vitamins and minerals, possibly promoting better health. So, what changed?

If we analyze anthropological records, we can see that the consumption of fruit was more common among the peoples that lived closer to the equator.[127] This is easy to understand, since only there would you have access to fruit year-round. For all other regions of the globe, fruit was more of a scarce seasonal delicacy. Not to mention that the fruits we consumed back then were possibly a lot less "meaty" and sweet.

Some authors also argue that, back in the day, fruit had the function of helping us get nice and fat to get through the "starving" winters. During those times of limited access to food, we would burn those summer-gained love handles and make enough energy to survive. Nowadays, we don't have difficulty finding food during the winter, nor do we have fruit only seasonally. I can eat berries, pineapples, and bananas every single day of the year if I want to. These fruits get flown from exotic locations, and in a couple of days they are on the shelves of your favorite supermarket. Just think about this for a second. If planes did not exist and you never left your country, you might never have eaten several fruits you now have access to daily.

Fructose has the same number of calories as glucose, but it has a different metabolic effect. Because most of our cells can't use fructose for energy, it is channeled to the liver, where it's converted into a usable form called pyruvate.[128] Since fructose is sent directly to the liver, it does not cause a spike in insulin—at least not right away.[129] In the liver, fructose stimulates lipogenesis (conversion of glucose and fructose into fat).[130] Glucose can also cause lipogenesis, but research shows that fructose stimulates lipogenesis at least twice as much as glucose does.[131] This excessive storage of fat in the liver can then cause nonalcoholic fatty liver disease (NAFLD).[132]

Once the liver is at max capacity, fat spills over into the bloodstream as triglycerides. This is why excessive fructose is one trigger of high triglyceride levels in the blood.[133] Fructose has also been associated with increased liver synthesis of the free fatty acids (FFAs) diacylglycerol, ceramides, and acyl-carnitines, which strongly contribute to development of insulin resistance.[134–138] Research also shows that fructose induces mitochondrial dysfunction and triggers oxidative stress and muscle cell death.[139] Finally, fructose also contributes to the formation of AGEs.[140]

HIGH-FRUCTOSE CORN SYRUP

Unfortunately, our fructose story does not end here. In 1970, high-fructose corn syrup (HFCS) was introduced in the food industry as a sweetener for processed foods.[141] HFCS results from the chemical processing of corn (usually GMO), which creates a sweetener combining fructose and glucose.[142] Because HFCS is much cheaper to produce, it easily replaced traditional sugar (sucrose) and conquered the food industry.[143] Even foods that traditionally would not contain sucrose or fructose are now, in their modern, processed versions, filled with HFCS.

Research has connected HFCS consumption to the same diseases triggered by high intake of simple sugars and fructose. HFCS in the diet is associated with a slew of health concerns, such as NAFLD, high triglyceride levels, insulin resistance, hyperglycemia, type 2 diabetes, gout, increased accumulation of AGEs, metabolic syndrome, heart disease, and even reduced life expectancy.[144–153]

Some of the most common foods that contain HFCS are bread, candy, canned fruit, cereal, chocolate, crackers, energy/sports drinks, fast food, fruit jams, fruit juices, granola/energy bars, ice cream, premade frozen foods, salad dressings, sauces, sodas, sweetened yogurt, and syrups.

Even knowing all this, I want to warn you that initially, you might have a hard time leaving these products or even replacing them with healthier versions. As it seems, this industrially processed fructose may be as addictive as alcohol, and perhaps even morphine.[154–156] Ouch!

HONEY

Honey, or as it's called in the streets, "bee barf," is many times considered the healthiest alternative to sugar. Historically, honey has been used both for nutritional purposes and for its medicinal properties, as documented in ancient civilizations such as those of the Babylonians, Egyptians, Chinese, Greeks, Mayans, and Romans.[157] This golden bee puke is composed primarily of water, fructose, and glucose, but it also contains trace amounts of enzymes, amino acids, antioxidants, minerals (including calcium, iron, magnesium, phosphorus, potassium, selenium, and zinc), and vitamins (B_1, B_2, B_3, B_5, B_6, and C).[158–163] Honey can also act as a prebiotic to help feed and support our beneficial gut bacteria.[164,165] Yes, honey still has sugar, but it also packs an incredible nutritional punch.

Sadly, not all honey is made equal. Commercial honey is heavily processed, and it's depleted of most of its benefits. An investigative article analyzed 60 samples of commercial American honey brands and observed that more than 75 percent of all samples were devoid of most nutrients and contained no pollen.[166] But isn't pollen bad? Some people do have pollen allergies, but the reality is that pollen can contain more than 250 beneficial compounds such as amino acids, essential fatty acids, minerals, vitamins, and antioxidants.[167] It's so powerful that in Germany, the Ministry of Health recognizes bee pollen as a medicine.[168] Bee pollen has antifungal, antimicrobial, antiviral, anti-inflammatory, immunostimulating, and even analgesic properties.[169,170] Finally, it's also known to fight inflammation, improve liver function, and protect against heart disease and stroke.[171]

Unfortunately, it seems most commercial honey doesn't have pollen. And that's not all, folks. Because of the demand for honey, commercial producers get creative and try to stretch their raw material. Studies have detected the adulteration of honey by adding sugar or other sweeteners like HFCS.[172–174] Always go for raw honey. Raw honeys are not pasteurized and skip the filtration process, so they retain pollen, enzymes, and their amazing nutrients.[175,176]

One of the most famous (and studied) honeys is New Zealand's own Manuka honey. According to Kiwi research, Manuka honey has unique antibacterial properties that might make it even more effective at killing bad bacteria.[177] Manuka honey also has antiviral, anti-inflammatory, and antioxidant properties, and it has been shown to work for wound healing (even in diabetic ulcers and wound infections caused by antibiotic-resistant strains like MRSA), soothing sore throats, killing *C. diff*, healing gastric ulcers, and improving digestive diseases like IBS and IBD.[178–185] Surprisingly, it may also help with oral health. Excess sugar and even honey are associated with cavities, but with Manuka honey, its potent antibacterial effects attack harmful oral bacteria associated with plaque formation, gum inflammation, and tooth decay.[186,187]

Although Manuka honey is world famous, there are many other rising stars worldwide. They probably just don't have as much research behind them yet. Either way, a good-quality local raw honey might even be more beneficial, since, as suggested by Dr. Josh Axe, it might be a great means of exposure to local beneficial microorganisms that can boost your digestive and immune systems.[188]

Before I turn into Winnie the Pooh, let me wrap up this section by sharing that studies show that raw honey is a strong anticarcinogenic agent and a valuable therapeutic tool for respiratory, gastrointestinal, and cardiovascular diseases.[189,190]

Word of caution: Honey is another fructose-rich food that probably should be consumed in moderation. The best way to take advantage of its benefits is to choose a high-quality brand and use it sparingly.

MAPLE SYRUP

Maple syrup, a.k.a. liquid gold in Canada, is a traditional sweetener made from the sap of maple trees. Just like cane sugar, maple syrup is about two-thirds sucrose. However, its glycemic index is only 54, compared to cane sugar's 65. Besides that, just like honey, unrefined maple syrup packs a ton of nutrition. Research shows that pure maple syrup contains as many as 24 different antioxidants.[191] And unlike honey, maple syrup is low in fructose, which makes it more tolerable by people with IBS.[192] Maple syrup is also known for having vitamin B_2, calcium, iron, manganese, potassium, and zinc.[193] These micronutrients are important for bone and tissue formation, blood clotting, fat and carbohydrate metabolism, nerve function, immunity, and sexual health. Furthermore, polyphenols in maple syrup have been shown to help reduce the growth of cancer cells.[194]

Maple syrups come in different colors and classifications. Grade A dark syrup is made from sap extracted later in the harvest season and has a higher nutritional content.[195]

Despite all these benefits, if your goal is to lose weight or improve your metabolic health, you're better off avoiding maple syrup and even honey. But once you reach a later stage in your health journey, it's okay to include them occasionally.

AGAVE

What about agave? It's sold in all the health stores—it must be good! Agave is a processed syrup that comes from the sap of the blue agave plant. Fun fact: The sugars in agave are also fermented to make tequila. Agave, the plant, seems to have some health benefits.[196] Unfortunately, agave, the syrup, is highly processed and during its preparation loses any health-promoting properties it might have had.

Agave syrup (or nectar) is often sold as a better alternative to honey because it has a lower glycemic index. While that is true, please don't be fooled. It has a low glycemic index because it's mostly fructose and not glucose. If you grab a couple of agave syrups, you'll find out that they are anywhere between 70 and 95 percent fructose, depending on the brand. That is a *looooot* of fructose. Do I need to remind you what all that fructose can do in your body? I rest my case!

ARTIFICIAL SWEETENERS

As the calorie-free fad grew, several "no-calorie" artificial sweeteners were introduced to the market. Because they are incredibly sweet, the amount needed is so small that you end up consuming almost no calories. No calories, no issues, right? According to the FDA, five artificial sweeteners (acesulfame potassium, aspartame, neotame, saccharin, and sucralose) are "generally recognized as safe."[197] "Generally recognized as safe" is like saying, "I'm pretty sure I didn't leave the stove on." You think everything is okay, but your house might also be about to burn down. Indeed, many authors argue that artificial sweeteners might have toxic effects in the body.[198,199]

Let's start with aspartame. Did you know that aspartame is broken down into formaldehyde in your body?[200] Yes, the embalming fluid formaldehyde. In animal studies, formaldehyde from aspartame consumption was linked to oxidative stress and even cell death.[201] In addition, while the body processes aspartame, it creates metabolic by-products such as phenylalanine, aspartic acid, and methanol. The excess of phenylalanine contributes to a reduction of important neurotransmitters like dopamine and serotonin, which can trigger neurological issues.[202] In high concentrations, aspartic acid is connected with degeneration of astrocytes and neurons.[203] Finally, methanol metabolites can cause vision disorders, depression of the central nervous system, and other symptoms leading ultimately to metabolic acidosis and coma.[204]

Sucralose, commercially known as Splenda, is no better. In fact, Splenda is more chemically similar to the commonly used pesticide DDT than it is to sugar.[205,206] Animal studies show that sucralose consumption decreases male fertility, negatively impacts the gut microbiome (promoting the overgrowth of *E. coli*), and reduces insulin sensitivity.[207–209] Similarly, further animal studies have also connected aspartame, acesulfame potassium, and saccharin to changes in the gut that led to glucose intolerance and weight gain.[210–213]

In human studies, despite not knowing exactly the mechanism behind these findings, researchers noted that people who eat artificial sweeteners have different (less beneficial) microbiome profiles than the individuals who avoid them.[214,215] Artificial sweetener consumption might even have effects farther out on the family tree. In studies with pregnant animals, these artificial sweeteners were associated with altered sweet taste preference later in life and metabolic dysfunction in the offspring.[216]

To be fair, there aren't many human interventional studies, and the ones that exist show conflicting results. We cannot conclude that humans will experience the same effects as animals. Nonetheless, several long-term observational studies support that human consumption of artificial sweeteners might actually contribute to the development of metabolic issues that lead to obesity, type 2 diabetes, cardiovascular disease, stroke, and dementia.[217–220]

Finally, we have the case of polyols (sugar alcohols) such as erythritol, isomalt, lactitol, maltitol, mannitol, sorbitol, and xylitol. Even though more research is needed, their excessive consumption has been associated with flatulence, abdominal discomfort, and laxative effects.[221] Moderate doses of polyols could also induce shifts in the gut microbiome in healthy people.[222] Of all the polyols, erythritol seems to be the one with the most research supporting its safety. Either way, it would be advisable to keep its intake low.

Artificial sweeteners can be found in most processed foods and beverages, especially in their light, diet, and calorie-free versions. You can also find them in toothpaste, mouthwash, and chewable vitamins.

ALTERNATIVE NATURAL SWEETENERS

Ideally, we should aim to desensitize our palate and slowly break the sweet-taste addiction. But I also understand that this takes time and you may benefit from a healthier alternative to keep your cravings controlled. Beyond the occasional use of honey and maple syrup, there are four other natural sweeteners that might assist you in this journey.

1. Stevia
Stevia is extracted from the leaves of a plant called *Stevia rebaudiana* and has been growing in popularity in the past few years. It's a good low-glycemic sweetener that does not seem to have direct or indirect effects on insulin.[223] Stevia is said to be 30 times sweeter than sugar, so a little goes a long way. This sweetener has a mild, licorice-like taste that's slightly bitter. But exact flavor seems to vary among brands, so try different ones. A word of caution: In animal models, excessive intake has been linked to reduced fertility and hormonal dysfunction.[224,225] Children with a history of allergies might also react to stevia.[226]

2. Raw Yacon Syrup
Yacon syrup (or yacon nectar) comes from the yacon root. This tuber is rich in prebiotics, such as inulin and fructooligosaccharides (FOSs). It's actually the FOSs that give the syrup its sweet taste while still keeping it at an incredibly low glycemic index.[227] Besides tasting sweet, the FOSs (and inulin) serve as food for our gut bugs. Studies also show that yacon syrup can help control weight, improve insulin sensitivity, and regulate cholesterol levels. Yacon syrup should be consumed raw. If processed at temperatures higher than 104°F (40°C), a good portion of the FOSs turn into sugar, making this sweetener no longer healthy. Choose high-quality raw syrup that's free of additives.

3. Chicory Root
Chicory is a perennial plant grown in different places in the world and commonly used as forage for livestock. In terms of human consumption, it is probably best known for being used as a caffeine-free coffee alternative. Similarly to yacon, chicory root is also rich in prebiotics, inulin in particular.[228] Since inulin also has a sweet taste, processed chicory root is now being used as a sugar substitute.[229] This low-glycemic sweetener is said to promote a good microbiotic profile and may also improve intestinal transit, insulin sensitivity, blood sugar control, and weight management.[230-234]

4. Monk Fruit
Monk fruit (a.k.a. luo han guo or *Momordica grosvenori*) is native to Southeast Asia but lately has been gaining popularity worldwide. The natural powdered extract from this fruit is free of calories and, similarly to stevia, gets a zero on the glycemic index scale. Once again, it's also incredibly sweet, so small amounts suffice. Research suggests that monk fruit may support good blood glucose management, decrease inflammation, and perhaps even slow the growth of some of cancer cells.[235-240] More long-term interventional studies on humans are needed, but so far all points toward moderate consumption being perfectly safe.[241]

THE VERDICT ON CARBOHYDRATES

Up to this point, I've presented several pieces of evidence against carbs, but I've also shared cases of populations following high-carb diets without apparent health repercussions. The carb question is not a linear one. Even though restricting carbs might be beneficial, the most important factors to consider are the quality of the carbs and even the timing of their consumption.

Carbs are not evil. We need sugar in our blood to stay alive. Without adequate amounts of carbs in the diet, many people can experience reduced levels of active thyroid hormone, elevated levels of cortisol, and reduced levels of testosterone. Appropriate carb intake can help us thrive! What we do not need is the insane number of refined sugars we are consuming.

Each one of us has a different tolerance to carbs. Some will thrive with one amount, while for others that same amount will be detrimental. It's believed that there's a tipping point at which your carb ingestion crosses over from being supportive of your health to making you sick. Later in the book, I will show you how you can determine your limit.

Besides quantity, we also have to consider the timing of consumption. As we saw, consuming a high-carb meal as soon as you wake up is not the best approach. That insulin spike will cause cortisol's fat-burning effect to shut down and give way to a muscle-burning effect (muscle loss). If instead you ate that same high-carb meal after a workout, when all your glucose and glycogen reserves have been used, the food will help you grow stronger with no fat-gaining effects.

Finally, we have the quality issue. You can take in the same quantity of fructose from a soda with HFCS or from a piece of fruit, but the effects on your body will be completely different. Fruit has fiber, antioxidants, vitamins, and minerals that can minimize the effects of the fructose and contribute to your health. The soda? Well, the soda has nothing good to offer you. Whole-fruit consumption is also self-limiting. While you can drink a gallon of orange juice in a day, I doubt you would eat the 48 oranges it takes to make that amount of juice.

The takeaway message is that our modern diet is filled with refined carb sources that are making us sick. For most of us, cutting back on our carb intake will help improve insulin sensitivity, reduce oxidative stress, decrease inflammation, and lower overall risk of disease.[242]

Reducing carb intake does not mean complete elimination. It means eating healthier carbs at the right times. And even treating yourself occasionally. Yes, it is okay to eat some sugar once in a while, as long as you have a healthy relationship with it and don't crave it to fill an emotional void.

METABOLIC EVOLUTION

Nowadays, it's hard to think of a time when carbohydrates were not our primary source of fuel. We look at the food pyramid and see that the base of the recommended diet is high-carb foods. You think of fast food and it's all grain-based baked goods. Even if you think of more traditional restaurants, you might imagine a dish significantly composed of either rice, pasta, or some sort of starchy vegetable or legume. Although it seems as if we've been eating like this forever, this is not the case. Carbs were incredibly rare (even nonexistent for some populations) for most of our human evolution. Looking back, scientists recognize that the fuel they used might have been more efficient for human performance.

When you eat carbs, you use glucose as fuel. After you digest the food, your body uses the glucose circulating in your bloodstream. As the level drops, your liver and muscle reserves break down glycogen into glucose to keep up with the demand. The problem is that your liver holds only about 100 grams of glycogen and your muscles about 400 grams.[243] That is not a big tank, but if you don't do much, it should be enough to last you for most of the day. But what happens when you exhaust your reserves and your cells don't have anything else to munch on? When your body doesn't have more glucose to use, it has to look to the other two fuel sources: protein from your muscles, and your body fat.

Through gluconeogenesis, the body can use protein from the muscles to create glucose. While this is a good survival mechanism, having our muscle eaten away is not the best way to stay strong and healthy for long. Your body fat, au contraire, is there almost exclusively to be used as fuel. And this fuel tank has almost unlimited capacity. When you run out of carbohydrates, you break down your accumulated fat (in a process called lipolysis), and your liver uses these resulting fatty acids to create ketones (a.k.a. ketone bodies), through a process called ketogenesis.[244] Then, the ketones leave your liver, enter your bloodstream, and are distributed throughout your body to be used as energy. Some authors consider ketones to be a better fuel than glucose and have even called them a superfuel.[245-247]

Ketones are considered a clean fuel because they create more energy per unit of oxygen, require fewer metabolic steps, and generate fewer waste products such as free radicals.[248] To add to that, research has shown ketones' ability to substantially increase body-produced antioxidants like glutathione.[249] In other words, these powerhouses help you clean up the mess from glucose metabolism's excessive ROS formation. This state of using ketones for fuel is known as ketosis.

Historically, humans used to be in ketosis most of the time. Think about it—carbs were not a major part of our ancestors' diet. Not to mention that they would sometimes spend days without eating because of food scarcity. Their only option was to use their fat for fuel. Ketosis was an important metabolic state for humans, so much so that even newborns appear to rely substantially on ketosis.[250-252]

THE KETOGENIC DIET

The ketogenic (or keto) diet focuses on high fat and an extremely restricted carbohydrate intake. This tells your body that it cannot rely on carbs for fuel and signals it to use fat instead. The traditional macronutrient ratio of a ketogenic diet consists of 60 percent to 80 percent of calories from fat, 15 percent to 35 percent from protein, and 5 percent or fewer from carbs.[253] That is to say, grains, starchy vegetables, and sweet fruits are not welcome.

Although this diet seems to be all the rage right now, it was initially studied as a therapeutic tool about 100 years ago.[254] Keto diets were initially designed to treat epilepsy in children, but with the introduction of antiepileptic drugs, the diets' use declined dramatically.[255,256] Fortunately, keto is on the rise, and recent research has linked this diet with:

- enhanced blood sugar and energy stabilization;[257]
- suppression of appetite and cravings;[258]
- improved weight management;[259]
- increased antioxidant production;[260,261]
- protection against oxidative stress;[262]
- reduced inflammation;[263]
- neuroprotection against seizures, Alzheimer's, and Parkinson's;[264]
- increased brain-derived neurotrophic factor (BDNF) levels, which are associated with improved mood, learning, and overall brain health;[265]
- improved memory in patients with mild cognitive impairment and early Alzheimer's disease;[266,267]
- enhanced mitochondrial function;[268]
- decreased growth and proliferation of cancer cells;[269,270] and
- elevation of compounds (sirtuins and NAD+) that are associated with longevity.[271]

Neo Note: Keto Flu

During the metabolic adaptation period, some folks might experience what is commonly called the keto flu. The keto flu can present itself in different ways, but some common symptoms are dizziness, headaches, irritability, mental fogginess, muscle cramps, nausea, and weakness. It's believed that the cause of the keto flu is electrolyte unbalance. During the first few days or weeks of a ketogenic diet, there is an increase in mineral wasting due to declining levels of insulin signaling. Obviously, your body ends up adjusting to this, but until then, it might be a good idea to increase your consumption of mineral-rich salt to compensate for the wasting.

THE KETOACIDOSIS CONCERN

Many people have negative beliefs about ketosis and ketogenic diets because they've heard they can lead to ketoacidosis. Ketoacidosis is a potentially life-threatening condition caused by incredibly high levels of ketones in the blood (around 10 to 20 millimoles per liter). The thing is, in a state of normal ketosis, your blood ketones only get to around 1 to 2 millimoles per liter, which is 10 times less than the amount needed for ketoacidosis.[272] Please be assured your body is more than capable of keeping you within a safe range. If levels are getting too high, your pancreas releases insulin to balance the ketone levels.[273]

Ketoacidosis can occur in cases of severe alcoholism, severe dehydration, excessive drug use (especially cocaine), misuse of insulin by people with diabetes, or acute major illnesses such as pancreatitis, cirrhosis, myocardial infarction (heart attack) or sepsis.[274,275] Although it is incredibly rare, there have been reports of ketoacidosis in women lactating while on a low-carb diet.[276,277] The reason for this is not fully understood, but it is recognized that breastfeeding women have higher glucose requirements.[278] Considering this, a traditional ketogenic diet is probably not the best choice for pregnant or lactating women.

Neo Note: Ketones and Brown Fat

In your body, there are essentially two kinds of fat: white fat and brown fat. White fat is the typical fat you think about—the kind in your belly, arms, and legs that serves as the fuel tank. Brown fat (a.k.a. brown adipose tissue, or BAT), however, is rich in mitochondria and is metabolically active. I know this will sound cannibalistic, but BAT helps you burn white fat to heat your body.[279] BAT is located deeper in your body and surrounds your heart, kidneys, neck, spine, and major blood vessels. Babies are born with a large amount of BAT to maintain their body temperature, but with age BAT becomes scarcer. Besides helping us burn white fat to produce heat, BAT also produces anti-inflammatory compounds.[280] What a nice combo!

One reason people lose weight on a ketogenic diet is because of BAT. Studies have found that while insulin inhibits BAT, ketones make it more active.[281] This possibly explains why keto diets tend to cause more weight loss than traditional calorie-restricted, low-fat diets, even while keto dieters consume significantly more calories.[282,283]

INSULIN RESISTANCE AND KETOSIS

I've already written plenty about the devastating consequences of insulin resistance, but there's more. Insulin resistance can make it really hard for you to burn your body fat and enter a state of ketosis. In situations of insulin resistance, insulin levels are chronically high. When insulin is high, it blocks glucagon and HSL, which are the main hormones triggering your body to go into fat-burning mode. This means that while insulin is elevated, you won't be able to transition to fat as fuel, and you will remain in fat-storage mode. It doesn't matter if you reduce carbs and start eating high fat; as long as insulin is still high, fat burning and ketosis are blocked. This is why so many people who try a keto diet crash and feel terrible. Even though they get plenty of fuel from food and have enough fat reserves, their still-high insulin levels don't allow them to burn fat. It's like dying of dehydration while surrounded by water because you can't open your mouth. This is why one should make a gradual transition into a keto diet, by slowly decreasing carb consumption and improving insulin sensitivity. Only when you are insulin sensitive will you be able to enter a ketogenic state and take advantage of the benefits of burning a "clean" fuel.

LONG-TERM KETOSIS

According to the US Institute of Medicine of the National Academies, "the lower limit of dietary carbohydrate compatible with life apparently is zero, provided that adequate amounts of protein and fat are consumed."[284] In other words, we do not need carbohydrates to survive. Using this argument, many keto advocates say you should eliminate carbs and stay in ketosis as much as possible.

But just because we can survive without carbs doesn't mean we will thrive without them. For example, there are several anecdotal reports of women experiencing mood issues on ultralow ketogenic diets and feeling much better with a small increase in the carb quantity. Likewise, some people eating low carb seem to undergo a decrease in T3 thyroid hormone production, which may be an issue for those with hypothyroidism.[285] And then we have the brain. Even though the brain loves ketones, it also needs some amount of glucose.[286-288] While the body can provide glucose through gluconeogenesis of protein, the brain still needs about 20 to 30 grams per day of carbohydrates from dietary sources.[289] Because many people "keto so hard," they don't even achieve this bare minimum, and the deficiency can have damaging long-term consequences.

Finally, we also want to have some carbs (100 to 150 grams will be enough for most) in order to have healthy leptin dynamics. As you know, leptin is not only a satiety hormone but also helps boost your metabolism. What you probably don't know is that when an insulin-sensitive person eats carbs, the secreted insulin will boost his or her leptin levels.[290] As Max Lugavere suggests, when combined with exercise, a weekly higher-carb "refeed" can increase energy expenditure, recalibrate mood, and speed up fat loss, especially for those who've seen their weight loss stall.[291]

Thriving is not being stuck in a macronutrient ratio forever. Thriving is having an antifragile body that can adapt to anything you throw at it. You should not have to pick between being a great carb burner or fat burner. You should have the flexibility to enjoy the benefits of both. For most of us, the goal should be to achieve intermittent ketosis but still take advantage of the occasional spike of insulin.

KETOSIS AS A THERAPEUTIC TOOL

You can use a tool like a hammer to build a roof over your head, or you can use that same hammer to bash someone's head in. The hammer is not good or bad. It's what you do with it that determines its meaning. Think of ketosis as a therapeutic tool. It's something that should be used at the right time for the right task. Similarly to any tool, it should be used with proper know-how and respect, so you can get the most out of it while not overusing it and causing harm.

As I just mentioned, a healthy individual does not need to and should not aim for constant ketosis. However, prolonged keto diets can be incredibly beneficial, addressing a wide range of health concerns. Some of the main conditions for which research supports the use of ketosis as a therapeutic tool are:
- Alzheimer's disease;[292–295]
- autism spectrum disorder;[296–299]
- cancer (brain cancers in particular).[300–308]
- epilepsy;[309–311]
- metabolic syndrome;[312–315]
- MS;[316–318]
- Parkinson's disease;[319–323]
- PCOS;[324–326] and
- type 2 diabetes;[327–330]

METABOLIC FLEXIBILITY

How can you remove the years of bad programming and reset your metabolism to its factory settings? You do this by regaining your metabolic flexibility. This resets your mitochondria to operate like they used to before they were compromised by all the crap food we shoved down our pieholes when we didn't know any better.

In his book *Two Meals a Day*, fitness author Mark Sisson states, "metabolic flexibility is the holy grail of all health pursuits."[331] This is one of the most important health attributes imaginable, since it allows you to burn a variety of fuels, especially stored fat, based on your body's needs at any given time.

Let's face it. Right now, you probably have a bunch of sugar-addicted mitochondria desperate for carbs because that's the only thing they've known how to process for the past few years. They no longer remember the days when they could burn all the fuels with ease and have you feeling great all the time. Now, if they don't get their carbs every few hours, they will make you have cravings and feel shaky, groggy, or "hangry." That's not how we should live.

As a healthy human, you should use the glucose from the food you just ate. And once you use all that energy, you should be able to easily transition to burning your stored fat—without crashes, cravings, or any signs of weakness. You should be able to forget that you haven't eaten for several hours because you still feel amazing.

I recognize all this sounds quite conceptual, and you might worry that there will be no practical application. Fear not. Soon enough, we will get our hands dirty, and I am going to show you how the Neo Diet puts all these concepts together in an easy-to-follow way. But before we get there, I still need to expose you to one of the biggest health lies we all have been told.

DIETARY FAT

How can I be recommending cutting back on carbs and bumping up your fat consumption? After all, we've all been told that dietary fat is bad. We've all heard that fat buildup in the arteries is the primary cause of heart attacks and strokes. Not to mention that overweight people have more health issues. It seems logical that the fat on our plates will turn into fat in our bodies and make us sick.

Fat has an evil reputation, but body fat is as important as any organ you have. Beyond serving as a never-ending fuel tank, fat also produces its own hormones, can help you increase your metabolic rate, and is part of all your cells. Yes, fat is needed to make and sustain the membranes of your cells. A healthy membrane provides structure and the ability to communicate with other cells, since it's in the membrane that all the receptors are located. About 60 percent of your brain is fat.[332] Your organs are also mostly fat. Myelin, which is the sheet around our neurons that makes the electrical signals super-fast, is also made of fat.[333] Many hormones are made of fat, and fat is also required for the absorption of crucial, health-promoting fat-soluble nutrients like vitamins A, D, E, and K.[334] Dietary fat is essential for our survival, and honestly, it deserves more recognition.

Let me make one thing clear. It's not the consumption of fat that makes us fat. We get fat because of the genetics-lifestyle dissonance. Our genes still carry the information of a world where you needed to pack as much fat as possible to face the hard times ahead. Our ancestors lived in cycles of feast and famine. But the life most of us live right now no longer presents those dietary hardships and periods of starvation. We are surrounded by food 24/7, but your cells still think that at any moment *winter is coming* and you need to be fat to survive it.

And then there's the entire situation of eating excessive carbs, developing insulin resistance, and having all the metabolic issues we've already discussed. Indeed, studies have shown that high consumption of certain fats did not increase blood levels of those fats. Ironically, the highest circulating levels of the fats were found after the study participants consumed a high-carbohydrate meal, while eating fewer carbohydrates led to lower circulating levels.[335,336]

BODY FAT

The main types of body fat are subcutaneous, visceral, intermuscular, and intramuscular fat.[337] The ones that interest us the most are the first two. Subcutaneous fat, or subcutaneous adipose tissue (SAT), is the fat that's right under your skin.[338] It's the soft and "wiggly" fat we can accumulate just under the surface of our arms, hips, and bellies.[339,340] Even though aesthetically it's the type we notice the most, biologically it's not the one that causes the most harm. That place is reserved for visceral fat.[341]

Visceral fat, omentum fat, or visceral adipose tissue (VAT) is the deep fat that surrounds the internal organs (kidneys, liver, pancreas, etc.) in the abdomen.[342] Because this fat is more internal, it can go unnoticed for years and cause surprise when doctors start seeing "thin" people showing symptoms usually associated with the obese.[343] This is what some researchers call "skinny fat" (or "normal-weight obesity").[344]

Researchers theorize that the specific free fatty acids produced by visceral fat can cause insulin resistance (hence metabolic syndrome), and the anatomical location of the fat is compressing and putting the organs and circulatory system at a higher level of stress (affecting their normal function).[345] Independently of the exact process, studies have linked this fat to greater risk of insulin resistance, diabetes, metabolic syndrome, NAFLD, systemic inflammation, cardiovascular disease, hypertension, and certain cancers.[346-357] Visceral fat is also associated with the severity of infectious diseases like COVID-19.[358] To compound the problem, once insulin resistance is in place, it will magnify the detrimental effects of visceral fat.[359]

WE USED TO LOVE FAT

There's no question that fat is essential for us to survive and thrive. So, why were we told that fat is evil? Why did our ancestors hate fat? The truth is that our ancestors did not hate fat. They actually prized it above all else. Anthropologists believe that our hunter-gatherer ancestors would immediately eat (the incredibly fatty) organ meats but many times would leave muscle meat uneaten.[360] Some researchers believe that this might have led to wasteful killing of mammoths simply to extract their fatty tongues, for example.[361]

In the 1930s, a dentist named Weston Price decided to travel the world in search of remote, "untouched" civilizations that still followed the diets of their ancestors. Dr. Price studied the isolated people of Lötschental in Switzerland, the Gaelics in the Outer and Inner Hebrides, the Inuits of Alaska, the Native Americans in different locations in the USA and Canada, the Melanesians and Polynesians in the South Pacific, several tribes in Eastern and Central Africa, the Aborigines of Australia, the Maori of New Zealand, and the ancient civilizations and their descendants in South America. When possible, he also studied the closest "modern" peoples, their diets, and their health. The initial goal was to study how their ancestral diets affected their dental health, but he quickly realized that the peoples with the best teeth were also the more muscular and the ones immune to several of our modern diseases, including heart disease, diabetes, cancer, depression, and obesity.

In his book *Nutrition and Physical Degeneration*, Dr. Price explains that the healthiest cultures heavily consumed fat, from either animal or plant foods.[362] For example, the Polynesian populations of Tokelau took in most of their fat through a coconut-rich diet.[363] All the healthy traditional peoples shared the characteristic that they ate a lot of fat. In Africa, the Masai, Muhima, Nuer, and Watusi were all cattle-keeping people, and their diets consisted largely of milk, blood, and meat. For the Nuer, fatty organs like the liver were so sacred that they could not touch the organs with their hands.[364]

In her book *Big Fat Surprise*, science journalist Nina Teicholz reports that in the early 1960s, Gerald Shaper, a South African doctor studying the Samburu, found that, depending on the season, a young Samburu man would drink two to seven liters of milk each day.[365] This represents more than a pound of butterfat per day. Professor George Mann from Vanderbilt University joined Dr. Shaper and found similar dietary patterns among the Masai. The men would drink three to five liters of milk daily. When milk ran low during the dry season, they would mix it with cow's blood. On special occasions, when cattle were killed, the Masai would eat four to ten pounds of fatty beef per person.[366]

Another example comes from the Australian Aborigines, who, except in times of famine, rejected kangaroos that were too lean since they were not worth carrying back to camp. According to the researcher, during periods of abundance, animal meat would be wasted because only the best and fattest parts of the game were eaten.[367]

Dr. Price also shared the story of Professor Vilhjalmur Stefansson, who lived for about a year with the Inuits of Alaska. Stefansson reported that when lean caribou was the only meat available, the natives would become anxious, since they believed that without fatty meats they would be more prone to disease.[368] Fat was so valued that the ancient Native American tribes would not eat female bison in the spring because when pregnant or nursing, the animals would have lower fat reserves.[369]

Even if we look at "less isolated" peoples, we can still see a traditional Northern European diet rich in fatty fish, meat, and fermented, full-fat dairy products. Similarly, we can trace the traditional Mediterranean diet and see that even though they go heavy on carbs, the Mediterranean peoples also take in plenty of fat through fish, meats, olive oil, nuts, full-fat milk, and cheeses.

Fat has been an integral part of our lives for many, many years. So, when did things change? When did fat become evil?

FAT LIES

The defamation of dietary fat, especially saturated fat, started in the mid-1950s. Around that time in the US, an increase in cardiovascular disease scared the population, and experts were looking for answers, since heart disease used to be incredibly rare. One of those experts was a pathologist from the University of Minnesota named Ancel Keys. Years earlier, Keys had created the K ration, a system of boxed meals delivered to soldiers during World War II. One can say that Keys had some reputation and was well connected. In 1956, with funding from the US Public Health Service, Keys began the study that would change the perception of fat around the world.[370] In his Seven Countries Study, Keys presented a positive association between the consumption of fat and death from degenerative heart disease.[371] This struck terror into the population, and thus fat suddenly became public enemy number one.

What was not publicly known at the time was that Keys had gathered data from 22 countries and then omitted the ones that did not fit what he was trying to prove. When the data of all 22 countries was considered, the association between fat and heart disease became much weaker.[372] One of the most obvious discrepancies was the case of France. At that time, there was no epidemic of heart disease among the French, despite their high consumption of fatty meats, cheese, and butter—the so-called French paradox.

Not everyone agreed with Keys. British physiologist and nutritionist John Yudkin publicly stated that the blame should not be put on fat but on sugar instead. His findings suggested that the countries where obesity, diabetes, and heart disease were becoming more prominent were also the countries with higher consumption of sugar and sugar-containing foods.[373] Fun fact: Many years later, the reanalysis of Keys's Seven Countries Study's data confirmed that sugar intake had a stronger correlation with heart disease risk than any other nutrient.[374]

If the media had gone with the findings of researchers like Yudkin instead of Keys, our perception of fat might not have been compromised, and our reality would probably much different today. Unfortunately, that was not the case. As explained in detail in the Teicholz's *Big Fat Surprise*, Keys's theories were in line with the interests of the food industry, so there was a lot of money involved in making sure he got the attention the food companies needed. With so much support from high places, Keys ended up becoming a celebrity and even made the cover of *Time* magazine in 1961.[375] Having the media and the food industry behind them, Keys's theories became facts, and unfortunately for us, we started to demonize all the foods that contained saturated fats. In fact, in 1977, the first edition of the *U.S. Dietary Goals* was published, and it recommended that all Americans restrict their intake of saturated fat.[376] This was music to the ears of the food industry. Now that saturated fat was evil, they could start selling thousands of brand-new, low-fat processed food products that would "save us" from disease.

THE TRANS FAT TWIST

In 1901, a German chemist named Wilhelm Normann discovered a way to transform cheap liquid vegetable oils into a semisolid, shelf-stable form (later called trans fats).[377] His discovery was important because it solved a market problem. There was an enormous demand for animal fats like lard and butter that was becoming more and more difficult to meet. But there was a growing supply of cheap by-product vegetable oils from industrial manufacturing that were going to waste. So, when Normann figured out how to make these oils into cooking-friendly fats, this changed the food industry forever.

By 1910, Procter & Gamble already owned the rights to Normann's patent in the US and created the first commercial partially hydrogenated fat, which they branded as Crisco. People loved their saturated animal fats, so Crisco struggled initially, but then everything changed. As Dr. James DiNicolantonio brilliantly explains in his book *Superfuel*: "Between marketing, the Great Depression, and World War II, animal fats were down for the count. Procter & Gamble, seeing an opportunity to propel their beloved invention even further into the spotlight, decided they would pay the American Heart Association $1.75 million dollars for an endorsement proclaiming that Crisco was healthier than animal fats. The American Heart Association accepted, and with that, the demise of animal fats in the American diet was inevitable."[378] Can you see now why Keys's findings were so good for the food industry?

During his heyday, Keys suggested that saturated animal fat was the culprit behind the rising rates of heart attacks, but it was later discovered that in his laboratory and human experiments, he wasn't using animal fats.[379] In fact, his test subjects were fed margarine made from partially hydrogenated vegetable oil. It was not saturated animal fat that was producing the poor results he was presenting to the media; it was vegetable trans fats.

People eventually questioned Keys's work—so much so that even Keys eventually waived his support for his own hypothesis.[380] Unfortunately, by then it was already too late. His diet-heart hypothesis that blamed saturated animal fats had spread like wildfire. With the support and marketing dollars from the food industry, Keys's theories were the "science-backed facts" the industry needed to promote its new wave of cooking vegetable oils and low-fat products.

Although the impact of these lies prevailed for decades, things are finally changing. In 2001, as a study from the Harvard School of Public Health stated, "the low-fat campaign has been based on little scientific evidence and may have caused unintended health consequences."[381] Moreover, the researchers concluded that the low-fat approach not only did not improve the epidemic of metabolic disease but actually made it worse. In a 2009 article, an expert panel held jointly between the Food and Agriculture Organization (FAO) and WHO concluded that saturated fatty acid intake was not significantly correlated with cardiovascular events or mortality. Similarly, the panel concluded that low-fat diets did not reduce the incidence of fatal coronary heart disease.[382] Finally, we also have a large 2019 meta-analysis of 43 studies, reporting that no correlation between total fat or saturated fat intake and cardiovascular disease was found.[383]

To recap, before Keys and food industry's tag-team fight, people ate a lot more saturated fat than we do today. Back then, heart attacks were incredibly rare, almost unheard of, even.[384,385] After Keys, our consumption of saturated fats plummeted to less than a quarter of what it had been, vegetable oil consumption rose tremendously, and heart disease became one of the major causes of death in both men and women.[386-388]

Beyond not having fear of dietary fat, I hope you understand the importance of adding more of it in your life. Healthy fats are the foundation of the Neo Diet because of their physiological importance but also because they taste amazing and are incredibly filling. This makes this diet super easy to follow and sustain. The right fats are a nutritious and clean-burning fuel that makes you function on all cylinders and brings you closer to your superhuman potential. Ready to learn more about each type of dietary fat?

ALL ABOUT FATS

There are several types of fats—some good, some bad. In this section, we are going to review them so you know which ones you should rely on to achieve your health goals. At a fundamental level, we can start by splitting fats into two categories: saturated and unsaturated. A fat is considered either saturated or unsaturated depending on the presence or absence of double bonds between the carbon atoms in the carbon chain. I know this sounds a bit too nerdish, but in the figure below you can easily see what I mean by that.

Fats are saturated when they don't have any double bonds. When they have one or more double bonds, they are unsaturated. If a fat has only one double bond, it's known as a monounsaturated fat (MUFA), but if it has more, it's called polyunsaturated (PUFA).

SATURATED FAT

Saturated fat is usually associated with animal fat, but as we saw not too long ago, coconuts (and also cocoa and palm fruit/kernels) are incredibly rich in saturated fat. To be fair, most animal fats comprise almost equal parts of MUFA and saturated fat, and even have a small amount of PUFAs.

$$H - O - \overset{\overset{\textstyle O}{\|}}{C} - \overset{\overset{\textstyle H}{|}}{\underset{\underset{\textstyle H}{|}}{C}} - \overset{\overset{\textstyle H}{|}}{\underset{\underset{\textstyle H}{|}}{C}} - \overset{\overset{\textstyle H}{|}}{\underset{\underset{\textstyle H}{|}}{C}} - H$$

SATURATED FAT (E.G. BUTYRIC ACID)

Within the group of saturated fats, we can subdivide them into long-chain, medium-chain, or short-chain fats. The length of the chain is basically the number of carbon atoms the fat has.

• Short-chain fatty acids (SCFAs) are fatty acids with five or fewer carbon atoms in each molecule.[389] SCFAs are found in foods like butter and ghee but, as you know, are also produced by our gut bacteria as they process prebiotics.

• Medium-chain fatty acids (MCFAs), or medium-chain triglycerides (MCTs), are fatty acids with 6 to 12 carbon atoms.[390] They are found in foods like coconut, palm oil, and goat's milk. Fun fact: capric, caproic, and caprylic acids are all MCFAs named after their primary source: goat's milk. In Latin, a female goat is a *capra*.

• Long-chain fatty acids (LCFAs) are fatty acids with 13 to 21 carbon atoms, while very long-chain fatty acids (VLCFAs) have 22 or more.[374,375] Since VLCFAs are less common and usually not a significant part of our diet, we will focus only on LCFAs. These can be found in foods like red meats, dairy, coconut, palm oil, and cocoa butter.

> **Neo Note: The Incredible MCTs**
> MCTs are metabolized differently than other fats. Instead of going to the lymphatic system and then into your bloodstream for distribution, MCTs travel directly to your liver to be converted into ketones. Because of this difference, fats containing MCTs are less likely than other fats to be stored as body fat, which makes MCTs a splendid choice for weight-loss regimens.[393] Since they go straight to your liver to be converted into ketones, adding them (in particular, caprylic acid, C8) while restricting carbs might be a great hack to speed your adaptation to using fat as fuel.[394]
> If you want to use MCTs while you're trying to regain metabolic flexibility,

remember that C8 is the most efficient one to induce ketosis. But please scrutinize the labels of MCT supplements, because the cheaper products usually have a combination of different MCTs, which makes them less powerful.

MCTs help us trim body weight, waist circumference, hip circumference, total body fat, and even the dangerous visceral fat.[395] There are different mechanisms behind these findings. First, MCT oil has been shown to increase the release of the hormones PYY and leptin, which, as you know, promote satiety.[396] Second, MCTs can boost your metabolic rate and your fat-burning ability, at least temporarily.[397,398]

But the benefits of MCTs don't stop with metabolic optimization and weight loss. Studies demonstrate that MCTs have antibacterial, antifungal, and antiviral abilities and support a healthy gut microbiome.[399,400] MCTs also boost brain health and improve memory, even in cases of mild-to-moderate Alzheimer's disease.[401,402] Finally, MCT consumption is associated with an increase in exercise performance, allowing individuals to train at a higher intensity and for longer periods of time.[403]

P.S. Please do not use MCT oil to cook. MCT oils mostly consist of capric and caprylic acids, which have low smoke points. Please consume your MCTs raw. A better cooking alternative would be "whole" coconut oil, since it also has lauric acid, which has a high smoke point. Besides that, coconut oil is low in unsaturated fats and thus is less likely to turn rancid with oxidation.

UNSATURATED FAT
Monounsaturated Fats

The fact that unsaturated fats have double bonds allows them to remain liquid at room temperature but also makes these oils more fragile.[404,405] MUFAs have only one double bond in the carbon chain. This means that although they're more unstable than saturated fats, they are more stable than PUFAs. MUFAs can be found in foods like olives, almonds, macadamia nuts, Brazil nuts, cashews, peanuts, avocados, duck, pork, tallow, lard, and certain types of cheeses, such as Cheddar and Colby.

MONOUNSATURATED FAT (E.G. OLEIC ACID)

A 2016 meta-analysis of 24 studies found that diets high in MUFAs can improve metabolic risk factors (reducing blood glucose levels and improving insulin sensitivity), in particular among individuals with type 2 diabetes.[406] And an 18-month randomized controlled trial published in the *International*

Journal of Obesity and Related Metabolic Disorders determined that the participants with the higher ratio of monounsaturated fats in their diet lost more weight, more body fat, and more inches off their waists than the low-fat group (which actually gained in all those parameters).[407] High-MUFA diets have been shown to lower blood pressure and the risk of heart disease, even in individuals with type 2 diabetes and metabolic syndrome.[408-410] Lastly, research has also uncovered that individuals who eat a Mediterranean diet high in MUFAs have significantly lower inflammatory markers.[411-413]

Omega-9s

Let's start with the most famous monounsaturated fats, the omega-9s. The main ones are oleic acid (OA), eicosatrienoic acid (ETE), and erucic acid (EA). By far the most beneficial, and honestly, the only one worth mentioning, is OA. OA is one reason why we consider olive oil so beneficial for our health. It has been found to have multiple positive effects on cardiovascular health, such as lowering the susceptibility of LDL to oxidation, reducing blood coagulation, and improving blood-vessel function.[414] Additional research has also linked OA with improved insulin sensitivity, decreased risk of type 2 diabetes, and significant anti-inflammatory properties.[415] The best food sources of omega-9s include olives, cold-pressed olive oil, avocados, pasture-raised meats, and sprouted nuts.

Polyunsaturated Fats

Some of the most famous PUFAs are omega-3s and omega-6s. Unfortunately, they are surrounded by controversy and misinformation. PUFAs are essential for our optimal health, but they are also incredibly fragile, and here is where the confusion starts. Because they're so fragile, if we don't know what we're doing, we can turn a health-promoting PUFA into something incredibly toxic. PUFAs' multiple double bonds make them more reactive and vulnerable to oxidation.[416]

POLYUNSATURATED FAT (E.G. LINOLEIC ACID)

Oxidation is the phenomenon in which oxygen interacts with certain "unstable" molecules, converting them into toxic (damaged) versions, creating more free radicals. With PUFAs, oxygen free radicals will "attack" these double bonds. The more double bonds a fat has, the more harmful it can become. When the oxygen free radical connects to the PUFA, it creates a toxic PUFA, and it releases an extra electron (a free radical). This electron is available to react with other unstable molecules, and this can set off a potentially never-ending chain reaction of oxidative stress. This oxidative stress will then cause inflammation, cellular damage, and all the diseases that can come from that.

The good news is that PUFAs in their wholesome form are combined with several antioxidants like vitamin E and phenolic compounds that protect them against oxidation.[417] The bad news is that most of our PUFA consumption is coming from refined vegetable oils. When seeds and nuts are processed to create vegetable oils, the heat and chemicals used destroy the antioxidants in these foods, and their PUFAs become defenseless to oxidation. This is the main reason for the bad press. They are not bad; they're just fragile. If we take good care of them, they will take good care of us. But if we process them, they become one of the major toxins in our food supply.[418]

Omega-6s
– Linoleic acid
Most dietary omega-6s are in the form of linoleic acid (LA). LA is considered an essential fat. In other words, it's a fat you cannot produce and need to get from your diet. Since it is an essential fat, one would assume that it's beloved by the health experts, right? Not really. LA has a pretty poor reputation in the nutrition world. Experts have put omega-3s on a pedestal and shoved omega-6s, LA in particular, into the trash. But why is that? After reviewing the work of several authors, I believe we are once again committing the same mistake. Our need for quick answers has made our experts reach rushed decisions and load different things into the same boat. If you learn nothing else from this book, please learn to question everything, and never to assume that things are as linear as many make them seem.

According to experts, omega-3s are anti-inflammatory, while LA omega-6s are inflammatory. But a 2012 systematic review of multiple trials concluded that there's "virtually no evidence available from randomized, controlled intervention studies among healthy, non-infant human beings to show that addition of LA to the diet increases the concentration of inflammatory markers."[419] Another systematic review published in 2017 also supports these findings.[420] So, what is the deeper story here? Nowadays, the big majority of LA in our diet is coming from vegetable oils extracted from canola, corn, cottonseeds, soybeans, and sunflower kernels. As you know, these were never part of our diet until recently. Do you want to know why? Do me a favor. Grab a kernel of corn and try to squeeze some oil out of it. Take your time, I'll wait.

Before the 20th century, we did not possess the technology to extract these refined vegetable oils. They only became possible once we created chemical solvents, oil mills, and the processes to purify and chemically alter these seeds and fruits. During the extraction process, these PUFA fats are exposed to three oxidation triggers: air, heat, and light.

Exposure to air is inevitable, but the high temperatures used during refinement increase oxidation rates exponentially. These heat-oxidized oils are then further refined (mainly, bleached and deodorized), which exacerbates the loss of nutrients and antioxidants, further increasing the oils' oxidative potential.[421,422] When processing is finished, the oils are bottled in clear (often toxic) plastic containers and then sit on the shelves of warehouses and stores where they're exposed to light and continue to oxidize, further surrendering the limited remaining nutrition they had.[423]

When you buy the vegetable oil, what you have is not an LA-rich food but a food full of oxidized "zombie LA" and other toxic compounds. During the processing and consequent oxidation of these oils, you also get compounds called oxidized linoleic acid metabolites (OXLAMs). Without boring you with details, what I can say is that OXLAMs have been linked with triggering or worsening many health problems, including chronic pain, cardiovascular disease, liver disease, and neurodegenerative diseases.[424] Besides OXLAMs, the industrial processing can also originate aldehydes like 4-HNE.[425] Aldehydes may lead to plaque formation in the brain, which is linked to Alzheimer's disease.[426] Research also shows that these compounds are toxic to mitochondria and disrupt cellular function, including in the central nervous system.[427,428]

Not-so-fun fact: When you use these oils for cooking, which ironically is the purpose they were created for, you rev up the oxidation process and increase the concentration of aldehydes by a factor of 10 or more.[429] *Ouch!* To make matters worse, most times these vegetable oils, like corn, canola, and soy, are made of GMO versions of these plants. Independently of our ability to process GMOs, as we saw before, they often are highly contaminated with pesticides and herbicides. Double ouch!

Remember trans fats? The ones that were causing all the health issues while the blame was being put on saturated fats? Well, trans fats are born when hydrogen is added to liquid vegetable oils to make them more stable (partial hydrogenation), giving them a semisolid texture and extending shelf life. The processing of these LA-rich oils creates trans fats. Research has shown that even bottles of organic, expeller-pressed canola oil contain as much as 5 percent trans fats.[430]

Neo Note: Trans Fats

Trans fats may have started with margarine and Crisco but quickly spread into most processed foods. They could even be found in "healthy" nut butters and vegan "cheese." This trans fat use can be justified because they are cheap and add a rich, buttery texture to foods, while extending shelf life. But, sadly, research suggests that trans fats can cause heart disease, diabetes, Alzheimer's disease, cancer, neurological disorders, depression, and even increased risk of all-cause mortality.[431-439]

After much controversy, many countries have limited trans fats in foods. However, depending on where you are in the world and depending on the exact type of food, you may still find them.

Is it possible that it's not LA omega-6 causing all the issues some studies show, but instead the problems are being caused by oxidized LA, OXLAMs, aldehydes, or even the trans fats? Most of the studies don't use wholesome sources of LA, which are also packed with antioxidants. Instead, they use refined, oxidized vegetable oils and all the harmful metabolites in them. As we saw, these toxins by themselves can cause all the issues attributed to LA. This is why, when we look at systematic reviews studying the effects of "whole" LA, we don't see these negative effects. It's not the unadulterated LA causing inflammation and disease; it's the refined vegetable oils.

LA is an essential building block for your cells and even entire organs like your brain.[440-442] In his book *PEO Solution*, Dr. Brian Peskin states that LA is one of the most important health-promoting fats we can consume. According to Dr. Peskin's research, LA is crucial for several biological functions, such as maintenance and proper permeability of cell membranes, improvement of cellular signaling, cell detoxification, synthesis and transportation of cholesterol, protection against cardiovascular disease, and brain function improvement.[443] Some of the best sources of unadulterated LA are hemp seeds, sesame seeds, sunflower seeds, Brazil nuts, pecans, pine nuts, walnuts, and grass-pastured dairy.

Please note that the roasted seeds and nuts are often covered in oxidized oils. Some authors suggest dry-roasted nuts, but since this still adds heat to the equation, I would opt for raw, soaked, and sprouted (to reduce antinutrients) when possible. Cold-pressed oils made from these nuts may also be an option, but you should always go with a trusted brand that does not use heat and chemicals.

Neo Note: The Ratio Issue
Many authors claim that our omega-6–to–omega-3 consumption ratio has increased substantially. What experts believed to be our normal in the past, between 2:1 and 6:1, is now hovering at around 17:1 or even 50:1 with the Western Diet.[444,445] Although this is completely correct, it does not account for the actual issue here. The problem is not that we are eating a lot more LA, in natural foods, than before. Foods like hemp seeds and walnuts, rich in LA, also have omega-3s, for example. And let's be honest, I am not seeing many people with nut/seed binge-eating disorders. These seeds and nuts in their natural form are filling, and one naturally doesn't overeat them.

The ratio problem has to do with the consumption of "zombie" omega-6s in processed foods or foods fried in refined vegetable oils. Even organic and so-called superfoods are filled with rancid, oxidized oils. Avoiding junk food is not enough. You also need to check the labels of some of these "healthy" snacks. Restaurants are also to blame. Most restaurants fry and sauté foods in cheap refined vegetable oils. They buy them in enormous quantities, which causes them to be exposed to air and light for weeks, even months, and then they are used several times. Imagine how oxidized they become. As Ann Louise Gittleman observes, we are consuming substantial amounts of omega-6s but are still omega-6 deficient. We are deficient in the real, healthy, functional omega-6s.[446]

To sum this up, I don't think you should obsess about the ratio. As long as you take in omega-6s in their wholesome form, you will be okay.

– Arachidonic acid

Arachidonic acid (AA or ARA) is a nonessential omega-6 fatty acid that also gets plenty of hate from the scientific community. For years, we have considered it an inflammatory fat because it is a precursor to several potent pro-inflammatory mediators. However, studies in healthy human adults have found that increased intake of ARA or LA does not increase the concentration of inflammatory markers.[447] Blaming ARA for causing the inflammation is like blaming the cops for doing the robbery. They were at the crime scene but did not rob the place. Similarly to LA, ARA is also an important constituent of our cells' membranes, conferring the fluidity and flexibility necessary for their function in muscular tissue, the nervous system, and the immune system.[448-452] Fun fact: ARA is an important component in human milk.[453] So, how bad can it be?

Research has shown that ARA is associated with lower levels of inflammation in the brain, decreased inflammatory markers in the bloodstream, improved athletic performance, protection against some potential parasitic infections, decreased risk of initiation/development of cancerous tumors, and lower risk of cardiovascular death.[454-457] Some of the best sources of ARA are animal organs and meats, poultry, fish, seafood, and eggs. Since it's a nonessential fatty acid, we can convert LA into ARA when needed.

– Gamma-linolenic acid

Here we have another nonessential omega-6 fatty acid. Not half as famous as the previous two, but incredibly powerful nonetheless.

Gamma-linolenic acid (GLA) was initially discovered in the plant evening primrose, which Native Americans used as a remedy for various ailments. Eventually, settlers took it to Europe, where it became such a popular remedy that it was nicknamed "the king's cure-all."[458] GLA has unparalleled fat-burning properties, increasing metabolic rate through the activation of brown fat.[459] Beyond weight loss, GLA has been found to reduce inflammation, lower blood pressure, quiet PMS, and improve conditions such as mastalgia (breast pain), diabetic neuropathy, eczema, rheumatoid arthritis, osteoporosis, ADHD, and autism spectrum disorder.[460–473]

Although we can convert LA into GLA, several factors might contribute to deficient levels in our body. Among them, I can highlight advanced age, alcohol abuse, smoking, insulin resistance, consumption of trans fats and partially hydrogenated oils, nutritional deficiencies (magnesium, zinc, and vitamins B_3, B_6, C, and E), and emotional stress.[474,475] Fortunately, you can get GLA from oils, such as evening primrose oil, black currant seed oil, borage oil, and hemp oil, and in lesser amounts from foods like hemp seeds, açai berries, and spirulina.

– Conjugated linoleic acid

Conjugated linoleic acid (CLA) is the last omega-6 fatty acid on our list. Technically, it's a trans fat, but since it is naturally occurring, there's nothing to worry about. Cows, deer, goats, sheep, moose, bison, buffalo, and other ruminant animals can convert LA into CLA, and we rely on their meat or their dairy to get CLA, since we can't make it ourselves.[476]

The total amount of CLA in these foods can vary substantially depending on the animals' diet.[477] Research tells us that CLA content is 300 to 500 percent higher in beef and dairy from grass-fed animals than in grain-fed ones.[478] CLA is usually known for boosting fat metabolism. Many animal studies have found that CLA has the potential to increase metabolic rate, boost fat burning, and inhibit fat accumulation.[479–481] But in human studies, the results have been mixed. A 2007 review of 18 controlled trials concluded that CLA might produce a modest weight loss.[482] This was also supported by the author of a 2019 study, who concluded that CLA "confers some degree of body weight loss" in humans.[483] Independently of its efficacy for weight loss, CLA might have other health benefits we need to consider. Studies have shown potential effects in lowering the risk of diseases such as type 2 diabetes, cardiovascular disease, and cancer.[484–487]

Despite the need for more interventional human studies, it seems reasonable to conclude that getting small amounts of natural CLA from food is beneficial. Some of the best sources of CLA are the meat of the pasture-raised ruminant animals mentioned before and even their milk, cheese, yogurt, and especially butter. Some CLA might also be found in vegan sources like white button mushrooms and pomegranate seed oil. Since CLA supplements are widely available, I need to make this warning: After reviewing the studies presented here, I've gleaned that a dose of three to four grams per day seems safe. Supplementing with higher doses may cause several side effects, including diarrhea, insulin resistance, inflammation, oxidative stress, and development of metabolic syndrome.[488–491]

Omega-3s
– Eicosapentaenoic acid and docosahexaenoic acid

While omega-6s are bullied, omega-3s are the beloved fatty acid celebrities. Omega-3 fats come in different subtypes. The ones you're probably most familiar with are alpha-linolenic acid (ALA), eicosapentaenoic acid (EPA), and docosahexaenoic acid (DHA). However, at least eight other omega-3s have been discovered. Since there aren't many studies or interesting findings about those eight, we'll focus on the main three. Fun fact: EPA and DHA molecules are longer than ALA molecules, so they are also known as long-chain omega-3s or even long-chain marine fats, since they come mostly from seafood.

ALA is the equivalent of LA for the omega-3s. It's the essential fatty acid that your body cannot produce, so you need to get it from your diet. EPA and DHA, on the other hand, can be created out of ALA. To be fair, even though we technically can convert ALA into EPA and DHA, this conversion process is like me keeping my office organized—not very efficient. In fact, most people can convert only about 5 percent of ALA to EPA and just 0.5 percent to DHA.[492] One exception to this, probably to favor fertility and the development of a child, occurs in women of reproductive age, who can convert 21 percent of their ALA to EPA and 9 percent to DHA.[493]

This raises one question. If researchers say that EPA and DHA are so important for our health, why are our bodies so bad at turning ALA into these long-chain omega-3s? One can say that if we're such bad converters, this might mean that they're not that biologically important. And in fact there are several authors who contend that we give EPA and DHA too much credit. Even though some of these articles present some valid points, I cannot ignore the tsunami of studies showing the benefits of EPA and DHA and how they outperform ALA in many physiological functions. Are EPA and DHA by themselves the best thing since sliced bread? Probably not. But it's undeniable that they are important for optimum health.

So, why do we suck at converting them? Researchers suggest that during Paleolithic times, ALA intake was extremely high, so even with such embarrassing conversion rates, the sheer amount of ALA was enough to give us all the EPA and DHA we needed. During those times, our direct consumption of EPA and DHA was also high (2,000 to 4,000 milligrams a day), so there was no need to produce more.[494,495] Use it or lose it, at its finest. Unfortunately, since then, our consumption of ALA, EPA, and DHA has dropped. That's probably why our modern human brains are 11 percent smaller than those of our Paleo ancestors. I wonder if with that extra 11 percent, I could make more intelligent jokes. Probably not.

It's important to note that some benefits attributed to omega-3s may come mostly from EPA and DHA, and not as much from ALA. Research comparing flax oil (rich in ALA) and fish oil (rich in EPA/DHA) concluded that

EPA and DHA were more powerful at improving markers for heart health.[496] Moreover, EPA and DHA are precursors of compounds called resolvins and protectins, which, as the names suggest, can resolve inflammation in the body and protect cells (particularly neurons in the brain) against damage and death.[497] Researchers have also uncovered that the individuals with the highest levels of EPA and DHA in their bloodstreams have the largest hippocampus (memory area of your brain) size and overall brain size, while the folks who had the lowest levels actually have smaller brains.[498] Unfortunately, this is not temporary, "the water is cold" kind of shrinkage. This is more like "I don't remember where I left my keys" long-term brain. As a matter of fact, these two fatty acids are so important for brain health that several clinical trials testing marine omega-3s found that DHA and EPA are as effective as prescription antidepressants in treating depressive disorders.[499-504] It's also been found that both children and adults with ADHD have lower levels of DHA and EPA, and that these deficiencies are linked with learning problems, poor conduct, hyperactivity, anxiety, tantrums, and sleep difficulties.[505]

One reason why EPA and DHA have such an impactful influence on the brain might have to do with a protein called brain-derived neurotrophic factor (BDNF). Both EPA and DHA have been shown to increase the supply of BDNF.[506-508] BDNF is recognized for boosting memory, mood, and overall brain plasticity (ability to reorganize its structure and function) in the long term.[509,510] To understand how relevant this is, research has shown that individuals with Alzheimer's may have half the BDNF of a healthy brain, and raising the level might slow progression of the disease.[511] Even depressive disorder may result from having low BDNF, since its increase seems to improve symptoms.[512]

These omega-3s are also important for your metabolism. DHA in particular seems to be determinant in boosting your metabolic rate and even the number and efficiency of your mitochondria.[513,514] Omega-3s are also linked with preventing loss of muscle mass and boosting muscle growth and strength.[515-517] Research has shown that DHA and EPA are indirectly associated with the reduction of tumors' growth and invasiveness, and a lower risk of all-cause mortality.[518-521]

EPA and DHA are great for everyone but may be especially beneficial for people with:
- ADHD;[522]
- Alzheimer's disease;[523,524]
- anxiety;[525]
- autism spectrum disorder;[526]
- autoimmune diseases;[527-530]
- bipolar disorder;[531,532]

- borderline personality disorder;[533]
- congestive heart disease;[534,535]
- depression;[536,537]
- schizophrenia;[539] and
- seasonal affective disorder.[538]

Want to get more of these superfats into your body? Some of the best food sources are algae, algae oil, anchovies, halibut, herring, krill, mackerel, oysters, salmon, salmon roe, sardines, and trout. You may also find some in egg yolks and grass-fed beef.

Neo Note: More Than Just Omega-3s

Dr. Gerhard Spiteller was one of the biggest contributors to our current knowledge about fats and their effects in our bodies, especially the harmful effects of oxidized PUFAs. During his research time, he noticed that omega-3s in natural sources were accompanied by a type of fat called a furan fatty acid (F-acid). It seems these F-acids are incredibly powerful at scavenging and neutralizing free radicals, consequently decreasing oxidative stress in the body.[540] Further studies by other scientists have concluded that F-acids present a higher anti-inflammatory action than the actual omega-3s EPA and DHA.[541] Other research has also shown that F-acids create a powerful antioxidant effect in the brain.[542]

Knowing this, some argue that omega-3s are overrated and that some effects attributed to them might actually be coming from compounds like F-acids and other molecules we have yet to discover. In a way, I tend to agree that we might have a bit too much hype around omega-3s, but that doesn't mean they're not important. They might not be the cure-all substance some claim them to be, but they are still essential for a healthy and thriving body.

My take on these findings is that there is a lot more to certain foods than we currently know. While the health industry gravitates toward isolating compounds and creating the purest form of the "next big thing," I think we are missing the bigger picture. It's not about determining whether it's DHA or F-acid that is causing the most significant health impact and trying to create supplements with isolated molecules. It's about realizing that whole foods have many compounds (some that we haven't even found out yet) that work together to nourish our bodies. Therefore, we should always favor whole foods over supplements.

– Alpha-linolenic acid

I have to recognize that ALA doesn't get nearly as much love from the scientific community as its fellows EPA and DHA. But just because ALA isn't as flashy doesn't mean it's not important. The ALA you consume is used for energy, and it is an important building block to incorporate in different tissues directly or through its by-products, EPA and DHA.[543,544] In fact, ALA is so important that its deficiency has been associated with dryness and scaliness of skin, muscle pain and weakness, and vision problems.[545-547]

Research suggests that ALA helps stimulate the burning of fat for fuel in both muscle and fat cells.[545] And in different interventional studies, increased ALA intake was associated with reductions in overall body weight, visceral fat, waist size, and blood triglycerides.[449,450] ALA may also be important for cardiovascular health. It has been shown to stabilize heart rhythm.[551,552] Large population studies have linked high amounts of dietary ALA with lower rates of heart disease, lower blood pressure, lower triglycerides, less arterial plaque, and fewer heart attacks and strokes.[553-558]

Research also shows that ALA may boost bone health, ease inflammation, and even play a role in the beneficial action of flaxseed on different cancers.[559-565] Some of the best sources of ALA are chia seeds, flaxseeds, pumpkin seeds, clary sage oil, sacha inchi, Brazil nuts, cashews, hazelnuts, walnuts, and greens such as broccoli, brussels sprouts, kale, and spinach.

– Docosapentaenoic acid

Earlier I said I was going to focus on only ALA, EPA, and DHA, but newer research has been exploring the benefits of docosapentaenoic acid (DPA), which is one of the other eight forms of omega-3s, so I've decided to briefly highlight it here. Even though DPA is the third-most-abundant omega-3 fatty acid in marine oils (after EPA and DHA), you won't find it in most fish oils, since it's unintentionally removed during industrial processing. But by eating natural sources of marine omega-3s, you will benefit from this fatty acid.

It's said that DPA can augment the effects of both EPA and DHA.[566] Studies show that DPA is more efficiently absorbed into the bloodstream than EPA and DHA, thus it might produce more results.[567] Besides being absorbed into the body efficiently through your diet, DPA can also be made in your body from EPA, and can also be converted back to EPA or even transformed into DHA.[568,569] In plain English, DPA can function as a reserve for both DHA and EPA in the body. Other findings support this theory of DPA working as an EPA and DHA "tank." Researchers found out that DPA is less actively oxidized for energy, so it seems indeed to be used as "omega-3 backup" in the body.[570]

Studies have shown that DPA acts as an important anti-inflammatory agent and protector of cardiovascular health. Data suggests that DPA-derived resolvins and protectins might be more efficient than EPA/DHA-derived ones in preventing and resolving inflammation.[571] Furthermore, DPA may also be more effective than EPA and DHA in inhibiting platelet aggregation (a key factor in the development of atherosclerosis) and reducing C-reactive protein and other markers of inflammation.[572,573] The best natural sources of DHA are fatty fish like halibut, herring, mackerel, sablefish, salmon, and sardines. It's also present in beef and pork brains.

Neo Note: The Dark Side of Omega-3s

Remember how PUFAs are the least stable of all fats? This is because they have multiple double bonds that can be compromised by oxidation. The oxidation of vegetable oils during their refinement is one reason most omega-6s still have a terrible reputation. But as we found out, "whole-food" omega-6s can be incredibly healthy as long as we respect their fragility and consume them in their natural form.

What's my point here? Omega-3s are also PUFAs and are also at risk of oxidation.[574] In fact, EPA and DHA are actually considered HUFAs—highly unsaturated fatty acids.[575] As you can figure out, the word *highly* is not a good thing in this case. Unfortunately, HUFAs are more easily oxidized than other PUFAs.[576] In other words, omega-3s are incredibly fragile, and if we don't take good care of them, they have the potential to be a lot worse than some refined vegetable oils.

By consuming fresh, whole-food omega-3s full of antioxidant compounds, you are getting the nourishment you need. But when you are obtaining your omega-3s from highly processed fish oils, you are consuming oxidized, antioxidant-devoid, toxic omega-3s. This is probably why there have been studies associating fish oil consumption with intestinal disfunction, systemic inflammation, cardiovascular disease, and various cancers.[577] Once again, it's not the omegas causing the issues, but the oxidized, zombie versions of them. [578,579] The bottom line is, focus on natural whole sources of omegas, and eat them fresh. And if you're using cold-pressed oils, please don't ruin them by exposing them to air and heat.

The Other Omegas

You might be surprised to learn that we also have omega-5s and omega-7s. They aren't as famous as the other omegas mentioned earlier, but they still have some interesting properties. Unfortunately, they did not make the final cut. However, if you are interested in learning more about them please go to my.neodiet.co/otheromegas or scan the QR code on the right.

SCAN ME

Neo Note: Hack to Clean Up PUFA Oxidative Damage

Vitamin E is recognized as a key essential antioxidant in humans, protecting lipoproteins, PUFAs, and cellular and intracellular membranes from damage. Research suggests that vitamin E requirements rise with an increase in oxidized PUFA consumption.[580] I am not saying that it's okay to consume oxidized PUFAs and minimize the damage with vitamin E; instead I am suggesting that vitamin E may help you clean up the damage of years of eating damaged fats. This theory gets further support from a study that shows that vitamin E can scavenge free radicals generated by lipid peroxidation of PUFAs.[581]

Eating foods rich in vitamin E like argan oil, red palm oil, black walnuts, English walnuts, pecans, pistachios, flaxseeds, pumpkin seeds, and sesame seeds might be an excellent strategy to help clear years of toxic PUFA buildup. But, for a short period, you might even benefit from a vitamin E supplement. Please note that most vitamin E supplements contain only alpha-tocopherol, but it's gamma-tocopherol that's believed to be one of the best free-radical scavengers, so read your labels.[582]

P.S. Dr. James DiNicolantonio also advises that supplementation with 20 grams of glycine (split into four servings of 5 grams each) and 2 to 5 grams of spirulina may also be an efficient strategy to clean up the effects of the oxidized oils.[583]

THE CHOLESTEROL MYTH

Cholesterol is a sterol, a type of lipid that is a precursor of many vital compounds in your body.[584] But most people use the word *cholesterol* to refer to the lipoproteins LDL and HDL. When the lipid levels in your blood are either too high or too low, this is called dyslipidemia.[585] When we talk about dyslipidemia, the main lipids we look at are triglycerides, low-density lipoprotein (LDL) cholesterol, and high-density lipoprotein (HDL) cholesterol. Most doctors focus on the two "cholesterols," and the common belief is that LDL is bad and HDL is good.[586] While one can definitely find data supporting this simplistic dual view, there is also a lot of research showing us that things are not this simple, as you are about to find out.[587-589]

Contrary to what you may have heard, cholesterol is not necessarily an enemy. In fact, even if you stopped consuming fatty foods that contain cholesterol, your body would still produce it, because we need it for many basic functions. In fact, most of the cholesterol in your body right now did not come from food. Dietary cholesterol accounts for around 25 to 40 percent of our daily turnover of cholesterol, whereas production in the body accounts for 60 to 75 percent.[590]

Every day, your body will make cholesterol for many important purposes, including the proper formation of all your cell membranes, production of all the steroid hormones (estrogen, testosterone, cortisol, progesterone, and aldosterone), preparation of bile acids, and synthesis of vitamin D—a molecule that's essential for bone and cardiovascular health, and may even play an important role in your immune function and protection against cancer.[591-595] Cholesterol is also vital for the brain, since 25 percent of the body's total cholesterol content can be found there.[596]

Why do people think cholesterol is bad? What if I tell you that the notorious Ancel Keys was nicknamed Mr. Cholesterol?[597] Does that work as a clue? Before blaming saturated fats, Keys first targeted cholesterol as the villain behind coronary heart disease. Keys spent a few years trying to prove his theory but ended up finding that no matter how much dietary cholesterol he fed volunteers in his studies, the levels in their blood remained the same.[598] Although he never pinpointed a direct relationship between dietary cholesterol and heart disease, his theory stayed within the medical community. Some later epidemiological studies also supported this theory around total cholesterol (and LDL), and we ended up believing that cholesterol caused atherosclerosis and heart disease.[599]

We know that cholesterol is deposited in the arteries' endothelium in cases of atherosclerosis, but it isn't the cause of the disease. When entering the endothelium, cholesterol and fats are benign. Indeed, like all other cells in the body, the cells that line blood vessels need cholesterol to maintain healthy function. Believe it or not, we have known this lack of association between blood cholesterol levels and atherosclerosis from studies as far back as the 1930s.[600]

Research shows that half of heart disease patients have perfectly normal cholesterol levels, yet they have an underlying risk of plaque buildup in their arteries.[601] According to a 2009 study, nearly 75 percent of heart attack patients who were hospitalized had cholesterol levels that would not put them in the high-risk category.[602] Ironically, it is *low* cholesterol that is associated with higher risk of mortality from heart disease, stroke, and cancer.[603] Even a gigantic research project like the China Study, which examined the health and diets of thousands of people in 65 rural Chinese communities, showed that there was no association between cholesterol levels and heart disease.[604] Let's make one thing clear: dietary cholesterol is not, and never was, a problem for most individuals, and science supports it.

LDL—LACKING DIETARY LOVE

As we saw before, when you eat carbs in excess, after your body takes what it needs for energy, the rest of the glucose is shuttled to your liver to be converted into fat—triglycerides in particular. LDL cholesterol is the primary carrier of these triglycerides to the various spots in your body where you are going to use or store them. By the way, LDL particles are not all the same. They differ in size and density. And even though these different types of LDL are the main carriers, the other lipoproteins are also part of this distribution operation.

When your body works well, triglycerides are properly distributed through these different-size carriers and are efficiently delivered. Problems arise when you remain in a state of overeating and your body is producing more and more triglycerides. When this happens, not only are your larger LDL particles being used to their maximum, but smaller and more dense lipoproteins are also being recruited to assist. It's almost like a delivery company the week before

Christmas not having enough space in their trucks and vans to deliver all the goods. When this happens, they have to pay ordinary people to deliver these goods using their cars or even their motorcycles. Suddenly, you have a guy carrying a 55-inch TV on the back of his bike, going at full speed on the highway. Eventually, the TV will fall from the bike and will cause an accident. It's inevitable. The TV was never supposed to be delivered by bike, but because the company was so overwhelmed, that was the only option. This is what happens in your body with the triglyceride distribution. Because you now have so many triglycerides being created all the time, smaller and denser lipoproteins are distributing triglycerides that in normal circumstances would have been delivered by the larger and denser LDLs.

HDL particles, in contrast, are more like recycling trucks. They basically have an opposite function to the other lipoproteins. Instead of taking triglycerides to be stored in the body, they collect them from the different tissues and lug them back to the liver to be converted into fuel. HDL is activated and produced whenever you are not eating and need to burn some of your accumulated fat as fuel. Not only is this good because you are burning some of your reserves, but it leads to a decrease in lipoprotein traffic in your vascular highways. Unfortunately, most people spend their lives in a state of constant eating, so HDL is not produced, since the body is getting an excess of fuel.

In summary, it is the excess of fuel that leads to the creation of too many triglycerides . This excess of triglycerides then lowers HDL, and increases LDL and the other smaller and denser "accident-prone" lipoproteins. Clearly, this is an oversimplified vision of what happens in your body, but the point is that the excess of triglycerides is one trigger for the cascade of events that can lead to atherosclerosis. In fact, high triglycerides are a far better predictor of heart disease than high LDL is.[605]

THE REAL CAUSES OF ATHEROSCLEROSIS

The excess of triglycerides definitely has its role in heart disease, but there is a lot more to this story. Initially, I thought I would keep things light and only share this version. But you know what? You deserve better. Contrary to Jack Nicholson's line in *A Few Good Men*, I know you can handle the truth!

Lipid Oxidation and Oxidative Stress

This first mechanism was extensively studied by Dr. Spiteller, whom I briefly introduce before because of his phenomenal research on lipids. In an article released in 2000, Dr. Spiteller explains that it is processed PUFAs, not saturated fat or cholesterol, that deserve the blame for atherosclerosis.[606] When you take in refined vegetable oils, these oxidized fats need to be transported by LDL to be stored. As the cholesterol lipoprotein is giving the oxidized PUFA a piggyback ride, the oxidation spreads and LDL becomes oxidized as well.[607] Once your LDL becomes "zombie LDL," your immune system identifies the threat and sends macrophages (immune cells) to gobble up the LDL. As the macrophages eat LDL particles, they fatten up and become a "foam cell." The more oxidized PUFAs in your LDL, the more foam cells are created and end up lying around. Eventually, this mix of foam cells and lipids can accumulate and become the core of the atherosclerotic plaque.

What could have solved this? Our friend HDL. Besides recycling lipids, HDL is also known for having antioxidant properties.[608] Between the recycling and antioxidant skills, it could have reduced the number of oxidized LDL particles and consequently quelled the formation of foam cells, and later atherosclerotic plaque. Unfortunately, because of our overfed state and high numbers of triglycerides, HDL numbers are kept low, which further aggravates this issue.

But there's more. Before your macrophages can eat all the zombie fats, the fats' free radicals cause damage wherever they pass. It's almost like a fire. They burn everything they come in contact with, including the arterial walls. The free-radical chain reactions weaken the walls and fuse molecules together, creating a kind of crunchy protein plastic. This "fried" artery can easily rupture and bleed.[609]

Many authors, including Dr. Paul Saladino, believe that cholesterol is used as a patch to repair the damaged arterial wall.[610] This could mean atherosclerosis may also result from these "cholesterol patches" created to fix the free-radical-fried arteries.

High Blood Pressure

One fascinating fact is that we do not develop plaque buildup in veins—only in arteries. Why is that? If the whole theory about cholesterol causing plaque accumulation were correct, one would expect that this would happen in veins, since they also carry cholesterol lipoproteins. Makes sense, right? Some researchers justify this by saying that arteries and veins are constructed differently and that arteries are more prone to plaque formation. Unfortunately, this is as true as saying that I am an amazing dancer. In cases of cardiac bypass surgery, where vein grafts are used to replace the damaged part of the artery, soon enough the vein graft also develops aggressive atherosclerotic lesions.[611] Moreover, when researchers transplanted arteries into the venous circulation, they did not develop atherosclerosis.[612] These findings prove that the type of vascular vessel is irrelevant to plaque formation, and that there is more to be uncovered here.

An interesting finding is that plaque buildup usually occurs at arterial branch points (the equivalent of a crossroads), where turbulent blood flow can damage the interior walls of our arteries.[613,614] Chronic high blood pressure might be the trigger we were looking for. Think about it. High blood pressure causes more tension in arterial branch points, which can lead to arterial wall damage, which then is patched by cholesterol. This would support not only this mechanism but also the theory of LDL being used to patch arterial wall damage.

LPS

LDL and other lipoproteins play an important role in the immune response against infectious invaders.[615-617] One band of these invaders is the lipopolysaccharides (LPSs). LDL particles have LPS-binding proteins that allow them to scavenge those "little pieces of shit."[618] In fact, when the liver senses that LPSs have entered the bloodstream, it boosts its production of LDL to bind and neutralize these endotoxins.[619] Knowing this, some cardiologists believe that atherosclerosis and heart disease can originate in the gut.[620] If you suffer from leaky gut, you could be under constant attack from LPSs, which will make LDL levels rise substantially. This, associated with the inflammation and oxidative stress caused by the remaining "free-flowing" LPSs, creates the perfect storm for plaque formation.

Insulin Resistance as the Superglue

Under normal circumstances, your LDL particles can float around in your arteries with no issues. But several studies have shown that in cases of insulin resistance, both the LDL particles and the arterial walls become "stickier."[621-625] This stickiness compromises the interaction between LDL and the arterial wall and increases the risk of plaque formation. This is why people with diabetes have such a high rate of developing atherosclerosis and having heart attacks, even with low levels of LDL.[626]

Neo Note: Insulin Resistance and HDL

Researchers have found out that HDL levels correlate directly with insulin sensitivity.[627-629] So, individuals with insulin resistance can develop metabolic dyslipidemia, a condition in which HDL levels fall and triglyceride levels rise.[630] What this means is that states of insulin resistance not only increase the "stickiness" of LDL but also lead to a reduction in antioxidant-recycling HDL and an increase in the troublemaking triglycerides, which only exacerbates the risk of heart disease.

FOCUS ON BETTER MARKERS

I've shared enough data to support that cholesterol in general, and LDL in particular, are not risk factors for atherosclerosis and heart disease. In fact, there are even studies suggesting that higher levels of LDL may be protective as we age, because of their role in immune function.[631-634] Furthermore, if you get your LDL to a "safe" 70 milligrams per deciliter, you still have nearly the same risk of heart attack you'd have at a dangerous LDL of 150 milligrams per deciliter.[635] In the danger zone, your risk is said to be about 20 percent, but in the safe zone you only decrease the risk to roughly 15 percent. Not to mention that this drop in LDL will significantly hike your risks of anxiety, depression, infections, severe kidney disease, stroke, and cancer.[636–641]

Clinical context is a lot more important than focusing on LDL in isolation. Do you have high blood pressure? Do you eat refined vegetable oils? Do you have signs or symptoms of inflammation? These parameters are much more important than LDL. As a matter of fact, if you want to focus on a marker, focus on HDL and triglycerides. Earlier in the book, I suggested the triglycerides/HDL ratio as an informal way to determine insulin resistance. This can also be used for heart disease risk, since they are so interconnected.

Earlier, I suggested a result of 2 or lower. However, for this specific case, Dr. Gundry goes even further and suggests a ratio of 1 or lower, which basically means that you're recycling more fat than you are storing.[642]

Neo Note: Statins

Back in the day, doctors paid little attention to LDL. As long as HDL was good, that was all they cared about. And it's easy to understand why. Statistically speaking, if patients had an HDL of 60 milligrams per deciliter, their risk of heart disease was less than 2 percent. Even the heart-attack risk calculator guidelines used by cardiologists don't ask for LDL levels.[643] Some authors maintain that the bigger push to look at LDL as a risk marker only began when Big Pharma introduced the cholesterol-lowering drugs called statins.

Since there are no drugs to raise HDL, the pharmaceutical industry had to focus on the best they could create, a drug to lower LDL. After that, it was just a matter of scaring people about LDL, and statins would sell like candy. It's no coincidence that statins are the most widely prescribed class of drugs in the world.[644]

How Do Statins Work?

Statins indeed appear to slightly reduce arterial plaque, but just not the way they were supposed to.

Initially, statins were to treat heart disease by lowering LDL levels. We now know that statins actually produce some results, but by lowering inflammation.[645] As we saw before, less inflammation means less probability of plaque formation and heart disease. The reduction of LDL should be seen more as a side effect.

The Dangers of Statins

For starters, statins have been shown to create major micronutrient deficiencies of copper, selenium, zinc, and vitamin E.[646–648] But to be honest, this might be the least of your concerns. As you know, cholesterol is needed for many essential bodily functions. By taking a medication that lowers your cholesterol levels, you incur the risk of developing serious issues. Research is still unclear, but there are studies showing likely connections between statin intake and higher risk of nerve and muscle damage, liver disease, diabetes, birth defects, endocrine dysfunction, and even cancer.[649–656]

You remember that the brain is 25 percent cholesterol, right? As it turns out, depriving the brain of cholesterol may have some nasty consequences. Using statins has also been associated with increased rates of cognitive impairment.[657] Furthermore, in large clinical trials using statins, mood worsened and even led to higher rates of death by violent crime.[658–661] Please do not take statins if you have an annoying boss!

RED PILL

I know that I may have been a bit too technical at times, and I'm not offended at all if you skipped some of the more complex parts. But because you took the red pill, I wanted to give you the whole truth, without manipulation or hype. The problem was never the wholesome fats; it was always the sugar and the refined oils.

Get something in your head. . . . You are fat! Oops. Sorry, this just sounded wrong. I didn't mean to call you names. I was literally stating that you are made of fat. If you want to be a healthy, top-performing human being, you need to add healthy fats back into your life. There is no way around this. Nor should there be. Fats are delicious, and you have nothing to be afraid of.

But what's most important is that you ditch all the bad fats you may have been consuming. Please do yourself a favor and throw in the trash all those "healthy" vegetable oils. Yes, even canola oil. Let me rephrase that. Especially canola oil. You are what you eat. And with fat, this is quite literal. You eat zombie fats, you develop zombie cells, and you get zombie health!

This also applies to my keto friends. Ladies and gents, it's not just a matter of avoiding carbs and eating everything fat. Vegetable oil is keto too. But I can guarantee that's not the keto you want. Focus on healthy foods. Eating highly processed, highly packaged foods, probably filled with trans fats, just to stay in ketosis is pure nonsense. You know better now.

While sugar is bad, you don't have any part of your body made of sugar. Not even your "sweet tooth." I googled it. What I am trying to say is that your body can take the occasional excess of sugar, but an excess of bad fats will literally become part of you. And it might take you months or years to get it out of your body. That's why I am anal about it.

Here is the great news! Healing doesn't require counting calories or getting stressed about ratios of different fats and other macronutrients. Honestly, that will just make you more stressed and turn your hormones against you. Healing starts with regaining your metabolic flexibility so you can reset your body to its factory settings. Metabolic flexibility is bliss. It allows you to live your days without the influence of cravings, low energy, or mood swings. Metabolic flexibility allows you to feel amazing all day long, staying sharp and focused, feeling happy, looking good, and performing at the highest levels you ever performed in all fields of life. And I mean all of them! In the next chapter, I am going to share with you the biggest hack there is to fix your metabolism in record time. I am really excited to share this with you.

NEO SUMMARY

• Processed foods were created to be hyperpalatable, causing insatiable hunger, food cravings and addiction.
• CICO is a linear concept that doesn't apply to our complex metabolism.
• Insulin stimulates fat storage and may be responsible for causing *hangriness*.
• Glucagon is the *antagonist* hormone to insulin, and it triggers fat breakdown to be used as energy.
• Leptin is produced in our fat cells and it's our main "satiety" hormone. Leptin resistance makes you hungry.
• Ghrelin is the *antagonist* hormone to leptin. Instead of creating the sensation of satiety, it produces the sensation of hunger.
• The stress hormone cortisol blocks the sensation of being full. That's why stress can lead to overeating.
• People following the western diet eat too many carbohydrates, especially the wrong kind (refined sugars).
• Excessive sugar consumption is linked to inflammation and increased risk of disease in all systems of the human body.
• Fructose goes straight to the liver and its overconsumption can cause metabolic syndrome.
• A high-fat, low-carb diet, and its occasional state of ketosis promotes an improved metabolism, and it has many health benefits.
• Fat is not the devil. Quite the opposite. It's incredibly healthy. You just need to choose wisely.
• Saturated fat is not bad. It's actually the best fat you can cook with.
• MUFAs and PUFAs are less stable but are incredibly powerful, stimulating many physiological processes in the body.
• Contrary to what you've heard, "raw" omega-6s are good for you.
• Cholesterol and LDL are not bad. They are protective. It's oxidized vegetable oils, inflammation, metabolic dysfunction, and high blood pressure that are the real triggers of heart disease.
• Metabolic flexibility is the key for a healthy and high performing life.

NEO ACTION

• Stay away from processed food. This is the best *neo action* in this book.
• Go for low carb and high fat in order to regain metabolic flexibility.
• Stay away from refined sugars, especially "refined" fructose.
• Don't combine high fat and high carb.
• Use saturated fats to cook.
• "Raw" MUFAs are great for your health and should be consumed abundantly.
• Remove the "zombie" omega-6s (refined vegetable oils and processed foods) from your diet.
• Increase your consumption of foods that are naturally high in omega-3s like wild-caught fish, seaweed, and pastured eggs.

NEO RECOMMENDATIONS

- *Alzheimer's Disease: What If There Was a Cure?* by Dr. Mary Newport
- *Boundless* by Ben Greenfield
- *Genius Foods* by Max Lugavere
- *Good Calories, Bad Calories* by Gary Taubes
- *Deep Nutrition* by Dr. Catherine Shanahan
- *Eat Smarter* by Shawn Stevenson
- *Fast Carbs, Slow Carbs* by David Kessler
- *Fat Chance* By Dr. Robert H. Lustig
- *Nutrition and Physical Degeneration* by Dr. Weston A. Price
- *PEO Solution* by Dr. Brian S. Peskin & Dr. Robert Jay Rowen
- *Primal Fat Burner* by Nora Gedgaudas
- *Radical Metabolism* by Ann Louise Gittleman
- *Sugar Crush* by Dr. Richard Jacoby & Raquel Baldelomar
- *Superfuel* by Dr. James DiNicolantonio & Dr. Joseph Mercola
- *The Big Fat Surprise* by Nina Teicholz
- *The Bulletproof Diet* by Dave Asprey
- *The Carnivore Code* by Dr. Paul Saladino
- *The Case for Keto* by Gary Taubes
- *The Great Cholesterol Myth* by Jonny Bowden & Dr. Stephen T. Sinatra
- *The Keto Reset Diet* By Mark Sisson
- *The Ketogenic Bible* by Dr. Jacob Wilson & Ryan Lowery
- *The Salt Fix* by Dr. James DiNicolantonio
- *Why We Get Sick* by Benjamin Bikman

my.neodiet.co/neorecommendations

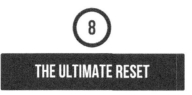

THE ULTIMATE RESET

When the Best Food Is No Food at All

"Everyone has a physician inside him or her; we just have to help it in its work. The natural healing force within each one of us is the greatest force in getting well. Our food should be our medicine. Our medicine should be our food. But to eat when you are sick is to feed your sickness."
Hippocrates

THE FASTEST WAY

Humans evolved and thrived in a lifestyle of feasting and fasting. This is easy to imagine when we consider our hunter-gatherer ancestors, since they would spend long periods of time without eating in between their hunts. But we don't have to go all the way back to the Paleolithic era to see examples of long periods without eating. The concept of several meals a day and "eating schedules" only developed after the Industrial Revolution. I don't have a crystal ball, but I am pretty sure that your great-grandparents did not have the luxury of grabbing a quick bite "before they crashed." It was normal for them to have empty bellies for extended periods of time.

Today the story is much different. Because of our refrigerators, processed packaged foods, fast-food joints, and even meal delivery apps, we have constant access to food. And while this might seem like a good thing, it's not. Those periods without access to food are actually important for us, since they trigger survival mechanisms that make us more resilient and improve our health. Keeping our bodies in a constant state of growth is not healthy. Do you know what condition is also characterized by a constant state of anabolism? Cancer. That's right. Overfeeding is not only making us fat but is also making us develop diseases that are taking us to our graves before our time. I don't know about you, but I am not done here yet. I intend to live a long and healthy life on this earth. Or even on another planet, who knows?

The fastest way to regain our health is to respect our genes and learn from traditions around the world, and start fasting. Fasting has been used as a therapeutic and spiritual practice for thousands of years. It's believed that in the sixth century BC, the Greek philosopher Pythagoras required his students to fast for 40 days in order to achieve the mental clarity needed to keep up with his teachings. Shortly after, the "father of medicine," Hippocrates, trusted that the body could heal itself and recommended that people fast to heal from illness.[1]

Fasting has also been an important part of Chinese traditional medicine and Indian Ayurvedic medicine. The same applies to the physical and spiritual practices of many indigenous peoples and ancient civilizations around the world. From the Incas to the Mayans to the Evenks of Siberia to the indigenous American cultures, all had fasting practices. Among the Cherokee, for example, fasting was one of the most important spiritual tools in their ceremonies.[2] Similarly, if we look at every world religion, most of them have some sort of fasting practice. The Buddhist, Christian, Hindu, Jewish, and Muslim religions all promote a period of fasting to cleanse the body and the soul. And even though now we look at this practice just for the spiritual aspect of it, fasting was also seen within the religions' core as an important tool to heal the body.

Fasting has also been a part of "modern" medicine. Back in the 16th century, the "father of toxicology," Paracelsus, believed that fasting allowed the body to heal itself, referring to it as "the physician within."[3] And in the late 1800s, the American physician Edward H. Dewey wrote of the power of fasting in his book *The True Science of Living*. He believed nearly every modern disease was caused by frequent and excessive eating, and he was probably one of the first to suggest intermittent fasting by skipping breakfast.[4] In the early 1900s, studies about fasting got published, and the practice was used not only to fight obesity but to treat convulsive disorders.[5–7]

Nowadays, even though there isn't a shared consensus within the medical community about fasting, countries like Russia and Germany use it as part of their medical approach. You can also find "less formal" medically supervised fasting clinics all over the world.

Fasting generates fear because of the lack of knowledge about it. In this chapter, we will focus on all its uses and the scientific data supporting its benefits.

WHAT IS FASTING?

Fasting is not starvation. Starvation is the involuntary absence of food. As much as people want to eat, food is simply not available. Fasting, on the other hand, is a choice. It's a voluntary decision that can be interrupted at any time. Even though these two are commonly confused, even in the scientific community, please understand that fasting is also not calorie restriction.

Calorie restriction means consuming fewer calories than you require to meet your body's physiological needs. With calorie restriction, the body is forced to lower its metabolic rate, down-regulating thyroid function, and your hormones will turn against you, making you feel intense hunger.[8-10] The combination of hunger and the decrease in metabolic rate is probably the reason more than 80 percent of people regain weight once they go off their calorie-restricted diets.[11] Instead, planned fasting seems to increase metabolic rate and lessen feelings of hunger.[12,13]

Fasting is an umbrella term, and there are several types of fasting. What we are going to discuss in this chapter is intermittent fasting. Well, according to its scientific definition, intermittent fasting relies on specific timings of fasting and feeding. To be honest, I prefer to keep things simple and use it as a broader concept, without the time restraints.

Intermittent fasting has also been called time-restricted eating or chrononutrition. Throughout this chapter, I'll use the terms *fasting* and *intermittent fasting* interchangeably.

HOW FASTING WORKS

Consider fasting as a tool to activate your survival genes. Independently of how metabolically inflexible you might be, if you fast long enough, you will eventually enter a state of ketosis and use your body fat as fuel. Obviously, it will take you longer if your body is addicted to sugar. But you should look at this practice like exercise. The more you practice, the more flexible your metabolism becomes, and the faster your body goes into ketosis.

Besides being a great tool to improve your metabolism, fasting also triggers autophagy. As you know, this is the orderly degradation and recycling of all damaged cells—an essential process for optimum health.[14,15] Think about it. As we live, our cells accumulate toxins, are invaded by pathogens, have oxidized fats incorporated into their membranes, or simply suffer the normal wear and tear of everyday life. The more damage they accumulate, the more dysfunctional they become, and the more issues they can cause. If we just left them unchecked, these damaged cells would continue to multiply and affect the function of tissues, organs, or even entire systems. Does this sound familiar? Yep, this is basically the modus operandi of cancer.

Autophagy really takes the recycling concept of "nothing gets lost" to the ultimate degree. Not only will autophagy help you rejuvenate your cells, it will also digest these "trash" proteins and then use them as fuel.[16] Instead of having to nosh on your muscle, through autophagy your body makes energy out of tissues that have been damaged and are no longer needed. This is probably why researchers have said that autophagy is required to maintain muscle mass.[17]

Let's reflect on that for a second. Even during ketosis, your body still needs a small amount of glucose to function. If you did not have the amino acids from the breakdown of recycled proteins during autophagy, your body would be forced to break down healthy muscle to get these aminos. Just to give you an idea, if autophagy were not taking place, just to support the brain's metabolic requirements alone, the muscle breakdown needed would most likely kill you within 10 days.[18] Fortunately, through autophagy, your body can collect enough amino acids to convert into glucose through gluconeogenesis and does not need to take apart your much-needed muscle.

There is also another protective mechanism to ensure that muscle loss is minimal. When we're fasting, our bodies produce growth hormone (GH).[19] GH has many functions (including making you grow when you're younger), but its key role in adults is to prevent muscle protein breakdown.[20] Intermittent fasting optimizes GH levels in two indirect ways. First, the drop in body fat caused by fasting promotes GH production.[21] GH then spurs more weight loss and reinforces this cycle.[22] Second, because you are not eating, you don't have insulin spikes. This is great news because insulin spikes can disrupt the secretion of GH.[23] Research performed on 24-hour intermittent fasting shows that patients could shed significant fat mass, improve cholesterol and triglyceride levels, shrink their waist circumference, and still keep their precious muscle mass.[24]

While researchers are still trying to figure out the intricacies of fasting and autophagy, one thing is certain: both are critical mechanisms to promote health and longevity, and we all should take advantage of them.

Neo Note: Recycling Skin

As you know, autophagy helps us recycle damaged cells and use the protein components as fuel to meet our glucose needs during a fast. In theory, when someone loses a lot of fat, the extra skin could be considered a tissue that is no longer needed. It would only make sense that the body would recycle that protein, right? Some authors believe this is the case. In their book *The Longevity Solution*, authors Dr. James DiNicolantonio and Dr. Jason Fung recount that in one of the coaching programs run by Dr. Fung, he had not found the need to refer his clients for skin removal surgery even when the clients had lost over a hundred pounds.[25] This lack of excessive "skin accumulation" suggests that the extra skin was being recycled during the intermittent fasts his clients performed.

FASTING, METABOLIC HEALTH, AND INFLAMMATION

As Friedrich Nietzsche said, "that which does not kill us makes us stronger." This perfectly describes the concept of intermittent fasting (IF). IF is a phenomenal hormetic stressor shown to produce many beneficial effects in the body.[26] The most obvious benefits of IF are metabolic. As mentioned before, while you are taking a break from eating, your body can finally leave the anabolic mode of growth and fat storage, and switch into recycling-and-repair mode. In this mode, not only does your body "cleanse itself" but it also finally has the opportunity to burn some of that accumulated fat. During this time, your body also keeps its blood sugar levels low, so your insulin levels can drop. In fact, IF helps reverse and prevent insulin resistance.[27,28] A 2021 literature review concluded that IF is effective at reducing body weight, decreasing fasting glucose, lowering fasting insulin, reducing insulin resistance, decreasing levels of leptin, and raising levels of adiponectin (a hormone that promotes the breakdown of fat).[29] Another 2021 review found that (IF-induced) autophagy could improve metabolic dysfunction and reverse diseases such as type 2 diabetes and sarcopenic obesity (low levels of skeletal muscle combined with high body fat), particularly in elderly people.[30]

As a result of our eating habits, we keep our immune system hyperactive and remain in a state of low-grade chronic inflammation. When you perform IF, you give your body a break from those inflammatory foods and, most importantly, you activate anti-inflammatory pathways in your physiology. As we saw before, IF stimulates the production of adiponectin, which, besides boosting fat breakdown, also has anti-inflammatory properties.[31] In addition, IF has been shown to turn off monocytes, which are immune cells that are often overactivated, causing inflammation.[32] Fasting also works as an inflammation antidote, not only for your dietary excesses but for chronic inflammation and autoimmune conditions as well. One study on asthma patients showed that following an alternate-day IF plan for a month reduced markers of inflammation and oxidative stress.[33] Other studies have also shown beneficial effects of IF in conditions such as fibromyalgia, IBS, MS, psoriasis, and rheumatoid arthritis.[34-37] Better yet, IF can break out these potent anti-inflammatory properties without compromising the immune system's response to acute infections.[38]

Finally, there is some research suggesting that IF may have a role in reducing the risk of developing cancer. More research is definitely needed, but this hypothesis is based on fasting's ability to assist the body in clearing out toxins and damaged cells.[39] At the very least, it's believed that fasting can be used as a possible complementary treatment, since it has been shown to increase the efficacy of chemotherapy and reduce its side effects.[40]

FASTING AND THE BRAIN

Fasting has important healing effects in the entire body, but the brain seems to be the organ that benefits most from it. Research shows that IF promotes the growth of neurons in the hippocampus, a part of the brain associated with learning and memory.[41] Remember brain-derived neurotrophic factor (BDNF)? Well, fasting is one of the best ways to boost BDNF, which leads to an uptick in brainpower (through an increase in mitochondria) and promotes the formation of more neurons.[42] Fasting also augments another protein named sirtuin 3 (SIRT3), which basically makes your brain cells' mitochondria (those in the hippocampus in particular) work more efficiently.[43] Fasting also activates the brain's self-repair mechanisms, which some researchers and authors believe might be important to improve neurological conditions like Alzheimer's disease, Parkinson's disease, MS, and stroke.[44-46]

> **Neo Note: Growth Hormone in the Brain**
>
> When we're kids, growth hormone (GH) helps us grow and develop. Once we're adults, it helps us build muscle, or at least preserve it. Unfortunately, our stressful lifestyles deplete our GH levels. And, since taking in carbohydrates immediately turns off GH secretion, our diet is also not helping us. Luckily, as we saw before, fasting is a great way to boost our growth hormone levels.
>
> Why is this important for the brain? GH, which by the way is secreted by the brain's pituitary gland, is also a strong cognitive booster. GH has been linked with brain processing speed and with mood.[47,48] In older adults, GH replacement therapy has been shown to increase cognitive function in patients with predementia and in healthy individuals after just five months.[49] Here is the great news! Fasting is your free, natural, and safe GH replacement therapy.

FASTING AND THE CIRCADIAN RHYTHM

Fasting is also connected with regulating your circadian rhythm. In a very simple way, your circadian rhythm is your internal biological clock. Fun fact: The term *circadian* comes from the Latin phrase *circa diem*, which means "around a day."[50]

All systems of your body follow your internal circadian rhythm, which is directly influenced by external factors, especially light (or the absence of it), which is why circadian rhythms are tied to the cycle of day and night. When your circadian rhythm is properly regulated, it can promote proper sleep, good health, and energy. But when this rhythm off, it can lead to the development of significant problems, including insomnia, diabetes, gut dysbiosis, obesity, cardiometabolic dysfunction, higher risk of alcohol/drug use, and behavioral disturbances including depression, aggression, and increased suicidal ideation.[51-55]

Researchers have found out that circadian rhythm is also influenced by the fluctuations and timing of feeding and fasting.[56] Your body expects a full stomach for a few hours a day and then an empty one for most of the day. By not giving your body enough fasting time, your internal clock gets the wrong feedback and can't properly activate all the physiological processes you need to function at your best.[57] A study by the famous circadian-rhythm researcher Dr. Satchin Panda demonstrated that reducing your eating period to 10 hours (leaving 14 hours to fast) was more beneficial than an eating window of 15 hours or more. Just over the course of a few months, the individuals observing the 10-hour eating window reset their cellular clocks, lost weight, had higher energy levels, slept better, and had improved moods and sharper thinking.[58]

FASTING, ENERGY, AND OVERALL HEALTH

Many people assume longer fasts will force the body to shut down and conserve energy. It makes sense, but once again there is more to it. Researchers have seen that even at up to four days of fasting, the body actually maintains a higher basal metabolic rate (resting energy expenditure) than in the fed state.[59] Fasting also helps your mitochondria increase the production of hydrogen sulfide, which works almost as an alternative fuel source that strengthens your mitochondria.[60-63] You know what this means? Stronger mitochondria, more energy!

Fasting has also been shown to boost cellular function, bump up the production of stem cells, heal the gut, and improve resilience against a wide range of stressors, including metabolic, oxidative, traumatic, and toxic stressors.[64-66] Fasting is the ultimate health reset tool.

Fasting's list of benefits is incredibly long, and I'm sure I've forgotten to mention several important ones. It really is incredible how much good can come from simply controlling *when* you eat. Your body has all it needs to repair itself. Sometimes, it just needs you to stay out of the way and let it do its magic.

> ### Neo Note: Fasting and Longevity
> Fasting might make you live longer. This conclusion is not a difficult one to reach, since fasting allows your body to repair, reduce inflammation, and improve metabolic health. It's like car maintenance. If you take your car to the mechanic often and everything is running smoothly, there's a better chance the car will last longer.
>
> It appears that researchers have found other biological mechanisms by which fasting might directly contribute to your longevity. The first mechanism has to do with adenosine monophosphate-activated protein kinase. Let's just call it AMPK. In a very simplified way, when your body is low on ATP (the body's energy molecule), as it is when adjusting to a fast or right after high-intensity exercise, your body activates AMPK. This enzyme, which is known as the "metabolic master switch," stimulates the recycling of damaged mitochondria and increased production of new ones. This, in turn, will boost fat burning, improve insulin sensitivity, decrease triglycerides, and reduce inflammation.[67,68] Since aging is deeply connected with metabolic health, it's believed that as AMPK improves metabolic efficiency, it also increases the chances of living longer.[69]
>
> Another mechanism that researchers are exploring is the mammalian target of rapamycin, or mTOR. *These names are killing me.* Increased mTOR is associated with accelerated growth and aging.[70] mTOR is especially stimulated by protein consumption, so when you are fasting (or following a fasting-mimicking diet like the ketogenic diet), your mTOR levels are lower, which promotes age deceleration.[71]

Fasting also leads to the production of ketones. Besides what we already covered about ketones, they also regulate the expression of molecules and proteins that play a part in aging, such as nicotinamide adenine dinucleotide (NAD+) and sirtuins.[72] With aging, NAD+ levels drop, and this affects cellular performance. So it's believed that by restoring NAD+ levels, you support cellular energy and preserve DNA health.[73] Then we have the brain-boosting sirtuins. They also play a crucial role in the body's cellular response to stressors like oxidative stress and DNA damage. Thus, research suggests that sirtuins might extend your life span.[74]

FASTING LENGTH

One could write an entire book about the different types of fasting. In fact, several authors have. As much as I love fasting, I'm trying not to get lost in the nitty-gritty. There is a lot more that can be said about various fasting protocols and even the different physiological phenomena that happen during the fasting timeline. But I'm going to keep things simple and focus on the fundamental concepts. If after this you're still interested in learning more about fasting, at the end of this chapter I recommend fantastic books on this subject.

In my opinion, there isn't a perfect "fasting way" that will work for everyone. We all are different, and most importantly, we all have different lifestyles. The point here is not to obsess over a specific concept but to find what works for you. Fasting should never be an obligation or something to stress about. Fasting should be a natural part of your lifestyle and something that brings you pleasure.

16:8 Intermittent Fasting

The basic concept behind IF is that you plan your periods of eating and fasting, following a specific timeline (typically keeping the fasting period longer than 12 hours).[75] These periods and their frequency during the week may vary depending on different fasting approaches. Some researchers promote 18 hours of fasting, some 24, some 36 plus. There is plenty of discussion and "politics" involved, but most authors seem to agree that even a 16-hour fast produces substantial results, so this is where we will start.

The 16:8 IF is considered the first stage of fasting. But just because it's the first stage, that doesn't mean it's not powerful. Consistent 16-hour fasts can build up to significant results. Most importantly, even if you aim toward doing longer fasts, this should be everyone's starting point. Let's face it. If you've never fasted before and you try to do a 24- or 30-hour fast, you will feel miserable. Your body is not prepared for it, and it will overreact to this time without food. It's like going to the gym after a long break. You need to start slowly, so your body gets used to it. With some practice, you can then easily transition to longer fasts and still feel amazing.

After 16 hours since your last meal, your body will have exhausted the energy from that meal and will have to go through the glycogen reserves in your liver and your muscles. As the reserves become depleted, the body breaks down some proteins in order to use their amino acids for gluconeogenesis and create more glucose. As this becomes insufficient and both glucose and insulin continue to drop, glucagon levels rise and activate glycogen breakdown. From here, we have the whole cascade of events that will lead to lipolysis and ketogenesis. Depending on how metabolically flexible you are, this metabolic switch may take 12 to 36 hours to start.[76,77]

The best way to do a 16:8 IF is by skipping breakfast. Please understand something. Morning breakfast is a marketing conception. *But breakfast is the most important meal of the day*—said the cereal industry, to make more money. The meal with which you "break your fast" is indeed important, but for most, considering our circadian rhythms, it should not be in the morning.

Here's another fun fact. In Brad Pilon's book *Eat Stop Eat*, I learned that the word *dinner* actually comes from the Latin *disjejunare*, meaning "to unfast," or break the fast. So, back in the day, the word *dinner* actually meant "breakfast." #mindblown

But I digress here. The point is, skipping breakfast makes the 16:8 plan incredibly easy. Let's say that you have dinner at 7 p.m. After that, you don't eat anything else until the following day (which is what most of us do anyway). While you're sleeping, you are obviously fasting. Then, you wake up, drink some water, tea, or plain coffee (no sugar, creamers, milk, etc.) so you don't break your fast, and go on with your day. Without thinking too much about it, when you reach your lunch hour, around noon, you have been fasting for 17 hours. Easy!

Neo Note: We Used to Skip Breakfast

Skipping breakfast now seems like a concept out of this world, but in fact, this was the norm for most people not that long ago. If you look at cookbooks or historical dietary literature from the time of your grandparents or great-grandparents, you'll realize that breakfast was very rare, and was recommended only for children, people with disabilities, and the elderly (because of their weak digestive systems).[78]

Historian Caroline Yeldham notes that the ancient Romans didn't eat breakfast. They consumed only one meal a day, usually around noon. In fact, breakfast was frowned upon because eating more than one meal was considered gluttony. According to Yeldham, this thinking influenced the way people ate for a very long time. During the Middle Ages, the monastic life had a significant impact on how people ate. It's believed that it was then that the word *breakfast* was first used, but just not the way we use it. Breakfast was the first meal of the day and was mostly eaten at what we think of as lunchtime, since record shows that monks consumed only lunch (at the time, breakfast) and supper.[79]

Another historian, Ian Mortimer, suggests that the timing of breakfast as a morning meal might not have appeared until the 16th century, while the House of Tudor was ruling the kingdom of England and its realms. At that time, especially in the cities, the concept of jobs appeared and people started to work for an employer, rather than working for themselves on their own land. Morning breakfast made sense then, since it allowed employees to work the long hours of the day without interruption.[80]

OMAD

OMAD is the IF concept of "one meal a day." Once you pass the 16-hour mark, your body really starts to get pushed into fat burning. Hormonal triggers force the body to protect muscle by blocking gluconeogenesis and prioritizing fat burning.[81] Here is where the magic happens. Until this point, you were *just skipping meals*; now you're in the fasting major league. Not to mention that saying you do OMAD sounds pretty badass.

During OMAD, you are eating only once a day. You have lunch or dinner and then eat again only when you have that same meal the following day. The thing to keep in mind is that since you're eating just one meal a day, it really needs to be a big, high-calorie, nutrient-dense meal. That one meal has to provide all the fuel and micronutrients you need to function at your best.

While some people do OMAD every single day, I am not a big fan of this. I feel that, for most people, this can cause nutrient deficiencies. The truth is that, for most, eating such an enormous meal is hard. They end up eating less than they should and not getting all the nutrition they need. If this happens two or three times a week, it's perfectly fine, since we can compensate on the other days. But if it happens daily, it can lead to malnutrition.

My personal experience is that if I eat such a big meal, I either go to bed with an incredibly full stomach and sleep like crap, or I can't perform at my best either physically or mentally while all my blood and energy are being channeled toward my digestion.

In his book *Fast This Way*, Dave Asprey states that if you do OMAD every day, there is a higher risk of having decreases in sex hormones, sleep quality, and even hair density.[82] The older you are, the greater the chances of your body having difficulty tolerating this consistent stressor. If you want to do OMAD consistently, you are probably better off with a daily 20-to-22-hour fast, which lets you squeeze in two meals during that small feeding window.

Nutrition expert Brad Pilon asserts that doing one or two 24-hour fasts during the week is the best way to get optimal results while still not having a significant impact on the lifestyle you're used to.[83] I also believe that the occasional use of OMAD, as suggested by Pilon, is an incredibly powerful tool. But I also think we could work in some 16:8 fasts on the other days, for example. But again, there are no rules here. You do what works best for you.

NOMAD

A small upgrade to OMAD is NOMAD—"no meal a day." This does not mean that you will never eat again. Instead, you are choosing not to eat for the entirety of one day.

Let me explain this better. Let's say you eat dinner at 7 p.m. (day 1), then you spend the whole next day (day 2) fasting, and only eat an early lunch on the following day (day 3). This adds up to a fast of about 36 to 40 hours, which further boosts the benefits of the OMAD approach. This particular type of fast is only to be done on occasion (e.g., once a month).

UMAD

Any fast over 48 hours I call UMAD. I believe I first heard this acronym from strongman and strength coach Elliott Hulse. UMAD stands for "Are you mad?" I think it's a brilliant way to describe this fast, since it is the exact reaction most people have when they hear about it.

Why would someone aim to do such a long fast? Most authors say that it takes about 48 to 72 hours of fasting to activate autophagy. Unfortunately, there is no way to objectively measure autophagy, so these are assumptions based on the time it takes, on average, to fully switch into ketosis and start producing ketone bodies. Once ketone bodies are running in your system, the body activates the mTOR and AMPK pathways that ultimately lead to autophagy.[84-86] These timings are subjective because it all depends on metabolic flexibility. For example, I can easily go into ketosis with just a 16:8 fast, while some people will need the full 72 hours to really make the switch. The important thing is that once you reach these longer fasting times, you can really get the benefits from ketosis and from the boosted levels of autophagy and detoxification.

Believe it or not, once you reach this point, the sensation of hunger vanishes for most people. And, curiously, you also experience more energy and a new sense of mental clarity that amplifies all your senses. It's a unique experience, but one that needs to be approached with caution. A UMAD fast should be done during a less-active time, like a long weekend, and should never be attempted right off the bat. Only when you feel comfortable with a couple of OMADs or NOMADs should you try to go that extra mile. This is a fast I like do two to four times a year as an ultimate reset for my body.

ULF

Finally, we have ultralong fasts (ULFs). Anything over 72 hours is considered a ULF. This type of fast has been described as having "miracle-like potential," but honestly, it can also be quite dangerous if not done correctly. It should be performed only under proper medical supervision. Some studies have shown that ULFs may amplify the effectiveness of chemotherapy for cancer patients.[87] Across the world, several "fasting clinics" are addressing all kinds of diseases through ULF, but despite some great anecdotal evidence, more research is needed.

> ### Neo Note: Fasting While You Sleep
> In the brain, you have the glymphatic system, which, among other functions, is also responsible for washing your brain with cerebrospinal fluid and clearing damaged proteins, toxins, and metabolites from your central nervous system.[88] This is a complex mechanism, but in simple terms, let's just say that this is a mechanism that occurs mostly while you're asleep.[89] If you deprive yourself of sleep and don't respect your circadian rhythm, you might compromise the efficiency of the glymphatic system. This can cause an accumulation of damaged proteins and toxins that can then lead to brain inflammation and disease.
>
> Research has found that insulin resistance or even higher levels of insulin after a meal can affect the efficiency of the glymphatic system.[90] This might also be an additional reason ketogenic diets promote brain health. Knowing this, some authors recommend that you have your last meal of the day at least four hours before going to bed in order not to have a negative effect on this waste clearance system.[91]
>
> One early dinner a week might be a good idea to make sure your brain gets a deep weekly cleanse.

MODIFYING YOUR FAST

Some authors suggest that you can get most of the benefits of fasting while still eating some foods. The key principle is that as long as you don't increase your insulin levels, your body continues to progress slowly toward ketosis. And, since it is ketosis that then promotes autophagy, it's believed that you can derive the same benefits. Unfortunately, researchers haven't confirmed this concept, but since it honestly makes perfect sense, I am going with it for now. Even if modified fasting does not promote the full spectrum of results of a "real fast," I think this can be an excellent way to make fasting easier, especially for people who are just starting.

The main author promoting this concept is the "father of biohacking" himself, Dave Asprey. Asprey suggests adding C8 MCT oil and grass-fed butter or ghee to your morning coffee in order to improve your energy levels and reduce hunger during your fast. Asprey asserts that since fat has no significant effect on insulin, adding these saturated fats to your coffee won't cause you to derail the metabolic benefits of the fast.[92] Yes, technically you're no longer fasting, but since there's no spike in insulin, your body is still on the same metabolic journey it would be on if you had not added those fats.

Adding MCTs to your coffee might be positive for two main reasons. First, ketones help regulate your circadian rhythm, so adding them in the morning will instruct your body that it is daytime, which in turn will "awaken" and energize you.[93] Second, C8 MCT oil is directly converted into ketones, and the caffeine in the coffee will double this ketone production.[94] High levels of ketones in the body might facilitate the metabolic switch to fat burning, and can also rein in the sensation of hunger, making the fast easier to sustain.[95]

What about the butter? Well, the practice of putting butter in hot beverages is not new. In fact, it's a Tibetan tradition to add yak butter to their tea. It's believed that the butter slows down digestion, decreasing the effects of caffeine sensitivity and reducing the famous "caffeine crash." However, I was not able to find any conclusive evidence to support this theory.

Beyond that, grass-fed butter or ghee promotes a sensation of satiety and, as a bonus, adds a creamy texture to the coffee or tea.

Another of Asprey's suggestions is to occasionally add some source of "pure" soluble fiber to your coffee. As we briefly discussed before, we can't digest fiber, so it does not cause a rise in blood sugar or insulin. But obviously the selection of the fiber is important, because some fiber supplements might also have regular carbs mixed with the fiber, which would affect insulin and defeat the entire purpose. By adding a "pure" fiber supplement to your coffee, you are providing food for your microbiome without affecting your insulin levels. In turn, your microbiome produces postbiotics that switch off the sensation of hunger, once again making your fast a more enjoyable experience.

HOW FASTING AFFECTS THE SEXES DIFFERENTLY

We forget this at times, but it is important to recognize that men and women have different physiologies and unique metabolisms. So it's important to look at some of these differences and determine how they can impact the fasting experiences of both sexes.

Biologically speaking, women are genetically programmed to have babies. Remember that our genetic code only cares about the survival of the species. And the species survives only if more babies are on the way. If a woman is depleted of nutrients, her genes recognize she is not healthy enough to build a healthy baby, and they remove her from the equation. This is why nutritionally deficient, extremely thin, or overly stressed women (those who are stressed mentally and physically because of an excess of exercise, for example) can have menstrual dysfunctions.[96] Their genetic programming does not allow them to get pregnant while they don't have the best chances of success.

This is so engraved in women's genetic coding that even if not pregnant, the female body always has to make sure that it has access to enough food and nutrients, or at least it has enough fat to "survive." If the body feels these basic conditions are not in place, not only can it cause havoc in the menstrual cycle, but it can also trigger anxiety and intense food cravings as a warning sign that things need to change.

This is probably why, when it comes to intermittent fasting, women tend to be more sensitive than men. Research has shown that women remain in an increased state of fat burning longer than men, even after the fast has been interrupted. Women have almost a temporary insulin-resistance response, since even elevated insulin levels do not push a woman out of fat-burning mode during the hours following a fast.[97] But don't worry. This insulin resistance is temporary and occurs only with longer fasts. During shorter fasts (12 to 38 hours), women actually seem to improve their insulin sensitivity better than men.[98-100]

So, women are better fat burners than men and are more sensitive to the effects of a fast. This is great news, right? In general, yes. Women appear to respond better metabolically and even seem to have increased protection against thyroid hormone (T3) level drops compared with men.[101]

The caveat here is that this whole situation inverts if women are very lean or are extremely active. In these situations, the genes kick in and try to protect women from the perceived starvation caused by fasting. Research on female athletes has shown that the combination of low body fat with large calorie deficits, as can occur during a fasting state, can cause amenorrhea (absence of their period), as well as decreased leptin and estradiol levels.[102] As you know, low levels of leptin will cause a metabolic slowdown and intense hunger. The low estradiol (which is the most active type of the estrogen hormone) can cause insomnia, depression, nervousness, headaches, brain fog, and fatigue.[103] Another study, this time with 72-hour fasts, also concluded that lean women (at the lower end of a healthy body mass index, or BMI) may be at higher risk of developing neuroendocrine and reproductive abnormalities when "nutrition is completely withdrawn for 72 hours."[104]

In other words, if you are an already-lean woman, shorter fasts or even modified fasts (with some MCTs) might be a better option. Another thing to consider is not to fast every day but to opt for alternate-day IF (every other day). That way, you are giving your body the input that there is enough food and that you are not in danger. Finally, please avoid strenuous workouts on the days when you are fasting. That is not a good combination and will definitely get your genes confused.

On average, women are also more carbohydrate-sensitive than men.[105] Although there hasn't been much research done on the subject, there is plenty of anecdotal evidence suggesting that women on a ketogenic diet feel better when they slightly increase their carb consumption. Ladies, with this point in mind, it might be beneficial for you to do a little carbohydrate refeed two or three times a week.

One more special note for my female readers: Please listen to your body. You have unique hormonal fluctuations throughout your menstrual cycle, and your appetite and cravings can change dramatically because of this.[106] If you experience more hunger some days, it does not mean you are "fasting wrong";

it might just be a hormonal response. If it doesn't feel right one day, don't force it. You can try again the next day.

HOW TO BREAK A FAST

The period after a fast is over should be the time to replenish your body with nutrient-dense foods. But these foods should be carefully selected. After a fast, you may want to prolong the state of ketosis in order to continue burning fat as fuel and get the metabolic benefits of it. While some authors defend going for vegetables and fruits, I recommend being picky about your choices. Eating starchy vegetables or high-sugar fruits will interrupt the metabolic changes you started during the fast and will bring your body back to glucose burning. You can still eat vegetables and fruits, but choose starchless leafy greens and low-sugar fruits like berries or avocados.

Especially after a longer fast, I recommend something light, just to get your digestive juices going. A soup, a fat-and-protein-based smoothie, or bone broth is an excellent choice for a lighter meal. In a way, these are already partially digested, so they cause little digestive burden. If you want something to chew, nosh on a handful of nuts. Then, after an hour or two, you can eat something more substantial. If you want to extend the keto benefits, opt for nutrient-dense fats such as fatty meats, fatty fish, nonstarchy plants, eggs, and butter.

WHO SHOULD NOT FAST

As much as I love fasting, there are certain people for whom I do not recommend this practice. Please do not fast if you

• **are pregnant or breastfeeding.**
You are trying to grow a human being. This is not the time to restrict calories.

• **have fertility problems or irregular periods.**
There is some controversy here, since some people claim that fasting can improve fertility. In fact, research presents mixed results here. Caution is needed and medical supervision is advised if you decide to explore this option.

• **are under 18 years old.**
Fasting at this age is generally not recommended because the child or teen is still developing. However, it might be something to explore in situations of obesity and metabolic dysfunction. Medical supervision is advised.

• **are underweight or malnourished.**
In this state, you do not need any caloric restriction or to send any starvation messages to your genes.

• **have an eating disorder.**
Fasting can cause an overfixation on food, trigger anxiety, and exacerbate the issues associated with the eating disorder.

WHAT TO EXPECT FROM A FAST
The First Fast

For most people, the first time they fast, the experience is not all rainbows and butterflies. It might really suck. I know I would sell a lot more books if I just said that everything is wonderful, but I would be doing you a disservice. I prefer to prepare you for the worst rather than surprise you with symptoms you aren't ready for.

The first time you fast, or even the first few times, you will most likely experience hunger. This hunger is not physiological, since you are not actually starving, or anything like it. You feel hunger because this may be the first time your body has spent more than 8 to 10 hours without eating. Your body may not be used to that, so it will try to trick you into eating because it does not want to leave its comfort zone. For most people doing their first fasts, this sensation of hunger is purely psychological. You are not hungry; you just emotionally need to eat something.

We are so conditioned to eat that the act of eating has become more than fueling the body. Our relationship with food is highly emotional, and we eat to deal with many feelings. Hunger then becomes a mental addiction and not a physical necessity for food. Because of this emotional addiction (and in part, the sugar addition), fasting can also cause feelings of withdrawal such as anxiety, anger, nausea, and headaches. You may also experience what I call "emotional hypoglycemia." You develop symptoms of hypoglycemia like shakiness, dizziness, brain fog, and weakness, but 9 times out of 10, you don't actually have low blood sugar. It's all in your head.

For the 10 percent who actually do experience physiological consequences from a fast, here are a couple of pointers. If you experience dizziness, it might stem from dehydration or lower blood pressure, which definitely can occur if you don't fast the right way. It is essential to stay hydrated and to replenish your electrolytes. Drinking plenty of water and adding a pinch of a good salt (e.g., Himalayan) every two to three hours does the trick. If you have a headache, it may result from actual sugar withdrawal. As we've seen, sugar can act like any other drug, and as an addict, you can suffer when your body doesn't get its next fix. Unfortunately, there is not a lot you can do about this besides drinking plenty of water and adding some salt. You just have to remember that this is temporary, and part of the much-needed detox process.

Tips Before Your First Fast

As always, there are hacks that you can use to improve your first fast. The best recommendation is not to jump straight away into fasting. This is a common mistake I see in most areas of life. People get excited and just go all in, even if their body is not yet prepared. With fasting, it's better to start slow and succeed than to go balls to the wall and not be able to stand the side effects of metabolic inflexibility and mental addiction. Start slow. One or two weeks before your first fast, start decreasing your consumption of carbs and shifting your diet more toward healthy fats. This will gradually train your body not to depend on carbs so much.

Aim to do your first fast during the weekend. You definitely don't want to experience a bad withdrawal while you're working and are supposed to be performing at your optimum. The good news is that after you've done a couple of fasts, you will actually start feeling sharper while fasting, and this will make you a lot more productive.

During your first few fasts, don't exercise on those same days. A workout can exacerbate some symptoms you might experience. As we are going to learn soon, exercising while fasting can be incredibly powerful, but only once you are metabolically adjusted.

To deal with the mental addiction, try to keep yourself busy during your first fasts. By doing something that requires some concentration or by simply having fun, you won't remember that you haven't eaten, and the emotional hunger won't show up.

Keep your stomach full, but not with food. Drink plenty of water. The more water you drink, the more you keep your stomach stretched (even if just for a couple of minutes). This tricks your body into thinking you are eating and will delay any physiological sensation of hunger. You can also drink mineral water, tea, or coffee, as long as they don't have any sweeteners or additives.

Another important thing to do is to keep your fast a secret. Yes, fasting is like the Fight Club. First rule of fasting: You don't talk about fasting! Well, "fasting club" has an exception. If you have other friends reading this book, they will understand, and it's actually a great idea to try these concepts together. But if the people around you know nothing about these nutritional concepts and are still stuck in the common junk information out there, they might give you a hard time if they know what you're doing. The last thing you need is to have to justify your actions and explain what you're doing, especially when you are still getting used to it. After you've adjusted to fasting, yes, please share with them how great you feel and invite them to join the fasting club. But until then, let's keep this just between the club members. #fastingclub

Issues with Waking Up

Folks who are too accustomed to their breakfast might suffer a little when they first start skipping it. A common complaint is that they feel like they are still half asleep for the first half of their day and feel low in energy. A great hack to solve this is to perform a modified fast with some grass-fed butter and MCT in your morning coffee, black tea, or matcha. This will give you the boost you need in the morning, and it may even make you forget that it's time to eat around lunchtime. Modified fasts are always a great place to start.

Issues with Falling Asleep

Fasting keeps your metabolism "on fire," and it will lead to the release of adrenaline. As you know, adrenaline is the hormone our bodies secrete in fight-or-flight situations, when we need as much energy as we can get. In a fasting situation, you will not have a big spike in adrenaline, but its levels might be higher than usual, which can create a sensation of more energy. This is a great thing during the day, but at night, when you want to sleep, it can be a pain in the ass.

The way to address this is by creating a simple relaxation routine before going to bed. You can stretch, meditate, or simply do a couple of mindful breaths. Do some box breathing. Lie down in a comfortable position. Inhale for five seconds. Hold it for five seconds. Exhale for five seconds. Then hold for another five seconds. And repeat the sequence until the revved-up feeling melts away.

Fasting Attitude

Some people interpret the idea of not eating as self-punishment for years of wrongdoing. Fasting should not be associated with feelings of punishment or even lack and emptiness. If you still use food to fill emotional voids, you first have to deal with those emotions in order to see fasting for what it is. Fasting is empowerment. Fasting is a practice that stimulates abundance—abundance of energy, abundance of time, and abundance of health. Adopt the right attitude and your results will be nothing less than amazing!

BACK TO THE FUTURE

As humans, we get so used to certain things that we are blinded by them and cannot see any other way. We've become so addicted to eating at all times of the day that thinking about changing that really challenges our comfort zone. But, as you know, there are other ways. In fact, these are actually what used to be our old ways. Along the way, because of our shiny-new-toy syndrome, we shoved these concepts to the side and forgot about them. That stops now. As they do in fashion design, it's time to bring what worked in the past back to the future!

One of the key health factors from the past is metabolic flexibility. *Have I mentioned this before?* By adopting a mostly lower-carb diet and combining it with regular periods of fasting, you will bring your body back to its factory settings and create a fresh start for a better future. The changes are not immediate, but as you regain insulin sensitivity and your body gets used to being in ketosis, your excess weight will melt off, your food cravings will disappear, you will feel stronger, your mind will be clear, and your energy will go through the roof, without the inevitable crashes of the past. This is the superhuman that has always been encoded in your genes!

THE NEO DIET IS NOT A KETOGENIC DIET

There are obvious benefits of a ketogenic state, but, as we've seen before, that does not mean you have to stay in ketosis all the time. If you have any of the health conditions that do incredibly well with ketosis, please be strict with your ketosis. But all others will benefit from purposely going in and out of ketosis. Combining strategies like fasting and a low-carb diet with planned carb refeeds can provide greater benefits than prolonged ketogenic diets. Not to mention that some carbs are delicious, and I am way happier if I can eat them once in a while.

In my opinion, "chronic ketosis" is a fragile state. Yes, it is a lot healthier than being a sugar addict, but you are an addict nonetheless. The same way your body was used to functioning only on glucose before, now it will only know how to function on ketones. When eventually you get kicked out of ketosis, you will not feel your best either physically or emotionally. But by cycling in and out of ketosis, you will benefit from it while still maintaining higher levels of insulin sensitivity, thyroid function, and overall metabolic health.

Later in this book, we'll learn about how humans are social beings and how being with people is a huge contributor to happiness and health. You do not need to be that person who awkwardly takes their own Tupperware to social events because of their restricted diet. Or, worse, the person who doesn't go out to social gatherings because of their diet. Some won't agree with me, but when it gets to that point, that is causing you more harm than good. Obviously, you are not going to go to the gathering and eat all kinds of junk food. You know better. But by being metabolically flexible, you can easily burn any fuel, and certainly can find something you can eat. That is the definition of an antifragile metabolism: being able to adapt to any circumstances and still feel amazing!

THE STRATEGIC USE OF CARBS

Metabolically speaking, the Neo Diet is a cyclical ketogenic diet. It comprises an initial phase of metabolic flexibility induction by combining strategic fasts with a low-carb, low-protein, and high-fat diet. Following the strategies in this book, you'll take between two and eight weeks to regain metabolic flexibility and conclude the initial phase. Then, in the second phase, now that metabolic flexibility is in place, we will increase protein content and add healthy carbohydrates two or three days a week, typically on days when we're exercising.

The strategic use of carbohydrates will not only make you more metabolically flexible but will also improve your health and performance. In his book *Intuitive Fasting*, functional-medicine expert Dr. Will Cole defends that strategic carb intake can help with what he calls the "3 S's": sleep, sex hormones, and stalled goals.[107] Adding some carbohydrates to your normal protein consumption may boost the amount of tryptophan in your brain. Tryptophan is then converted into serotonin.[108] As you'll remember, serotonin is a neurotransmitter that helps relax the brain, prevents anxiety, and promotes feelings of positivity.[109] What's more, serotonin is then converted into melatonin, which is the main circadian rhythm regulator and sleep inductor.[110] And if you have a better night's sleep, everything else will be better too!

Neo Note: Carbs and the Menstrual Cycle

This suggestion comes from Dr. Will Cole. According to him, some women feel improvements in energy, mood, and PMS symptoms when they ratchet up their carb intake around the time of their periods and ovulation. Physiologically, this makes sense, since during that time there is an increased stress in the body that should benefit some extra carbs. Everyone's cycle is different, and there is nothing like experimentation and seeing what works best for you.

Beyond relaxing you and helping you sleep, serotonin also helps suppress appetite.[111] This is why when you are having a lot of fun, you don't even remember to eat. But when you cut carbs for too long, you risk dropping your serotonin levels to a point where you feel anxious and hungry all the time.

While we're on the appetite-suppression subject: In people who are lean but still want the other health benefits of ketosis, a continuously carb-restricted diet can trigger a drop in leptin levels, which will make you feel hungry all the time, as you already know. These hunger signals tell your body that you are "starving," so the priority goes into conserving fat instead of burning it. This is the part Dr. Cole refers to as stalled goals. Having healthy leptin dynamics is important for controlling both hunger and metabolism. And there's more. Leptin is also deeply connected to your sex hormones. By following a cyclical ketogenic diet with strategic carb intake, you will keep your insulin and leptin sensitivity optimized, which will also keep your sex hormone levels regulated.

Insulin sensitivity and even the occasional insulin spike are also important to help you put on some muscle. Insulin has an important role in muscle hypertrophy. Following exercise, insulin will inhibit muscle protein breakdown and promote the production of new muscle protein.[112] That being said, the ingestion of some carbs post-workout will help you build that much-desired muscle.

Finally, research has shown that by having a couple of "carb days," participants were a lot more compliant, following a new diet while not suffering any metabolic consequences.[113] In other words, having some occasional "good" carbs will not affect your metabolic flexibility and will make you healthier and happier with your diet. That's a win-win to me.

TIMING YOUR CARBS

The time of day when you choose to eat your carbs has a significant impact on your metabolism. If you decide to load up on carbs in the morning, you are basically switching your metabolism into sugar burning for the rest of the day. Research shows that people who eat a higher-carb breakfast experience hunger sooner because of this metabolic change.[114]

For example, a six-month study compared participants eating a similar number of carbohydrates but dispersed differently throughout the day. The group who consumed about 80 percent of their carbs at dinner lost more weight, had greater reductions in waist circumference, improved their fasting blood glucose, and exhibited better insulin sensitivity, more favorable cholesterol ratios, reduced inflammation, and improved levels of leptin and adiponectin.[115] Reviewing these two studies, we can conclude that the old maxim "eating carbs at night makes you fat" is complete BS. By avoiding carbs in the morning, we continue enjoying the benefits of ketosis (or at least increased fat burning) for the rest of the day, and later we can give our bodies some carbs to replenish the reserves. Not only is this better metabolically speaking, but it also allows you to perform better both mentally and physically during the day.

Another option, as hinted before, is to take in your carbs right after your workouts. During this time, you have certain receptors in your muscles (GLUT-4 receptors) that become exposed because of the muscle contraction. While exposed, they open the "cellular gates" and invite your muscle tissue to absorb as much glucose as it can. What this means is that for a little while, your muscles become sugar sponges, and you don't need as much insulin to get rid of all that sugar from the carb meal. Thus, these carbs are less likely to promote fat storage, and you will transition sooner into a fat-burning state.

Whenever I have a social event where I know I'm going to eat more carbs than usual, I try to get a workout done right beforehand, or at the very least I go to the bathroom and do a couple of "toilet squats" to minimize the impact of those carbs. Especially on days of excess, remember to "earn them"!

> **Neo Note: Exercising in a Fasted State**
> Exercising in a fasted state is another controversial topic. Some believe that this can lead to increased muscle breakdown and not growth. Others contend that it reduces training performance, so they consider you are wasting your time training in that state.
> Even though both of these points have some validity, what makes them true or false is your state of metabolic flexibility. If you are not metabolically flexible, you won't have much energy for the workout, and you might even lose some muscle. But a metabolically flexible person might have a different response. In ketone-adapted individuals, during the fasted state, you have low insulin and mTOR but have increasing levels of GH, which are preserving your

muscle mass. Considering that you eat your meal with protein after the workout, your body will have an uptick in insulin and will transition into a fed (anabolic) state and rebuild all the proteins broken down during exercise.

Now, in the fed state, the body has high insulin, high growth hormone, high amino acids, and abundant glucose. In other words, it has all the components it needs to build even more muscle. Studies not only confirm that exercise in a fasted state will indeed promote the repair and growth of lean muscle tissue but suggest that it will also produce greater fat loss than "fed" training.[116-118] What's important to remember is that to maximize muscle building, especially if it's done on an empty stomach, you should eat or drink some post-workout protein.[119]

CARB QUANTITY

Fats and proteins are satiating macronutrients. There is only so much you can eat before you feel full. Carbs, on the other hand, do not produce the same satiating response, so we need to be more careful. As you become more metabolically flexible, you will slowly become more in tune with your intuition. I'm not saying you'll magically know that you need 164 grams of sweet potatoes. Being more intuitive is being able to read your body better. It's knowing when you've eaten too much because now you feel sleepy or are experiencing brain fog. It's feeling that after a certain amount of starch you feel hungrier than if you had had less. It's noticing these little hints that your body gives you. Until you reach a point where you can trust that innate intuition, the best approach is to follow some guidelines.

How many carbs you eat during these refeed days truly depends on your goals. If you are trying to lose weight, you're better off staying between 50 and 100 grams of carbs. On the other hand, if you are lean and are looking to build some muscle, you can consider 500-plus grams of carbs.

I hate measuring food, so this is just a guideline to be used initially so you can see what 50 grams of white rice looks like, for example. Once you know that, you test it out. For a couple of weeks, start slowly increasing the quantity and see how you feel and how your body reacts. The main thing here is to test, evaluate, and retest to establish what works for you while still promoting your metabolic flexibility. Contrary to what most diet plans suggest, please realize that everyone is different and there are no absolutes that work for everyone.

NEO SUMMARY
• Fasting has been part of our lifestyle for millennia.
• Fasting is not starvation nor calorie restriction.
• Contrary to what you've been told, eating every 2-3 hours is not beneficial.
• Fasting promotes ketosis.
• Fasting stimulates autophagy which is your body's recycling system.
• Fasting reduces the risk of most chronic diseases.
• Fasting reduces inflammation, lowers oxidative stress, and slows aging.
• Fasting boosts your emotional state and improves your relationship with food.
• Fasting is the ultimate metabolic flexibility switch.
• Except for people fighting specific diseases mentioned in the ketogenic diet segment of this book, most people will benefit from cycling in and out of ketosis.
• Carbs are better after workouts and later in the day.

NEO ACTION
• Start with a short modified fast and slowly progress until reaching the 16:8 fast.
• After a couple of 16:8 fasts, please progress toward OMAD and eventually NOMAD.
• Once metabolic flexibility is established, please aim to do 1-2 weekly carb refeeds, especially at night or after a workout.
• If you are going to eat more carbs than usual, excuse yourself to wash your hands, and do some toilet squats.

NEO RECOMMENDATIONS
• *Eat Stop Eat* by Brad Pilon
• *Energy Paradox* by Dr. Steven Gundry
• *Fast This Way* by Dave Asprey
• *Intuitive Fasting* by Dr. Will Cole
• *Metabolic Autophagy* by Siim Land
• *The Complete Guide To Fasting* by Dr. Jason Fung & Jimmy Moore
• *The Longevity Solution* by Dr. James DiNicolantonio & Dr. Jason Fung
• *Two Meals A Day* by Mark Sisson

SCAN ME

my.neodiet.co/neorecommendations

THE BUILDING BLOCKS OF LIFE

Protein—Broscience and the Vegan-Carnivore Debate

"If someone wishes for good health, one must first ask oneself if he is ready to do aways with the reasons for his illness. Only then it is possible to help him."
Hippocrates

THE SCOOP ON PROTEIN

Protein is a macronutrient, like carbohydrates and fat, but it's the popular one of the bunch. If macronutrients were the boy band NSYNC, protein would be Justin Timberlake. In fact, just like Justin, protein went solo for a while. For two or three decades, every single fitness magazine had articles telling you how important protein was for you. *Want big muscles? Eat protein! Want to lose weight? Eat protein! Want to be rich? Eat your protein!* Okay, that last one was not in the magazines (as far as I know), but you get the idea. The bottom line is that every article would tell you to eat at least 30 grams of protein every two to three hours and to never miss a post-workout protein shake.

Protein was and still is the epitome of "broscience." If you have ever been to the gym and spoken with a few old-school personal trainers, you'll know what I mean. If you're not making progress, it's obviously because you aren't consuming enough protein. *You are ruining your gains, bro!* The "bropothesis" (bro hypothesis) states, the more protein you eat, the more muscle you build and the more fat you will burn. It's a fact!

The goal of this chapter is to discover whether protein's reputation is just a mix of broscience and marketing, or if there is actual truth behind the claims we've all heard. Let's find out.

There are between 250,000 and one million protein molecules in the human body.[1] The protein we consume is broken down (in our digested system) into amino acids. These amino acids are then used as the building blocks to create thousands of different proteins used by the body in its physiological processes. Of the 20 amino acids, 11 are deemed nonessential because we can make them, and 9 are essential, since we have to get them from food.[2] Unfortunately, the body cannot store a lot of amino acids. What this means is that we need to have a daily influx of them to avoid deficiencies.

When you overconsume protein and end up with more amino acids than you need, these can be used through gluconeogenesis to create glucose, as we saw before.

These amino acids allow you to create and repair muscles, organs, and connective tissues. They are also responsible for the development of red blood cells, skin, hair and fingernails; the regulation of hormone secretion and digestion; the protection against disease; and the transport of nutrients and oxygen. In other words, protein is indeed really important for us. The question now is, do we need as much protein as we've been told to eat?

HOW MUCH PROTEIN DO WE NEED?

This is really the million-dollar question. In fact, scientists all over the world cannot agree on the answer. Even though there is no clear number, there are some broad assumptions and estimates. So, considering all the available data, I'll give you the best "guesstimation" I can.

The recommended daily allowance (RDA) set by the Institute of Medicine of the National Academy of Sciences is 0.8 gram of protein per kilogram of body weight.[3] This basically represents a recommended consumption of 60 grams of protein for a person weighing 75 kilograms (165 pounds). Please note that I am talking about 60 grams of actual protein, not 60 grams of beef, for example. Keep in mind that protein represents only 19 percent to 33 percent of the weight of meat, depending on the type and the leanness.[4]

This RDA was established using the nitrogen balance method. To make a long story short, this method does not seem appropriate for this measure.[5] Even the Food and Nutrition Board acknowledged that using nitrogen balance to set the RDA for protein was a mistake, because, and I quote, "this method does not measure any relevant physiological end point."[6]

As much as we love definite numbers, we have to accept the fact that our bodies work in complex ways, and protein metabolism might be one of the most complex ones. Defining a specific RDA becomes almost impossible considering that the protein requirements will vary depending on age, physical condition, and health. Not to mention that your body also recycles endogenous proteins created by your body.[7] These proteins come from your saliva, gastric juices, pancreatic enzymes, and other body fluids that end up in your intestines. Another example I gave you before was the case of Dr. Fung's patients who did not need skin-removal surgery because their bodies, through autophagy, were "recycling" the extra skin after they lost large amounts of weight. That extra skin is broken down into various compounds, including amino acids that can then be arranged in different configurations to be used elsewhere.

Remember that your microbiome produced postbiotics? Well, postbiotics can be the famous SCFAs but can also be other metabolites like protein.[8] This means that by eating prebiotics, you might end up with an increased amount of protein in your gut. Can you see how all these variables make it so difficult to assign a specific protein consumption?

Your body can up-regulate or down-regulate the amount of protein that is absorbed from the intestinal tract after a meal depending on what is already going on inside, and how many amino acids you already have available. Researchers have shown that when you suddenly start eating high protein, your body burns more amino acids as fuel.[9] If things were as linear as "more protein, more muscle," we would not have an obesity issue, we would have a swollenness epidemic.

To get a clearer idea about numbers, I reviewed several articles and books. I found recommendations ranging from at least 2 grams of protein per pound (454 grams) of body weight, to as little as 3.5 grams of essential amino acids per person. WTF?!

Then we have the acceptable macronutrient distribution range (AMDR), established by the Food and Nutrition Board of the Institutes of Medicine (IOM) in 2005.[10] The AMDR is defined as "a range of intakes for a particular energy source that is associated with reduced risk of chronic diseases while providing adequate intakes of essential nutrients." According to the IOM, the AMDR is 10 percent to 35 percent of a person's total calorie intake. Honestly, this does not help us much either. It does not account for any physiological differences between individuals, and it gives such a wide range that for the same person to eat 100 grams or 350 grams of protein a day is completely accepted within this theory.

Should we just go for a high intake of protein, just to make sure we get enough and keep things simple? Unfortunately, chronically high protein intake has been associated with several health conditions. Excess protein stresses the kidneys and liver, and might lead to the accumulation of the by-product ammonia, which is toxic and can cause dangerous brain swelling.[11] Other studies have found that long-term high-protein diets may be linked with disorders of bone and calcium homeostasis, renal and liver function disorders, and higher risks of coronary artery disease and cancer.[12]

Considering all I read, I will have to go with Brad Pilon's recommendation of a range between 70 and 120 grams of protein a day.[13]

This recommendation incorporates a slightly higher number than the RDA but supports the work of other authors who recommend higher protein intakes, like that of Drs. Michael and Mary Dan Eades in their book *Protein Power* and several authors in the Paleo and keto diet niches. Some might think that an upper limit of 120 grams is not high enough. However, research suggests that protein intakes above 120 grams do not confer any additional benefits.[14]

What about people who are working out? Interestingly, there is growing evidence suggesting that resistance training boosts the recycling rate of the amino acids within your body.[15-17] What this means is that the longer you've been working out, the less likely you are to need extra dietary protein.

Please follow this 70-to-120-grams recommendation, but as you restore your metabolic health, feel free to adjust your protein consumption depending on how you feel. If you are craving more protein, eat more. If you feel you are going to puke if you have to eat one more egg, please eat less. Once you heal your body, it will talk to you. You just have to listen.

VEGAN VS. CARNIVORE

When writing a chapter on protein, it is impossible not to go into the whole vegan-versus-carnivore beef (yes, I guess that was a pun). Traditionally, people associate protein with animal products, but plants also contain protein. Protein gives plants structure and function. To be fair, all protein actually comes from plants. Animals ultimately get their protein from either eating plants or eating animals that eat plants. However, plant protein differs from animal protein in many ways, and that's what we are going to discuss.

Time to answer the ultimate question: Who is right? Plants or meat? Drumroll, please. . . . Looking at the evidence . . . both are right and both are wrong! Not the answer you were looking for, I know. But please stay with me and I'll explain what I mean by this.

Let's look back 100 years and analyze the evolution of the research on nutrition in the Western world. Before the 1940s, we used to see meat, fat, and animal foods as healthy, empowering foods. Then, around the 1950s, because of all the bad science and great marketing, the narrative changed to "animal products and fat are giving us heart disease and we all need to eat more plants and vegetable oils." Nonetheless, during the past decade, a scientific shift toward plant-based diets has boomed with plenty of research supporting this trend.

Who is right? "Old" science or "new" science? Before I answer that question, I feel it is important to realize that one needs to have the humility to be open to different points of view. Only by listening to opposing views and having open discussions can one grow and find a more truthful answer. Unfortunately, we live at a time when everything is taken to the extreme. You are either with me or against me. There is no middle ground. This is something you see in religion, politics, sports, etc. Nutrition is no different. Sadly, this has become such a cult-like phenomenon that both sides are losing their credibility because of the actions of some.

In an effort to be as impartial as possible, I read some of the "biggest" books on both sides of this argument. After my research, I was able to understand why we have such division. If you read a vegan book, you will never want to eat meat again. If you read a carnivore book, you will never want to eat a single plant again. But if you read both, like I did, you realize that both camps see the tree but miss the forest. What do I mean by that? Both cherry-pick studies and present only information that conveniently supports their cause.

For example, carnivore authors point out how all the antinutrients in plant foods are terrible for our health. But as we already discussed, when taken in the correct dosages, some of these plant antinutrients activate a hormetic response, which can make you healthier and prolong your life. At times, the meat proponents also focus too much on in vitro studies and forget how complex our bodies are and that a substance that can be harmful in our blood may never get to our blood because of its interaction with our microbiome.

On the other side, vegan authors grab on to large observational studies and assume that correlation equals causation. C'mon, guys, you're better than that! Yes, there are also interventional studies stating that meat leads to bad health outcomes, but in those same studies, there's no consideration of how the animals were raised, whether the meat was processed, or even how it was cooked. Think of green beans. We can agree that they are pretty harmless, right? Now, eat them fried in vegetable oils every day and see what happens!

The truth is that you can be healthy or sick on either a vegan or a carnivorous diet. Both diets are good in a way because they are supposed to eliminate a bunch of junk from your diet. If you follow the wholesome versions of these diets and get proper supplementation to compensate for some deficiencies, you can definitely be healthy. On the other hand, you can also be incredibly sick on either of them. Carnivores can eat a bunch of antibiotic-filled, grain-fed, arsenic-poisoned meats and other ultraprocessed animal products, while vegans can go nuts on ice cream, french fries, herbicide-infected GMO plants, and highly processed meat-replacement products made with soy and vegetable oils.

COGNITIVE DISSONANCE

When you have well-formed beliefs and someone presents evidence that contradicts what you believe in, this creates cognitive dissonance. Cognitive dissonance is the mental stress or discomfort you experience when confronted with new information that conflicts with your existing beliefs, ideas, or values. At times, we can be presented with superb research, but because it contradicts our opinion, we may refuse to accept it. We do this because suddenly not only are our beliefs being questioned (and no one likes to be wrong) but our entire identity is also getting a huge slap in the face.

Imagine that one day, a bunch of aliens land on earth and say that all the religious figures most religions believe in were actually aliens. And that their miracles were, in fact, caused by advanced technological equipment we did not comprehend. The whole world would fall apart because beliefs held for thousands of years would be shattered completely. Thousands of people would literally kill themselves because they could no longer identify their roles in this world.

This is an extreme example, but in a way, this is what's happening with the whole vegan-versus-carnivore dispute. Neither side wants to accept anything that challenges their beliefs. And they end up adopting the "if I ignore it, it doesn't exist" approach. Or, worse, attacking each other.

This was not an easy chapter to write, and for some of my readers, it won't be an easy chapter to read either. I understand that for some, this chapter might feel as if I am questioning not only your lifestyle but also you as a person. This might lead to frustration and anger. I get it. But please remember something. I don't know you, and I am not trying to attack you in any way. I wrote this book for my family and friends. For the people I love. I want them to be healthy, and I am just sharing the best evidence I've found. To track down and analyze the available data, I had to put my own beliefs aside.

That's all I ask. Please try to keep an open mind. If, after you've read all my points, they make sense to you, perfect! If this is too much for you to process, or you simply don't agree, I'm not here to convert you or to force you into believing what I do. I truly respect your decision. All I can say is that, beyond this chapter, there is still plenty of great information you can use to improve your health tremendously. Sound good? So, let's go right in!

THE VEGAN DIET

While everyone has different motivations, I think we can agree that there are some common beliefs people probably share to make such a lifestyle change. I, myself, followed a vegan diet for a while, so I understand that there are strong emotional reasons for making such a choice. Even though I no longer have the same views as before, I completely respect your point of view, and I am not here to judge. I am here to share my findings. That's it. What you do with this information is up to you.

In 2015, while I was in the initial stages of my healing journey, there was this tremendous boom in vegan nutrition. Books were being published and documentaries were blowing people's minds. I remember very clearly that there was one documentary in particular that really shook me and made me want to try a vegan diet. I decided to do this not only for my health but for the health of the planet. Many of my vegan and ex-vegan friends share similar stories. All made this move for very compassionate and honorable reasons. After all, according to those books and documentaries, beyond getting sick, we are also killing innocent animals that did not need to die, and we're destroying our planet, one steak at a time.

In summary, one can say the reasons behind adopting a vegan diet are nutritional, political, moral, or even religious ones. Obviously, I will not discuss religion here, but I think it is important to uncover some political and moral facts that you might not be aware of. But where I am going to focus most of my writing will be on the nutritional reasons. After all, this is a diet book. Let's start by seeing what our physiology has to say about this.

HUMAN EVOLUTION AND PLANT CONSUMPTION

During our time on earth, humans evolved differently than our primate cousins. As we saw before, as we favored nutrient-dense animal foods, our bodies changed dramatically. We evolved to have larger brains, shorter large intestines, and longer small intestines. This is justified by the expensive-tissue hypothesis proposed in 1995 by scientists Leslie Aiello and Peter Wheeler.[18] According to this hypothesis, as we ate more fatty animal foods, our brains could develop more and more. Bigger brains allowed us to develop in social, cultural, and technological complexity, which led to group hunting and the development of tools with which to kill and cook these animals, thus further promoting this feedback loop.

As the brain needed more and more power, the body had to cut what was not needed. Since we were no longer fermenting pounds and pounds of leaves, like our gorilla cousins, our long large intestine became dispensable. Use it or lose it, right? The large intestine shrank and the small intestine grew longer in order to absorb these nutrient-dense foods to power the brain.

Some authors say that since humans have flat teeth and do not have claws for hunting, we were not biologically designed to eat meat. What these same authors forget is that as we evolved into omnivorous animals, we never really needed those claws or sharp teeth because we had access to stone tools, arrows, and fire, for example. We could easily hunt and prepare foods without needing to change our anatomy to make that work.

Our bodies have evolved for us to be omnivorous beings. Let's look at our mouth, for example. We have canine teeth (for eating meat) and flat molars (for grinding plants).[19] We also have a highly acidic stomach and a long small intestine designed to process and extract nutrients from animal foods.[20] Even though we no longer have huge colons and are not able to process certain plant fibers the way our primate friends do, we can still digest vegetables and fruits. Biologically, there is no reason we should not be eating a mix of plants and animal foods. In fact, researchers believe that many of the hunter-gatherer tribes of the past might have eaten 45 percent to 65 percent of their calories from animal foods and the rest from plants.[21] Several studies show that these same hunter-gatherers (the ones that didn't get eaten by wild animals, of course) did not experience the chronic diseases we face today and could live quite long lives, even with no access to health care.[22-26]

Fast-forward a couple of thousand years and we have the work of Dr. Weston Price. One thing Dr. Price noted in his research was that not one culture was thriving eating an exclusively plant-based diet. In his words, "it is significant that I have as yet found no group that was building and maintaining good bodies exclusively on plant foods."[27] He also concluded that animal fats (especially from fatty cuts and organs) were a staple of the healthiest tribes and cultures around the world.

VEGETARIAN STUDIES

Independently of our evolution and traditional eating, it's also important to understand whether it is possible to be a healthy person while following a vegan diet. At a very fundamental level, our bodies require different quantities of different amino acids in order to fulfill our biological needs. Proteins from animal products are considered complete because they contain all nine essential amino acids. That is not the case with most vegetables, since they are missing a few amino acids. Nonetheless, it is perfectly possible to obtain all the essential amino acids by planning your meals and eating the right variety of plant foods. Research has also shown that vegetarian and nonvegetarian diets were equally good at building muscle as long as equal total protein intake was maintained.[28,29] And of course plants are also important because they contain dozens of vitamins, minerals, and phytochemicals associated with many health benefits.

Several epidemiologic studies claim that vegetarians are generally healthier and live longer than meat eaters, but as you know, correlation doesn't imply causation. We can easily imagine other health-related practices vegetarians adopt that are not being considered. Think about it. In the past few decades, who were the people following vegetarian lifestyles? They were the ones worried about their health and listening to the mainstream nutritional advice. Most likely, these same people were also following other health recommendations, like avoiding junk food, exercising, not smoking, reducing alcohol intake, meditating, and making sure they got adequate sleep. It is quite possible that it was the combination of some of these other factors leading to healthier lives and not the meat avoidance per se. To support this, studies show that health-conscious meat eaters have similar health outcomes to those of vegetarians.[30]

Another thing we have to consider is that vegan authors commonly select epidemiologic studies from Western researchers. If you look into Asian research, the picture is much different. In one study, researchers studied almost 300,000 people in Bangladesh, China, Japan, and South Korea for an average of 11 years and concluded that there was no evidence that meat and fish consumption would lead to a higher risk of mortality. Quite the opposite. They found that intake of red meat, poultry, and fish was associated with less cardiovascular-disease-related death in men and a lower risk of cancer mortality in women.[31]

VEGETARIAN ANECDOTAL EVIDENCE

One thing is certain: the boom of veganism also fed on the immense influence of TV and social media. For a while, every other day, there were news stories and posts about another celebrity adopting a vegan diet. These same celebrities would reach millions, sharing with the world how great they were feeling with the diet change. This, of course, had a huge influence on many people, especially the teens who idolize these famous people. I am not saying that these celebrities were lying about their health in any way or form. I am certain that they actually felt fantastic and were just trying to spread the word and help people. But I feel that it's important to note that most of these celebrities have nutritionists and coaches who are able to properly prepare their meals in a way that minimizes nutritional deficiencies. Not to mention that the rich and famous have the financial means to purchase the very best supplements on the market to address the nutritional gaps caused by a vegan diet. Sadly, many of their social media followers do not have the same means to make such transition in a healthy way.

You don't have to look hard to find recently "converted" vegetarians or vegans claiming to thrive on their new diet. They will tell you how they have lost all this weight, how their minds are sharp, and how their skin is clear. And while all this is true, it is very difficult for most people to maintain over the long term.

When I adopted a vegan diet, initially I shared this same feedback. I was losing some weight, and my skin really improved. But what I later found out is that I was improving not because of my avoidance of animal foods, but because I had eliminated all the processed foods I was eating before. I had a really positive experience for the first two months or so. Then, I noticed I was also losing muscle mass because I was not properly planning my meals to incorporate enough protein sources like legumes and soy. As I tried to fix that issue, my intestines inflated like a balloon. It was so bad that I am pretty confident that if I'd pressed my belly and squeezed my butt cheeks the right way, I could have played "Scotland the Brave" like a professional bagpiper. Fart jokes aside, I really started to feel terrible. My mind was getting foggy, I was feeling dumb, anxious, and depressed, and I had no energy whatsoever. Even my sex drive was in the gutter. I felt like a gay monk in a convent full of nuns.

Probably I wasn't going vegan enough. I needed to go harder! I studied my diet and found out that even with the best food arrangements, I was still missing several key micronutrients. The solution was supplementation. I ordered some of the supplements the vegan coaches recommended, but these products were incredibly expensive. I could not afford this long term. Then, I tried to buy cheaper supplements (the ones I could afford), and I felt slightly better but never like my old self. After about nine months, I had to give up. In my mind, I felt guilty because I thought I was being selfish and I was failing the planet (more on that soon). But I could no longer live like that.

There are thousands of stories like mine. Even some of those celebrities who months ago were promoting veganism have now given up on that change. Feel free to google it.

In her book *Sacred Cow*, nutritionist Diana Rodgers makes a fantastic point about all the teenagers being influenced to become vegans. She writes, "parents whose children announce that they're giving up meat often feel compelled to support them, yet they might not know the right way to follow a vegan diet. Most parents aren't educated enough on the importance of protein and critical micronutrients (vitamins and minerals) to help their kids maximize their nutrition when removing animal products."[32] This is really concerning. Most of these kids do not supplement or follow whole-food plant diets. They eat "fake meats" and processed carbs. It's easy to see why these teenagers then perform poorly in school, are always sick, and develop hormonal issues that affect their development. The harsh reality is that most people will have substantial difficulty staying healthy on a vegan diet over the long term.

NUTRITIONAL DEFICIENCIES OF A VEGAN DIET

Fortunately for our health, the narrative is finally changing. Recent studies have noted that there are several important deficiencies associated with a poorly planned vegan diet. The most notable deficiencies are of calcium, iodine, iron, zinc, vitamins B_{12} and D, omega-3 fatty acids, and protein.[33-40] Many people don't realize that they can have calcium, iron, and zinc deficiencies on a vegan diet, because in theory, several vegetables are great sources of these minerals. Unfortunately, these people do not know about antinutrients like oxalates and phytates that can dramatically reduce the absorption of these minerals. The minerals are in the plants, but the body can't absorb them.[41-46] Therefore, it's important to learn about these deficiencies and understand their health consequences.

B_{12} Deficiency

Probably the most problematic and most prevalent deficiency in vegetarians and vegans is that of vitamin B_{12}. Research suggests that about 60 percent of vegans and 40 percent of vegetarians might be deficient in B_{12}.[47,48] In adults, B_{12} deficiency is linked with depression, psychosis, and cognitive impairment.[49] In children, it may lead to severe, sometimes irreversible neuropsychological damage and developmental delay.[50,51]

Seaweed contains B_{12} analogues.[52] These are molecules that are chemically similar to real B_{12} but do not produce the effects that real B_{12} produces in the body. In fact, B_{12} analogues actually have detrimental effects. They have been called "antivitamin B_{12}."[53] And while fermented soy tempeh does contain the real vitamin B_{12}, you would need to take in 300 grams of tempeh daily just to reach the RDA.[54]

Iron Deficiency

Studies have shown that even vegans who do supplement can have iron deficiencies.[55] A 2019 article reveals that in New Zealand, iron deficiency hospitalizations doubled over the preceding decade as red meat consumption declined.[56] Some of the earliest signs of iron deficiency are fatigue, shortness of breath, lightheadedness, and headaches.[57,58] Iron deficiency is associated with chronic diseases such as type 2 diabetes, chronic kidney disease, IBD, congestive heart failure, and cancer.[59,60] In children, iron deficiency has been linked to developmental delay, impaired behavior, diminished intellectual performance, and decreased resistance to infection.[61]

Calcium Deficiency

As mentioned earlier, there are several vegetables that are rich in calcium, but they also contain antinutrients that block its absorption. This causes significant issues because people assume they are surpassing their RDA, when in truth they are far from reaching it. Just as a curiosity, research suggests that you'd need to eat five to six cups of cooked spinach to get the same amount of calcium found in a single glass of milk.[62] Studies show that vegans have 30 percent higher bone fracture rates than those who consume animal products.[63,64]

> **Neo Note: Veganism and Baby Development**
> In May 2019, a group of doctors from the Belgian Royal Academy of Medicine proposed that feeding babies a vegan diet should be illegal. These doctors stated that a vegan diet is unsuitable for unborn children, children, and adolescents, as well as pregnant and lactating women, because it creates serious deficiencies, including low protein, vitamins B_{12} and D, calcium, iodine, iron, zinc, and DHA.[65,66] Is it really worth it to cause harm to a child just to honor personal beliefs that might be based on questionable "facts"?

Other Nutrient Deficiencies

• *Carnitine:* This nutrient is exclusive to animal products. Carnitine has been shown to boost our ability to use fat for energy, possibly even facilitating ketosis.[67] Some studies suggest that because of carnitine's antioxidant properties, there is some promise in its application as a treatment option for women facing infertility disorders.[68]

• *Carnosine:* Another meat-exclusive nutrient, carnosine has been shown to enhance antioxidant activity in the brain and to protect it against oxidative damage.[69] Carnosine is also associated with a reduction in the formation of advanced glycation end products (AGEs).[70]

- **Choline:** Mainly found in meat, poultry, fish, dairy products, and eggs, choline is essential for proper methylation, which is needed for optimal health.[71,72] Deficiencies of choline are associated with nonalcoholic fatty liver disease, neurodegenerative diseases, and heart disease.[73] Choline deficiencies in pregnant women are linked to increased risks of neural tube defects and other fetal development complications.[74,75]

- **Creatine:** This substance is usually associated with muscle growth but also has important effects on brain health, as well as hormone optimization.[76,77] The body can produce some creatine, but for optimum levels, we need to get it from animal foods.

- **DHA:** Usually found in marine sources, DHA has many significant health effects, such as controlling inflammation and regulating proper cognitive development and cell membrane function.[78]

- **Taurine:** Apparently the best sources of taurine are "red bulls"—*get it?* Taurine can be found in chicken, beef, and salmon, for example. Taurine plays a vital role in energy metabolism.[79] That's why it's commonly used in energy drinks. It has also been shown to possess anti-inflammatory properties that improve diabetes and support the cardiovascular system.[80]

> **Neo Note: Meatless Diets and Mental Health**
>
> Several studies around the world suggested that in general, people who did not consume animal products were "less happy." Since this is a very controversial claim, let's take a look at some of the research. In a 2018 French study looking at more than 90,000 people, the researchers concluded that depressive symptoms were substantially more common in vegetarians.[81] In Germany, studies demonstrated higher rates of mental disorders in vegetarians.[82] In Finland and Sweden, researchers noticed that vegetarians were three to four times more likely to experience seasonal affective disorder.[83] And finally, in Australia, studies concluded that vegetarians were twice as likely to suffer from anxiety and depression, and were more likely to be taking prescription or nonprescription medications for mental health issues.[84,85]
>
> This all should be taken with a grain of salt since correlation does not mean causation. However, it's definitely to keep in mind.

HEALTH CONCERNS ABOUT EATING MEAT

Despite recent data supporting the consumption of animal products, we still have a very strong anti-meat message being spread in the Western world. This anti-meat movement's adherents present plenty of scientific evidence supporting their cause, but we have to question what they've been presenting to us. In fact, a 2019 systematic review of the research used in vegan propaganda concluded that the evidence against meat is of inferior quality, and that there is no actual evidence that would justify public health recommendations to limit meat consumption.[86]

The truth is that most of the misconceptions against meat come from bad science. There is one study in particular that has been referenced repeatedly. This is a 2015 study from the WHO's International Agency for Research on Cancer (IARC), through which a group of 22 scientists from 10 countries compiled a report after considering 800 epidemiological studies. The researchers concluded that red meat increased the risk of cancer and that it should be classified as "probably carcinogenic to humans."[87] Once this got to the media, it was game over!

First, all these studies were epidemiological (observational), and as you know, such studies show only correlation, not causation. Second, in 2018, it was uncovered that, from the total of 800 studies, the researchers considered only 14 studies in their review. Of these 14, only 6 showed some correlation, and of those 6, only 1 actually presented a *statistically significant* correlation.[88] In other words, they said that meat is probably carcinogenic because they saw that claim in a single observational study about colon cancer.[89] Good job, guys!

What about the other 799 studies? Well, there was that huge Asian epidemiological study we discussed earlier that concluded that meat eaters had a lower risk of cancer mortality.[90] Another forgotten piece was the large study of more than 60,000 vegetarians and nonvegetarians in the UK that concluded that rates of colon cancer were actually higher in vegetarians.[91] And what about the 2007 study that suggested that meat consumption was actually associated with *lower* rates of oxidative stress and inflammation?[92] I could continue dumping studies on you, but I'm sure you get the point. Sloppy research can have dangerous consequences.

In case you still have any doubts after all this information, please consider a 2019 review of 61 studies on a total of four million people that found no link between eating meat and higher risks of disease or death.[93]

COMMON ARGUMENTS AGAINST MEAT FROM VEGAN AUTHORS

Many authors supporting a vegan diet share several common arguments against eating meat. Although I won't focus on every single one of them, I would like to briefly debunk the main ones.

AGEs

It's said that consumption of meat leads to higher accumulation of advanced glycation end products. AGEs may be produced in meat through sugar-protein bonding (the Maillard reaction) that occurs during cooking. This same reaction also occurs when you're toasting bread, but you don't hear anyone doing TED Talks about toast causing cancer. The vast majority of AGEs are formed in your body because of chronic carbohydrate consumption, as we saw before. In fact, research has shown that vegetarians, because they consume more carbs, have more circulating AGEs than people who eat meat.[94] Also, cooking meat with acidic ingredients, such as vinegar, tomato juice, or lemon juice, seems to reduce AGE production by up to 50 percent.[95]

Polycyclic Aromatic Hydrocarbons (PAHs) and Heterocyclic Amines (HCAs)

When meat is cooked at high temperatures, PAHs and HCAs are produced. Chargrilled chicken breasts in particular can have high levels of these compounds.[96,97] Research has shown that high levels of PAHs and HCAs in the body substantially increase the risk of several cancers.[98] This is why many authors still associate meat with cancer. But here's the thing. Research also shows that our bodies have plenty of mechanisms to deal with these substances in moderate quantities.[99] And only chronic high levels are suggested to increase the risk of cancer.[100,101] In other words, we would need to eat charred, burned, and massively overcooked meats with some frequency.

Science also shows us that there are several ways to minimize the formation of PAHs and HCAs. Strategies such as marinating the meat (e.g., in beer, Korean red pepper paste, white tea, or lemon) for as little as 30 minutes, continually turning meat over the heat source, and avoiding overcooking have been shown to substantially decrease the formation of these compounds.[102-107]

As a final note, I think it's important to share with you that whenever anything is cooked at high temperatures, be it coffee, grains, bread, or other foods, carcinogenic compounds are formed. It's not just meat. In truth, I would be a lot more concerned about grilled vegetables than grilled meats, since we tend to overgrill the veggies.

mTOR

Next on the list is mTOR (remember? mammalian target of rapamycin). Some authors suggest that eating meat can lead to an overactivation of mTOR, which can then trigger accelerated aging, cellular growth, and possibly cancer development. We've already seen that keeping mTOR levels on the lower side might be beneficial for longevity, but this does not mean that mTOR is bad per se. I also explained how mTOR was important in protecting muscle mass, for example. During childhood and puberty, mTOR activation is essential for proper development. In adulthood, I can compare it with insulin. It works the best when it is kept on the lower end but with occasional spikes. You don't want to have constantly low mTOR signaling.

Why do researchers overblow its effects? It's mostly because of some studies on people with Laron syndrome. In a nutshell, individuals with this syndrome have lower mTOR signaling. And because they also have an incredibly low incidence of cancers, it's said that lower mTOR signaling is the way to go. Unfortunately, people with Laron syndrome also have serious growth deficits (dwarfism), low blood sugar, and sleep disturbances.[108] I really have a hard time with this argument. I don't believe we have to choose between growth deficits and muscle atrophy, and cancer. In my view of things, if you are healthy, mTOR will promote health. If you're sick, mTOR can promote disease. Not to mention that this entire theory on mTOR with meat is fundamentally wrong. mTOR takes part in the anabolic signaling process of cells in response to four signals. These are insulin-like growth factor-1 (IGF-1), insulin, protein (mostly mediated through the amino acid leucine, which is present in larger percentage in meat), and exercise.[109]

Let's ignore meat protein and exercise for a second and focus on the other two. IGF-1 is produced in response to eating, sleeping, and exercising. Insulin, as you know, is triggered by protein but not as much as by carbohydrate consumption. If we were to really make a big case out of this mTOR situation, we would also need to make a recommendation against carbs, sleeping, and exercising. In fact, activation of mTOR increase by insulin is much stronger, and lasts three to four times as long, as its activation by leucine.[110] So tell me. Why are we vilifying meat protein? Are we also supposed to stop exercising and sleeping? Case closed!

TMAO

Finally, we have the case of trimethylamine-N-oxide (TMAO). This argument has been gaining more popularity as of late because researchers found that bacteria in our digestive system can convert carnitine (found in red meat) into TMAO.[111] Since TMAO had been previously associated with atherosclerosis and metabolic disease, it was assumed that eating red meat would lead to plaque-lined arteries. Again, there are several things wrong with these conclusions.

For starters, most of the studies associating TMAO with cardiovascular disease are observational. As you know, correlation isn't causation. Furthermore, there are studies suggesting that it's much more likely that the high insulin levels (from those suffering from metabolic diseases) are driving the exacerbated production of TMAO (and increased risk of cardiovascular disease) rather than TMAO causing the issue.[112]

Second, many species of fish have TMAO in higher levels than the ones presented in these initial studies.[113] I've heard no one associating fish consumption with atherosclerosis. Then, too, we have the fact that gut bacteria can also ferment vegetables into TMAO.[114,115] As a matter of fact, humans eating fish and vegetables have been observed to have higher levels of TMAO than those eating meat.[116]

If you are still concerned about TMAO, please note that there are polyphenols in red wine and olive oil that suppress your microbiome's ability to make this compound.[117,118] In other words, just eat your steak with some olive oil and a glass of red wine, and you'll be okay.

I tried not to go into full science mode and debunk all the concerns presented in vegan-diet-promoting books, but I believe I've properly addressed the main ones. If you have more questions about the topics mentioned above, or even about iron oxidation and Neu5Gc, I recommend reading Dr. Saladino's *The Carnivore Code*, since it goes into detail explaining these theories.

CARNIVORE DIET

Meat is an incredibly nutrient-rich food, and eating it is important for a healthy human. In fact, because of all the benefits associated with meat consumption, some people are choosing to completely stop eating plants and eat only animal foods. This Carnivore Diet has been getting a lot of attention lately, and many authors have shared incredible health transformations from people adopting this lifestyle. And it's easy to understand why this diet can be very powerful, since it is the ultimate elimination diet. Not only are you eliminating all the processed foods, but you are also avoiding all the antinutrients associated with plants.

Many of these authors point out that some ancestral populations were carnivorous. While I agree that there were indeed several *mostly* carnivorous peoples, there is also evidence that they would take advantage of some plant foods. For example, the Gaucho would supplement their diet with yerba maté; the Masai, Rendille, and Samburu also consumed herbs, tree barks, fruits, and tubers; the Canadian Inuit ate not just animal foods but wild berries, lichens, and sea vegetables; and the Russian Chukotka also consumed local roots, leafy greens, berries, or seaweed.[119-122] While there are more examples, my idea here is not to say that some carnivore authors are being imprecise, but to say that plant foods have their place in a healthy diet.

There are several low-sugar fruits and vegetables that, besides tasting really good, also contain useful vitamins, minerals, antioxidants, fats, and protein. By properly preparing some of these plants, we can make them more digestible and decrease their antinutrient content, safely taking advantage of some of their nutrients. Indeed, there are nutrients—such as vitamins B_9, C, and E, magnesium, manganese, potassium, selenium, and betaine—that are more abundant in plants than in most animal sources. And, as we've seen before, many plants also contain plenty of "good" antinutrients with powerful antioxidant effects.

Moreover, in my opinion, being limited to a carnivorous diet long term doesn't make us as antifragile as we can be. Even though there are obvious benefits from a temporary elimination diet like the carnivore diet, staying on it constantly will make our bodies less resilient in dealing with plant foods. With time, your body won't be able to digest them properly or to neutralize some of their antinutrients. Then, if you eat any plant food later, you will have an exacerbated reaction and feel terrible. Don't get me wrong, if you want to commit to never eating a single plant food ever again, sure, you will feel good, and you won't have to go through these "plant incidents." But you have to really commit!

I can't read your mind, so I can only share my vision of things. And I honestly do not want to make such a commitment. I enjoy some plant foods and the benefits they bring me. I enjoy being with family and friends and being able to eat most of the foods they prepared with love for me. I do not want to be the person they feel bad about inviting since they don't know what to cook for me. I continue to believe that the best long-term option is to remain an omnivore.

But let me emphasize *long-term*. Following a carnivore diet as a therapeutic tool can be incredibly healing, and I'm all in favor of it. At the end of this chapter, I recommend some fantastic books on this subject in case you're interested in learning more.

This is my take on eating meat. Nutritionally, there is no question that a diet-conscious omnivore can be far healthier than most vegetarians and vegans. Now it's time to move on to other ethical concerns against meat consumption. Although I won't go into detail about the morality of eating meat, as someone who did follow a vegan diet, I feel it is important to briefly present that side of the story. Sadly, a side that most of us have never learned about.

DIET AND DEATH

One reason I adopted a vegan diet was the idea of not having to "take an innocent life." I felt that by choosing a vegan diet I would not cause more harm, and that really made me feel good about that decision. The truth is that CAFOs have no consideration for animal welfare, and their practices are nothing less than cruel. There is no question that we all should fight for all animals to be raised in appropriate conditions, and for them to have good lives and humane deaths. We need to make our politicians accountable for what they are allowing to happen in farming operations and slaughterhouses. We have to make a stand!

I understand that some choose to make their stand by eliminating meat from their diets. At one time I also thought that was the best way to support this fight. But in order to have a truly educated debate on the morality of eating animals, we need to better understand food production and the alternative means of raising animals. Most of us are disconnected from this reality, but it was once common (and it still is in some places) for families to raise their own animals and have small vegetable gardens. Ruminant animals were pasture raised, and pigs and chickens would take over the backyard. These animals were raised with respect and were killed humanely. The families did not use any chemicals to grow their vegetables, and the manure from the animals made for healthy soils and nutrient-rich plants.

Unfortunately, this all changed with the introduction of industrial farming and industrial agriculture. And what most people don't realize is that industrial agriculture causes more death than animal farming.

As the world modernized, we lost the connection with our roots and forgot some basic facts. Life is not possible without death. No matter what you choose to eat, something has to die in order for you to be fed. Most people who choose to eat only plants have noble reasons, but unfortunately they also have blood on their hands. Industrial agricultural processes like digging, stirring, overturning, shoveling, hoeing, and raking destroy vast areas of land that animals previously called home. Plowing and harvesting directly kill millions of small mammals, lizards, and snakes. According to a 2011 research article, it was estimated that the production of grains killed 25 times more animals per kilogram of usable protein than red meat.[123] Additionally, from 1961 to 1975, the Environmental Protection Agency reported 31 million fish deaths because of pollution, of which 6 percent were directly linked to agriculture.[124] Pesticides are also linked to millions of bird deaths yearly.[125] Then we have the so-called secondary deaths of animals that die because of eating other, poisoned animals. These are completely impossible to measure.

Some will say that we cannot compare the killing of the small mammals, birds or reptiles to the death of a cow or a pig because the latter are such intelligent beings. What I can say is that during my lifetime I've met a lot of "not-so-clever" people and never thought it was okay to kill them because they weren't intelligent enough. As human beings, we are hypocrites. We have the god complex and think we can determine what should live and what should die. But who are we to say that the life of a mouse that died in a field is less important than the life of a cow? We really need to reflect on our beliefs.

Neo Note: Plants Have "Feelings"

Not-so-fun fact: Plants know when they are being eaten, and, as you can imagine, they don't get very excited about it. Research has found that certain plants detect the vibrations made by insects feeding on them. The plants then try to fight these bugs by producing mildly toxic mustard oils and delivering them to the leaves to deter the predators.[126] Another example is the *Mimosa pudica* plant. This plant defends itself from being eaten by folding its leaves.[127]

Plants also have circadian rhythms, just like we do. In fact, they have a gene that lets them know when it's daytime, so they can produce more natural insecticide to keep bugs away.[128]

I recognize that I could easily cut a plant from the ground but would have a hard time killing an animal. But once again, we also have to accept that plants are alive and we are choosing to kill them.

Before we move on to other subjects, I still have to answer the question about our planet. I'm certain that most people have seen documentaries, or at least read articles, about how animal farming is destroying the planet. We all know that every time a cow farts, we are one step closer to doomsday. At least that's what we've been told. But are things really like that? Or have we once again been told an incomplete (and possibly incorrect) story? I am truly concerned about the planet, and what I am going to share with you will most definitely surprise you!

MORAL RESPONSIBILITY

Let's go straight to the point. Cows do not fart greenhouse gases. They actually burp them. In reality, it's only one gas, methane. Cows belch methane as part of their digestive process. It's because of this that the mainstream media has deemed livestock to be a more serious factor for global warming than fossil fuels. This message has spread so widely that people think that going plant-based will save the planet. If you've read this far, you already know that unfortunately most of this mainstream information lacks proper scientific evidence. Is this the case with cows aggravating global warming?

Methane is only one of the three greenhouse gases (GHG) associated with agriculture. The other ones are carbon dioxide (CO_2), which is released through plowing soil, cutting trees, and burning fossil fuels, and nitrous oxide (N_2O), which mostly comes from the use of fertilizers.

The media have focused on methane because it has a bigger greenhouse warming potential (GWP) than CO_2. Methane has a GWP of 28 to 36, while CO_2 has a GWP of 1. What the media don't tell us is that N_2O has a GWP of 265 to 298—far higher than that of methane.[129] But as you can imagine, there are strong financial interests behind the chemical industry producing these fertilizers, so let's blame the cows!

Then things get a little trickier. It seems these gases remain in the atmosphere for different amounts of time. According to the Environmental Protection Agency, methane lasts about 10 years, N_2O about 100 years, and CO_2, and I quote, "thousands of years."[130] That's right, we are so worried about a cow burping, when the burp vanishes in a decade while CO_2 stays there for thousands of years.

Industrial farming with manure lagoons is a substantial source of methane, but manure lagoons are mostly from the pork, egg, and dairy industries. Independently of that, as I've said before, CAFOs should be completely forbidden. They are an abomination for animals, for our health, and for the planet. On the other hand, properly managed pasture raising of cattle tells a completely different story. Let me give you an example. It's estimated that before the mid-1800s, in North America, there were 30 million to 60 million bison, more than 10 million elk, 30 million to 40 million white-tailed deer, 10 million to 13 million mule deer, and 35 million to 100 million pronghorn and caribou.[131-135] That represents a whole lot of belching. However, it's believed that during this time, methane emissions represented only about 82 percent of the emissions from farmed and wild ruminants.[136] How is that possible?!

The truth is that the information disseminated in those documentaries and shared by the media is based on bad science. In fact, most of the bad press cows have received came from a 2006 report from the United Nations' Food and Agriculture Organization (FAO) titled *Livestock's Long Shadow*.[137] In summary, the report stated that livestock produced 18 percent of all GHG emissions, which was more than produced by the transportation sector. Ooh la. The media had a field day with this one! Not surprisingly, when other researchers looked at the data, in particular how it was gathered, they found serious methodological errors. It was so bad that even the FAO released updated reports with far different numbers. One of those reports, released in 2008, was titled "Belching Ruminants, a Minor Player in Atmospheric Methane."[138] Can you detect the "subtle" change in direction? In this new report, researchers concluded that cattle had been unfairly blamed for their methane emissions as a significant contributor to GHG emissions. More recently, a 2018 study led by NASA concluded that the largest contributors to methane are fossil fuels, fires, and wetlands (e.g., rice farming).[139] That's right. Production of rice is far worse for global warming than ruminant animals are.

Before we finish, please don't forget that N_2O from fertilizer use has a GWP of 265 to 298, and it lasts 100 years in the atmosphere. And even though carbon dioxide has a GWP of 1, it will accumulate in the atmosphere for thousands of years. So, yes, some of the carbon dioxide creating the greenhouse effect has possibly been there since the time aliens built the pyramids. #justmessingwithyou

My point is, we can blame climate change on many things, but blaming ruminants is not knowing what really is going on.

INDUSTRIAL FOOD PRODUCTION

Probably I'm too much of an optimist, but I believe we are finally seeing the beginning of the end of CAFOs. It might still take a couple of years, but governments across the globe have started to introduce new legislation to better regulate these operations and hopefully start shutting them down. Animals raised in CAFOs are made sick with their unnatural diets of corn, soy, ground-up animal parts, chicken excrement, candy, antibiotics, and hormones. Not only are these businesses destroying the health of the animals, but they're destroying the health of the people working there, and that of the millions feeding on these sick animals. I said this before, and I'll say it again: we all need to stand together and stop industrial animal farming.

But, to be fair, it's not just animal farming. It's also industrial agriculture. As we've seen before, tillage practices are destroying our soil, and the heavy use of chemical fertilizers, pesticides, and herbicides is killing plants and animals, polluting our rivers and oceans, and making us sick. How much more of our topsoil will we turn to dust while insisting on these destructive monocrop agricultural systems?

REGENERATIVE AGRICULTURE

Fortunately, there is still plenty we can do to turn this around. One of those things is supporting regenerative agriculture. Regenerative agriculture is guided by several principles such as restoring a healthy relationship between people and land, building soil health, reducing or eliminating the use of harmful chemicals, growing diverse crops, managing livestock in a holistic and humane way, using resources innovatively and efficiently, and maintaining equitable labor practices. Not only is this good for humans, animals, and plants, but it's also great for the planet. As we are now learning, when the soil is healthy, plants can sequester greater amounts of CO_2 from the environment.[140,141] Using methods like adaptive multi-paddock (AMP) grazing, in which ruminant animals pasture on grass and are moved frequently, allows plants to recover and protect the soil. Pasturing animals this way also serves to enrich the soil with organic matter and increase its carbon-carrying capacity.[142] In fact, the AMP system results in a net GHG decline of 3.59 metric tons of carbon per hectare, per year.[143] What this means is that instead of sending CO_2 into the atmosphere, the plants and soil are actually absorbing substantial quantities of it.

A study by White Oak Pastures reviewed the entire life cycle of 100 percent grass-fed beef at the company's regenerative farm in Georgia and concluded that the net total carbon footprint was the equivalent of −3.5 kilograms of CO_2 per kilogram of fresh meat.[144] In other words, by raising animals in a regenerative fashion, we are actually reducing the carbon footprint. This is even better than the numbers claimed by "climate-saving" Beyond Burger and soybean production, which averages 2 to 4 kilograms of CO_2 per kilogram of product.

Another meta-analysis studying carbon sequestration in soils from livestock grazing in South American countries concluded that grazing lands not only will sequester the carbon from the farm but can even partially or totally offset the carbon from nearby urban emissions.[145] After reviewing 80 science-based methods to mitigate climate change, the NGO Project Drawdown (an organization that identifies the world's most effective ways to "draw down" carbon from the atmosphere) reached the conclusion that regenerative agricultural practices are the number one solution to reverse climate change.[146]

Regenerative agriculture goes beyond climate change. These practices of using grazing animals can increase plant diversity, shrink bare spots in pastures, and trigger the return of pollinators, birds, and other wildlife. Using animals in regenerative agriculture also allows the lands to be fertilized naturally, eliminating the need for chemical fertilizers and their disastrous consequences.

As Dr. Mark Hyman states in *The Pegan Diet*, "regenerative agriculture is recognized as critical to achieving food security, reversing climate change, restoring biodiversity, and improving health. The UN estimates if we converted two million of our five million hectares of degraded agricultural lands to regenerative farming, we could stop climate change for 20 years."[147]

We still have some way to go, since regenerative practices represent less than 1 percent of all agricultural production. But the data leaves no doubt. Regenerative practices with the use of grazing animals help us build topsoil, produce natural fertilizer, conserve water, replenish ecosystems, and sequester greenhouse gases. Whether you choose to eat meat or not, the path is clear. We need more animals grazing this earth.

THE BENEFITS OF PASTURE-RAISED ANIMALS

As the old saying goes, you are what you eat. A more accurate saying would be "you are what you eat and also what your food ate." I think it's easy to figure out that the meat of a cow raised on pesticide-covered GMO corn and pumped with hormones will be substantially less nutritious than the meat of a cow who had a happy life and grazed on organic pastures. Same applies to its milk, or in the example of a chicken, its eggs. Not only are you doing the right thing for animal welfare and the environment by choosing pasture-raised animal products, but you are also doing yourself a huge nutritional favor.

Research has shown that pasture-raised meats are far superior to "conventional" meats, since they pack higher levels of vitamins A, B_1, B_2, and

E; minerals; omega-3s; CLA omega-6s; omega-7s; and the antioxidants catalase, glutathione, and superoxide dismutase.[148-150] A 2021 study found that pasture-raised meat contained phytochemicals such as carotenoids, phenols, terpenoids, and antioxidants with anti-inflammatory, anticarcinogenic, and cardioprotective effects.[151] In that same study, it was seen that the dairy from these cows carried up to 23 times more powerful anticarcinogenic, antiviral, antioxidant, and anti-inflammatory compounds called monoterpenes than that of conventional dairy cows. Finally, these researchers also uncovered that the dairy from goats raised on pasture have the same number of phenolic compounds as green tea and contain the phytonutrients quercetin (found in onions) and caffeic acid (found in coffee), which have strong anti-inflammatory and immune-boosting properties.

Pasture-raised animal products are not only more nutritious but also safer. Commercial cuts of conventional meats have been found to be more frequently contaminated by E. coli and other pathogenic bacteria.[152] In addition, the bacteria on conventionally raised cattle demonstrate a greater resistance to antibiotics.[153] What this means is that by eating conventionally raised meats, you have a higher chance of developing food poisoning and experiencing more serious symptoms than usual.

As a final note, please be aware that there are farmers who start cattle with grass and then "finish them" with grain to fatten them up before slaughter. Unfortunately, this completely reverses the superior nutritional content usually found in grass-fed meats. Research shows that just 80 days of grain feeding was enough to destroy the omega-3 and CLA content of the beef. The longer the animal ate grains, the lower the quality of the meat.[154] It is important to make sure that the beef is not only grass fed but grass finished.

Neo Note: The Different Meat Terminologies

It's very easy to get confused by all the meat terminologies used by stores when you are trying to buy some healthy protein. It would be impossible for me to give you all the different terms, because they vary from country to country. That being said, I am going to present the ones that are most commonly used.

Pasture-raised: This is the gold standard for superior animals, dairy, and eggs. *Pasture-raised* means that the animals were raised outdoors, which is better for the land, the animals, and you. The animals eat what they are supposed to eat, and it shows in their nutritional content.

Grass-fed: It's quite common to think this is the same thing as pasture raised, but *grass-fed* tells us only that the animals were fed grass; most likely they were not raised in the outdoors. Within this category, it's important to distinguish just grass-fed from 100 percent grass-fed or grass-fed/grass-finished beef.

Organic: This simply means that the animal was fed organic food. If the package does not clearly say that it is organic pasture-raised or organic grass-fed, please be aware that the animal was fed grains. Organic grains are better than conventional grains, but they should never be a part of a ruminant's diet.

Natural: There are several variations of the term *natural.* Please stay away from these. Producers use these meaningless terms just for marketing, to trick consumers into believing they're buying something healthy when in fact they're buying the conventional stuff.

What should you aim for? Look for pasture-raised, 100 percent grass-fed and grass-finished beef, ideally organic and from local farms.

PROTEIN SOURCES
Grazing Animals

My favorite source of protein is pasture-raised animals like cows, lambs, goats, and bison. These red meats have healthy fat in them and are filled with vitamins (A, B_1, B_2, and E), iodine, iron, zinc, antioxidants, carnitine, carnosine, CLA, creatine, omega-3s, and taurine. The cholesterol in the meat also helps us absorb and use vitamin D for many processes in our bodies.

Please remember that processed meat products are bad for your health and you should stay away from them. It's because of them that meat still has a bad reputation. But it's not just processed meats. Avoid preseasoned boxed meats, since you have no idea what was added. Focus on the real stuff: some good organic (if possible), pasture-raised meat.

If you have a limited budget, please favor quality meat instead of organic vegetables. It's far more important to choose pastured animals that did not eat grains filled with pesticides and herbicides. If the animals were raised on toxic grains or grasses, these toxins accumulate in their fat as they grow (the principle of bioaccumulation). In turn, the vegetables will contain lower levels than meats do because of the absence of bioaccumulation of toxins. Also, it's essential that you trust the farmer you are getting your meat from or, if buying in store, aim organic. It is well worth the difference.

I understand that the higher cost is a common concern. I could say what most authors say, which goes something along the lines of "you can pay a higher price for organic now or pay a much higher price for being sick later." Although I agree with that 100 percent, I can see how people dismiss clichés. But this is more than a cliché; it's a matter of putting things in perspective. When you compare the prices of organic, grass-fed beef with those of some pre-seasoned and processed meats, you can easily see that per pound, they cost about the same. Not to mention that in most countries, the ultraprocessed fake meats like Beyond Burger are even more expensive. And I don't see many people complaining about fake meat's price.

Additionally, as author Diana Rodgers says in *Sacred Cow*, "Per ounce, organic grass-finished beef is cheaper than many common foods like potato chips, red wine, name-brand cookies, popular coffee drinks, donuts, and even fresh strawberries."[155]

As more and more people buy pastured beef, the prices will go down. This happens because this consumer preference will trigger many farmers to switch to regenerative practices in order to stay in business. A perfect example is organic produce. Ten years ago, it was incredibly expensive. Now, because of increased availability, the price is much lower.

Quite honestly, the best way for you to buy affordable pasture-raised meat is to find a local farmer. The farmer probably will not have official organic certifications because of their cost (and the bureaucracy involved), but once you get to the farm, you can easily understand whether the animals are being raised humanely on pastures free from pesticides. Buying in bulk is also a great option to save money.

Pork

Pastured ruminant meats are nutritionally superior to pork or poultry, but that doesn't mean you shouldn't eat pork and poultry as well. Pork is a good source of protein and also has several important B vitamins and minerals. The biggest issue with pork is its fat. In the wild, pigs will eat anything they can find: grass, roots, leaves, grubs, nuts, fruits, and insects. This type of diet creates a "healthier" fat. In contrast, factory-farmed pigs are fed almost exclusively on corn and soybean meal. As you now know very well, this leads to the accumulation of very high levels of oxidized omega-6s and other toxins in their fat. Additionally, factory-farmed pigs have higher levels of fecal matter contaminations (that's right, there might be poop in it) and higher chances of *Salmonella* poisoning.[156-158]

The good news is that this changes substantially with truly pastured pigs. Depending on their diet, these pigs can actually be fine sources of healthy omega-3s and MUFAs. In countries like Portugal and Spain, we can still find farmers who follow the traditional methods of feeding pastured pigs with acorns. It's a true win-win. The pigs love them, and their fat profile improves substantially.[159]

In my opinion, it is healthier to favor ruminant animals, but pastured heritage pork is still a fantastic option. Maybe just don't eat it as frequently.

Poultry

Who doesn't love chicken? The tuna of the land. *Or is it the other way around?!* Unfortunately, chickens are one of the most "poisoned" meats in stores. Conventional chickens are pumped up with corn and antibiotics so they can grow and get fat in record time. In the US, commercial broiler chickens are slaughtered at an average of 47 days of age and a weight of 6.26 pounds (2.8 kilograms).[160] In the EU it's not much different, with an average slaughter age of 42 days and a weight of 5.51 pounds (2.5 kilograms).[161] Over the past 80 years, chickens have been growing so much faster that they reach slaughter in half the time while weighing more than before.[162]

Most of these birds are raised in CAFOs and live in terrible conditions. In the US, less than 1 percent of chickens are raised as "free range."[163] And even the free-range ones might not have better lives. The USDA defines *free range* as a "system that provides access to the outdoors," but this term is unregulated.[164] In simple terms, this means that you can just have a tiny door to the outside open for 5 minutes a day, and that still counts as free range. These animals live in crammed warehouses with very unsanitary conditions. It's no surprise that they bear higher risks of carrying dangerous pathogens like *Salmonella* and *E. coli*.[165]

To add to that, studies estimate that about 70 percent of the nine billion broiler chickens produced annually in the US are fed a diet containing roxarsone, which is an arsenic-based drug.[166] Factory chickens and pigs routinely receive these arsenic-based drugs to make them grow faster and improve the color of the meat. In humans, chronic arsenic exposure causes lung, bladder, and skin cancers, and it has been linked with cardiovascular disease, type 2 diabetes, cognitive deficits, and adverse pregnancy outcomes.[167-172]

It's also no secret that workers in chicken CAFOs often experience terrible working conditions. Not to mention the already-known impact these operations have on the environment. For everyone's health and to protect the environment, please stay away from conventionally raised poultry. This also applies to any all-natural, vegetarian-fed, or grain-fed labels you find for poultry or eggs.

On the other hand, truly free-range, heritage chickens are a different story. They can eat their preferred diet of grass, leaves, and bugs, which makes them happier and healthier. Although inferior to ruminant meat, poultry presents good levels of B vitamins and minerals like phosphorus and selenium. Poultry doesn't have as much fat as red meats, but it still contains saturated fat and MUFAs like palmitoleic acid, which has significant antimicrobial properties—probably one of the reasons chicken soup has traditionally been given to fight colds.[173-175]

Once again, eat poultry in moderation and choose the pastured variety. By the way, I used several chicken examples, but please note that this applies to all poultry (turkeys, geese, ducks, etc.).

Eggs

Eggs are one of the most complete and nutrient-rich foods nature offers. It's easy to see why, since the egg has to contain all the nutrients the embryo needs to develop and thrive. The yolk is rich in fats, good cholesterol, proteins, and minerals, as well as choline, lecithin, lutein, phospholipids, and zeaxanthin.[176-179] Another great thing about eggs is that you can buy the ones that come from organic, pasture-raised chickens at still very affordable prices. Eggs from hens raised on pasture provide as much as 10 times more omega-3s than conventional eggs, and they also pack higher levels of vitamins A, B$_9$, B$_{12}$, D, and E.[180-182]

Please remember that most of the nutrients are in the yolk, so, to preserve them, aim to eat yolks either lightly cooked or, better yet, raw. Frying or boiling oxidizes fats, denatures proteins, and destroys several micronutrients.

Yes, eating raw eggs carries some risks (e.g., Salmonella contamination). But, to be fair, this applies to most raw foods. As you might be aware, even lettuce has been recalled a bunch of times in the US due to bacterial contamination. This is another reason why you should get your eggs from regenerative practices and not from "egg factories."

Some people, especially children, have egg allergies, though. The albumin in egg whites seems to be the main allergen and can lead to symptoms such as watery eyes, hives, rashes, redness, swelling, stomach cramps, vomiting, and asthma.[183] If you have a sensitivity to chicken eggs, try eggs from other birds, like ducks or quail. Studies support this, since it's been shown that people respond differently to distinct types of poultry eggs.[184]

Neo Note: Stubbornly Afraid of Eggs

I know some beliefs are hard to overcome. Many people still avoid eating eggs regularly because they think it will increase their "bad cholesterol" and contribute to heart disease. I hope by now I've done enough to show you that these cholesterol myths are BS, but in case you still have some concerns about eggs, I just wanted to give you some data. Several studies and meta-analyses have refuted all claims linking egg consumption with increased risk of coronary artery disease.[185-187] To add to that, another study has shown that individuals who eat more eggs have a 25 percent lower risk of having a hemorrhagic stroke.[188] Finally, a 2016 study done in Finland concluded that egg intake was not linked with higher coronary artery disease risk, even in ApoE4 carriers (people with a genetic predisposition).[189] That's *eggcellent* news!

Dairy

Dairy is one of the most controversial topics in nutrition, but I'll try to keep this as simple as possible. One common thing you read everywhere is that we are the only species that continues to drink milk beyond childhood, or something like that. There are such brilliant arguments against dairy, but this one is just lazy. We are also the only species that drives cars and builds houses, and I don't see people complaining about that. The truth is that dairy has been in our diets for a very long time and it was never known for causing issues, but over the past few decades dairy has slowly become one of the most inflammatory foods out there. In fact, milk consumption has been dubbed a contributing factor to a wide range of conditions, ranging from acne and autism to diabetes and MS.[190-196] Is it possible that we have another "gluten situation" here?

Milk can be broken down into four main components: water, protein, sugar, and fat. Dairy sensitivities are usually linked to the sugars or proteins. I'm sure you have heard about lactose intolerance. Lactose is the main sugar in dairy, and when people are missing the enzyme lactase, they cannot digest it and thus can develop inflammatory symptoms. Besides lactose, another common trigger is casein, which is the main protein in dairy.

Milk Processing

Back in the day, the milk your great-grandparents enjoyed differed greatly from the milk we buy in stores. For starters, the cows producing milk had much different diets and lives. Second, the milk did not suffer the processing it does today. In fact, in countries with traditionally high milk consumption like Norway, Sweden, and Denmark, the switch from raw to processed milk can justify the substantial increases in the rates of osteoporosis and degenerative arthritis.[197]

In truth, we have ruined milk. When I wrote "processed milk," I was referring to the pasteurization of milk. Pasteurization is a process made famous by the illustrious Louis Pasteur in 1856. As you probably guessed, it was named after him, but there are records of similar processes being used by Chinese cultures as far back as 1117.[198] The pasteurization process was introduced and sold as a way to reduce the risk of milk contamination and to make it safer for human consumption. But some authors contend that there were other interests behind this. Pasteurization allows small family farms to produce milk like the "big guys." Since all milk is being boiled and "disinfected," sanitary measures and milk quality are no longer as important. This allows farmers to have more cows in the same space, and to use grains as the cows' main diet. But while pasteurization reduces the risk of milk contamination, it also kills off the beneficial probiotics in the milk, destroys digestive enzymes, and denatures milk proteins. In other words, it transforms a nutrient-rich food into a hard-to-digest, inflammation-promoting food.

Pasteurization also reduces vitamin content and morphs milk's lactose into beta-lactose sugars that are absorbed faster, causing higher blood sugar spikes.[199] During this process, calcium fuses with the fatty acids and forms a type of milk-fat soap that creates GI tract inflammation. This saponification reaction also makes calcium and phosphate much less bioavailable and more difficult to absorb.[200,201] And the heat used in pasteurization triggers glycation and oxidation, which leads to the formation of inflammatory compounds like N-carboxymethyl-lysine, malonaldehyde, and 4-hydroxynonenal.[202] Let's just say they are not good guys.

Besides pasteurization, milk processing also has another step called homogenization. In raw milk, cream naturally rises to the top, but this makes milk less stable. Homogenization blocks this natural cream separation and increases milk's shelf life. This is great for business but bad for your health. One thing that makes raw milk special is the presence of milk fat globule membranes called gangliosides. These molecules have strong prebiotic, anti-inflammatory, antimicrobial, and antiviral properties.[203–205] Sadly, homogenization significantly reduces gangliosides in milk.[206] Other studies further support that milk processing denatures proteins, alters milk's digestibility, decreases its probiotic value, and triggers intestinal inflammatory reactions.[207–210]

One might think that we're only finding out about this now, but the truth is that we have known that raw milk is superior for a long time. In fact, this was known as far back as the 1920s and '30s. Studies back then comparing the intake of raw and pasteurized milk revealed as much as 40 percent improvement in bone growth on the raw milk, along with less tooth decay, improved mood, greater disease resistance, and more.[211–213]

Casein

It's believed that sometime in the past, a mutation occurred in Northern European cows, which altered the casein protein in their milk. The protein mutated from casein A2 to casein A1. What seems to be just a simple name change actually carries significant health consequences. During digestion, casein A1 can turn into beta-casomorphin-7, which is an opioid and inflammatory peptide linked to the development of type 1 diabetes, celiac disease, Hashimoto's thyroiditis, ulcerative colitis, cardiovascular disease, and other autoimmune illnesses.[214–217] Patients with schizophrenia have been found to have higher levels of beta-casomorphin-7 in their blood. Furthermore, these patients experienced improvements in their symptoms after dialysis (when this molecule is removed from the blood) or through casein-free diets.[218]

The good news is that Southern European cows, water buffalo, goats, and sheep continue to produce casein A2 milk. The bad news is that "A1 cows" like Holsteins, Friesians, and Ayrshires are the most commercial milking cow breeds, since they produce more milk. As of the time of this writing, it's not common practice to label milk as A1 or A2, but I believe this is something that will change soon, since people are getting more educated on this subject. For reference, the cows that still produce milk with A2 casein are the Guernsey, Jersey, Brown Swiss, Scottish Highland, Limousin, Piedmontese, and Belgian Blue breeds.

> **Neo Note: Goat and Sheep Milk**
> One way to never go wrong is to go for goat's or sheep's milk, since they always contain casein A2. Organic raw or fermented goat or sheep's dairy is incredibly nutritious because it contains probiotics, omega-3 fatty acids, protein, calcium, magnesium, and the rare-to-find vitamin K_2. Goat's milk is naturally lower in lactose than cow's milk, which is also a plus. When fermented, it may not contain any lactose at all. Goat's milk is also incredibly rich in MCTs. Sheep's milk is not too different from goat's milk but is harder to find. However, there are several cheeses that are traditionally made with sheep's milk, such as Feta, Roquefort, and Manchego.

Farming Methods Matter

The quality of dairy and its ability to be a promoter of either health or disease also has to do with how the animals are raised. As we've seen before, cows grazing in grass not only have more nutritious meat, but their milk is also substantially richer. For example, studies have found that milk from pasture-raised cows had 500 percent more CLA than conventional milk.[219] But the nutritional content is not the only concern here. Research has shown that most of the stuff cows get injected with goes straight into their milk. One study published in the *Journal of Agricultural and Food Chemistry* uncovered that a single glass of pasteurized milk can contain up to 20 different drugs such as diclofenac, flunixin, ibuprofen, ketoprofen, mefenamic acid, and niflumic acid.[220] This is important to know because the milk from these medicated cows will carry these chemicals into your body. One more reason why regenerative farming practices are essential.

Fermented Dairy

If you can't find a good source of fresh raw milk, your best alternative is to get raw cheese, yogurt, or kefir from organic whole milk. During the fermentation process, damaged proteins are rejuvenated, sugars and proteins are partially digested by bacteria, and the micronutrients become more available. Fermenting diary has been used in many cultures around the world, not only to preserve dairy during the winter months but to make it more digestible. Research shows that during the fermentation process, *Lactobacilli* proliferate in the milk while breaking down sugars and proteins (i.e., lactose and casein) and inhibiting putrefying bacteria.[221] In this same study, it was seen that proteins in yogurt are digested twice as fast as proteins in unfermented milk.

Please note, though, that some fermented dairy can have mold contamination.[222,223] Cheeses such as Camembert and Roquefort intentionally contain mold and are said to be safe in low doses. However, for someone already facing health issues, increasing their exposure to mycotoxins is not the best way to go. Other cheeses, even though they aren't exposed to mold on purpose, can develop mold growths, so it might be a good idea to avoid them as well.

I personally favor kefir and yogurt, but I still eat some cheese once in a while. The anecdotal evidence I found suggests that fresh cheeses, such as ricotta, farmer cheese, cottage cheese, and fresh mozzarella, are easier to digest and less reactive than aged cheeses for most people. Don't get me wrong, aged cheeses also have their benefits, such as lower lactose and a better nutritional profile, but they can trigger allergy symptoms because of their histamine content (more on that in chapter 11).

Whey Protein

Most people associate whey protein with the fitness industry, but its use originated many years ago. Some say that the ancient Egyptians used whey to restore their vitality and boost their immune system.[224] Others mention that Galen, the "father of sports medicine," "prescribed" it as well.[225]

What is this "magical" whey? Whey is the liquid part of fresh milk that is left over from the making of cheese. Nowadays, the supplement industry filters this liquid, removes the water, and sells it in powdered form. Most manufacturers then add artificial flavors, sweeteners, and preservatives, and completely ruin this healing food.

Whey contains a mixture of proteins (e.g., lactoglobulins and lactalbumin) that boost the production of the antioxidant glutathione, improve your immunity, and have antiviral and antitumorigenic properties.[226–228] As hinted before, the less processed the whey is, the better its effects. Studies have shown that undenatured whey has greater antioxidant, anticarcinogenic, and immune-boosting effects compared with the (denatured) whey found in most supplements.[229,230]

You can purchase whey in liquid form from local farmers, or you can find a couple of good raw whey powder supplement brands. Another option is whey cheese. That's right! Even though casein is used for 98 percent of cheeses, there are a few cheeses made with whey, such as authentic Italian ricotta and Norwegian gjetost (or geitost), primost, and mysost. Depending on where you live, these might be difficult to find, but they are a wonderful source of protein and are much easier to digest than regular casein cheeses.

Neo Note: Toxins in Protein Powders

As of the time of this writing, the supplement industry is largely unregulated. Because of this, there are many companies with questionable practices selling dangerous products. In 2020, the US nonprofit Clean Label Project did a study on several protein powders available on the market.[231] The organization screened 134 products for 130 types of toxins and uncovered that many protein powders contained heavy metals (arsenic, cadmium, lead, and mercury), bisphenol-A, pesticides, and other toxins. In some products, the substances were in negligible quantities, but in many others they were present in concerning concentrations.

This is another reason to focus on nutrient-dense whole foods most of the time. When supplementing, it is essential to choose companies that actually care about the quality and safety of their products.

Dairy Alternatives

I'll go straight to the point here. I do not recommend most "fake milks," since they have either high sugar content, harmful additives, or toxic antinutrients. The only one I recommend is coconut milk (although macadamia milk is okay). Unsweetened coconut milk has a similar texture to that of cow's milk and is very low in sugar. Coconut milk is gut friendly and filled with healthy fats, such as the MCT lauric acid, which has antibacterial, antifungal, and antiviral properties.[232] Since coconut milk is completely free of dairy, soy, nuts, or grains, it's the very best option for someone with severe gut issues who still wants some "milk" while going through an elimination stage.

Neo Note: Carrageenan

Carrageenan is a food additive derived from the red seaweed *Chondrus crispus* (Irish moss or carrageen moss). In the past few years, it's become a popular additive used in milk alternatives like almond, rice, soy, and coconut milks, but also in ice cream, cottage cheese, yogurt, creamers, and many other processed foods. Research performed in 1982 cleared food-grade carrageenan as safe to use as a food additive.[233] But more recent research suggests that carrageenan may be a bowel irritant and a potential carcinogen.[234,235] More research is definitely needed, but it might be a good idea to stay away from this additive until we gain a better understanding of its safety.

Organ Meats

Eating organ meats, or offal, seems a very exotic concept to most people in the Western world. The idea of eating brains, kidneys, livers, or lungs might make you gag, but these have been important foods for humans through history. As we learned before, fatty organ meats were the favorite part of any kill and were considered incredible sources of health and vitality. Hunter-gatherers would crack open bones and skulls to reach the bone marrow and the brain.[236] In fact, animal brains contain more DHA than salmon, and eating this organ allowed us to develop larger head and body size.[237]

As a matter of fact, we don't need to go as far back as the Paleolithic era to see organ meats as part of our diet. Cookbooks from the 1940s and '50s have recipes teaching readers how to prepare meals using brain, liver, kidney, tongue, heart, and thymus.[238] In many countries, to this day, offal meats are part of their traditional cuisines. Growing up in Portugal, it was pretty common to see dishes made with stomach, intestines, liver, or chicken hearts and gizzards being offered at restaurants. But as the cuisine across the world became more westernized, these traditional dishes slowly became less popular.

Fortunately, organ meats are on the rise again, since they are rich in healthy fats and incredibly abundant in vitamins and minerals. If you eat organ meats often, I guarantee you will not experience micronutrient deficiencies. Organ meats are the best multivitamin one can take. More good news: Because they're still not in high demand, butchers sell them cheap. The bad news is that they are an acquired taste and you need to know how to prepare them properly. But fear not! At the end of this chapter, I recommend a fantastic cookbook with amazing organ meat recipes.

Liver

Among all the organs, liver may be the most nutritionally powerful. Throughout history, raw liver was considered a cure-all and was recommended to anyone feeling under the weather. Nowadays, I don't recommend raw liver unless you are very familiar with the source and you've frozen the meat for two weeks before consumption, to kill parasites.

Some people think that because the liver is a key player in the detox process, it is full of toxins. This is not correct. The liver is not like an air filter that accumulates airborne pollutants and needs to be changed every 90 days. We do not replace livers, do we? Sure, there are liver transplants, but you know what I mean. The liver coordinates the detox operation but does not retain the toxins. They are either sent for elimination through the sweat, urine, or feces, or stored inside fat cells. If an animal is exposed to heavy metals, for example, the liver will accumulate some of these toxins, but so will other parts of the animal. This is why it is essential to know where your meat is coming from.

Authors have called the liver the "nutrient savings bank." What this means is that if there is an excess of protein, sugar, vitamins, and some minerals, part of the excess is stored in the liver until it is needed. This is probably why the liver is so rich in micronutrients such as vitamin A; vitamins B_2, B_3, B_5, B_6, B_9, and B_{12}; copper; iron; phosphorus; selenium; and zinc.[239]

Other Organs

Several cultures around the world had the belief that by eating a specific organ, they could boost the health of that same organ in their own bodies. "Like cures like." The logic behind this belief is that the organ meat contains all the nutrients that organ needs in order to thrive. While this never has been fully supported by research, one can see several examples where this concept makes sense. For example, the brain has omega-3s, essential for brain development and healing, and the liver contains several vitamins essential to the liver's detoxification processes. Again, this is not hard science, but I think it's an interesting concept to explore as you consider other organ meats.

Here are some of the most commonly eaten organ meats and their nutritional benefits:[240]

• *Brain and nervous tissues*: These are a phenomenal source of DHA, phospholipids, BDNF, vitamins B_{12} and C, and iron. Word of caution: Beef brain consumption has been linked to mad cow disease outbreaks in humans, so it's probably best to be confident in your source or simply choose brains from other animals.

• *Eyes*: This organ is rich in the nutrients usually recommended for healthy vision, such as vitamin A, lutein, and zeaxanthin. The eye is also an excellent source of DHA and zinc.

• *Heart*: Hearts taste very similar to muscle meat. The heart is a great source of coenzyme Q10; vitamin B_{12}; and collagen, elastin, and other proteins.

• *Kidneys*: These organs are great for people with food sensitivities, allergies, or other autoimmune reactions, since kidneys are an excellent source of diamine oxidase (DAO), an enzyme that helps break down excess histamine (which modulates inflammatory response) in your body.

• *Lungs*: Similarly to the heart, their flavor is on the softer side. They are a fine source of B vitamins and a superb source of minerals such as copper, iron, phosphorus, potassium, selenium, and zinc.

• *Pancreas*: This organ is fantastic for people with digestive problems because it is a natural source of digestive enzymes such as lipase, protease, trypsin, and amylase.

• *Spleen*: Clearly the best source of bioavailable heme iron, the spleen also contains the peptides splenin, splenopentin, and tuftsin, which have been linked with improved immune function.

Bones, Marrow, and Connective Tissue

Most people look at bones as the "holders of meat" and don't realize how much they are missing out on. Probably the main thing to talk about is bone marrow. This is the spongy tissue in the center of bones. Bone marrow has been seen as a delicacy in many traditional cuisines, and for good reason.

Although it is not rich in vitamins and minerals, marrow is an excellent source of chondroitin, collagen, glucosamine, and glycine, which help decrease inflammation and contribute to bone, joint, and skin health.[241-248]

Beyond bone marrow, we also have the rest of the bone, cartilage, and connective tissues. These are not consumed directly but can be used to make bone broth. During the simmering of these animal parts, many nutrients are dissolved in the cooking water, making the broth incredibly nutritious. Bones are rich in calcium, magnesium, phosphorus, potassium, and other trace minerals, while cartilage and other connective tissues provide glycosaminoglycans, or GAGs (especially chondroitin sulfate, glucosamine, and hyaluronic acid); collagen; and gelatin (hydrolyzed collagen, the "cooked" form of collagen). GAGs are all the rage in the supplement and cosmetic industries because of their many benefits in fighting inflammation and promoting tissue regeneration. Several studies have also linked GAGs to improvements in inflammatory conditions such as osteoarthritis, atherosclerosis, IBD, and psoriasis.[249,250]

Bone broth is one of the best natural sources of collagen, and this protein is essential for the body. In fact, collagen is said to be the most abundant protein in the body, representing one-third of its total protein.[251] It's part of your bones, skin, muscles, tendons, ligaments, and also blood vessels, corneas, and teeth. Sadly, most people don't get enough collagen in their diets, and this can have damaging consequences in many facets of life. I first learned about collagen deficiencies while in college, reading articles about how individuals with poor collagen content experience more injuries.[252-255] Collagen deficiency may be another reason behind the epidemic of severe osteoarthritis people are experiencing at younger and younger ages. I believe we are not taking in enough collagen, and our joints are screaming for raw materials to lubricate and repair themselves. Collagen will not only help you move better and stay away from a knee replacement, but it will also keep you looking your best for longer. Proper collagen in the body improves blood circulation, facilitates wound healing, and prevents skin wrinkling.[256-258] The combination of GAGs and collagen makes bone broth an essential part of the diet of any human being. I cannot stress this enough.

Neo Note: Cellulite

Most people associate cellulite (dimpled-looking fat) with excess weight or aging, but there is more to this story. Irregular cellulite forms in fat deposits that lack adequate connective tissue to support a smooth shape.[259] This suggests that the body might not have enough glue (collagen) to connect everything uniformly. In her book *Deep Nutrition*, Dr. Catherine Shanahan suggests that "to get rid of cellulite, combine exercise with a diet full of healthy, natural fats (including animal fat) and collagen-rich stocks. This will send the message that you want your body to replace the saggy fat pockets with smooth, toned curves.[260] Not happy with your cellulite? Hit the gym and drink bone broth!

Insects

For most westerners, eating insects is unthinkable, but in several cultures around the world, insects are seen as great sources of nutrition. In fact, a 2013 UN report estimated that two billion people worldwide eat bugs as part of their diet.[261] Organic dried insects such as ants, bees, beetles, caterpillars, crickets, grasshoppers, spiders, and even wasps pack more protein, pound for pound, than most traditional meats, and they are also rich in fiber, vitamins, and minerals.[262] Research has shown that consumption of cricket powder may have positive health benefits such as promoting the growth of probiotic bacteria and reducing inflammation.[263]

Entomophagy (the practice of eating bugs) might also be a good way to help feed our growing population, especially in more densely populated areas, since this is food one could easily grow at home. Not too long ago, eating sushi was considered disgusting, and now we have sushi places everywhere. Insects might be the next sushi. If you're curious, in the book's resources I share some websites where you can purchase your dose of bugs.

Seafood

We humans have a tendency to ruin great things. Fish is one of those things. Seafood used to be one of the healthiest foods we could consume, and it helped many cultures not only survive but thrive. Unfortunately, during the past 150 years, we've wrecked this amazing dietary staple. We have polluted our bodies of water with industrial chemical discharges, nitrogen fertilizer runoff, and trash from our unconscious lifestyles. Fish are now full of mercury (and other heavy metals), pesticides, microplastics, dioxins, polychlorinated biphenyls (PCBs), and other contaminants.[264–267] These ultimately end up in our bodies and can contribute to developmental, reproductive, immunotoxic, and carcinogenic issues.[268] This situation has gotten so worrisome that several studies do not recommend the consumption of fish (especially bigger fish because of the phenomenon of bioaccumulation) by select groups of the population such as children, women of childbearing age, pregnant women, and nursing mothers.[269,270]

Then we have the whole ecological impact that industrial fishing is having on our planet. Our current, improperly supervised fishing practices are causing overfishing and depletion of entire fish populations. For example, as of this writing, we have extinguished 97 percent of all Pacific bluefin tuna.[271,272] Depending on when you are reading these words, we might have taken care of the other 3 percent just so we could feed our sushi cravings.

We need to take better care of our oceans, not only for the marine life, but also so we can live. Scientists believe the oceans absorb four times the amount of CO_2 the Amazon forest does.[273,274] Moreover, up to 85 percent of the world's oxygen may be produced by the phytoplankton in our oceans.[275-277]

Some look at farmed fish as an answer, but instead of thinking of regenerative ways of doing this, fish farmers are simply repeating what we have done to animal production on land. Fish are raised in overcrowded spaces where disease can easily spread. They are fed soy and grain feed, which you already know the consequences of. To add to this, the grain pellets used to feed the fish may contain antibiotics, as well as other drugs to fight the buildup of bacteria and fecal matter in these overfilled ponds.[278] There are even reports of farmed fish developing anemia, heart disease, lice infestations, and infectious diseases.[279-282]

Recently, investigative reporters have also questioned the practices of the agencies that are supposed to regulate sustainable fisheries. Allegedly (I learn this from American lawyer shows), by selling fishing companies the "sustainable" label, these agencies are significantly financed by the very companies they are supposed to regulate.[283] If that's true, it represents a big conflict of interest.

What's the solution? I honestly don't know. I wish I had the answer to such a complex issue, but this goes beyond my research and what I set out to do in this book. What I can say is that there are many things that need to be done on a political level, such as establishing and enforcing "no-take zones" (no-fishing zones) and stopping government subsidies for these industrial fishing companies.

To be honest, I'm a bit torn about specific fish consumption recommendations, since there is a lot I still don't know. Some researchers say that the contaminants in seafood outweigh the benefits of their omega-3s.[284-286] And, as I mentioned before, even though fish omega-3s are important, there are other sources of these omega-3s, like algae or even some offal.[287,288] Should we stop eating fish? I wouldn't go that far. There are many parts of the world where people rely exclusively on fish as their main sustaining food. What I think most of us can do is to reduce fish consumption and favor smaller fishing companies that really care about doing things the right way. I know this is easier said than done, but those in coastal cities can definitely try to do this.

In terms of the fish you eat, stay away from bigger fish like shark, swordfish, king mackerel, and tuna. Remember, the bigger the fish, the more bioaccumulation of toxins and microplastics. Instead, prioritize fish like wild-caught anchovies, herring, mackerel (not king mackerel), pollock, salmon, sardines, and trout, which are lower in heavy metals and other contaminants.[289]

Slowly, we are also seeing the growth of the regenerative ocean farming movement. As Dr. Hyman notes in *The Pegan Diet*, "mixed aquacultures of seaweed, scallops, oysters, mussels, and clams require zero inputs (fertilizers, cleaning agents, additives, feedstuffs) while sequestering carbon (think of seaweed as underwater rainforests). The seaweed can be eaten or turned into bioplastics, animal feed, fertilizer, and more."[290] Not only are these regenerative ocean farms creating sustainable omega-3 foods like seaweed, but they're also promoting the growth of sustainable and nutrient-dense foods like shellfish.

Neo Note: Shellfish

People usually group crustaceans, bivalves and other mollusks (even if they don't have a shell) as shellfish. These animals are recognized as bottom-feeders and, as such, they are "known" for consuming decomposing animals, feces, parasites, and trash accumulated on the floor of our bodies of water. Some of the most known ones are clams, crabs, lobsters, mussels, octopus, oysters, scallops, shrimp, and squid.

Some religious practices condemn the consumption of these foods, stating they are toxic. But, is there scientific evidence supporting this claim?

The truth is that many of these animals are scavengers and they do eat all the nasty stuff I just mentioned. Furthermore, research support that many bottom-feeders accumulate harmful bacteria, viruses, toxic chemicals, and biotoxins.[291,292] Finally, around three percent of the population is estimated to be allergic to crustaceans and/or mollusks.[293]

Does this mean we should stop eating these foods completely? Not necessarily. Bivalves, for example, are some of the most nutrient-dense foods you can find.[294,295] And, most of them, being filter-feeders, are not scavenging the ocean floors, eating trash. You also have to consider that in most developed countries, bivalves are subject to purification (depuration) processes where most harmful contaminants are expelled. Yes, they can still have some biotoxins even after depuration, but that is why you should only buy bivalves from trusted sources (preferably from regenerative practices).

I recommend the consumption of bivalves, but I suggest reducing the consumption of all other shellfish. As you move down your healing journey, it is ok to eat shellfish once in a while (like I do in a social setting) but this should be the exception, not the norm.

P.S. Just a last note on shrimp, since it's one of the most consumed types of seafood in the world. I eat some shrimp sporadically, but I am very selective about what I buy. Obviously, we have the whole bottom-feeder issue. And, sadly, most shrimp comes from toxic and inhumane farming practices. If you decide to buy shrimp, make sure it's certified as wild caught.

Vegan Protein Sources

As you have figured out by now, I am not a big fan of vegan protein sources. Most of the plant-based foods with a higher content of protein are rich in carbs and antinutrients, which can be disastrous for most people. Even so, I will try to give my take on the most common plant proteins.

Legumes

Legumes are rich in protein, but they are carb heavy. You have to be wise in selecting legumes to avoid overconsumption of carbohydrates. Legumes also need to be properly soaked and pressured-cooked in order to minimize their antinutrient content. Finally, beans are also rich in fiber, which can be challenging, especially for people who are still trying to heal their gut from dysbiosis or SIBO. Among all the legumes, probably the most "Neo Diet compliant" are lupini beans. These are high in protein and have zero net carbs (carbs you can actually digest and absorb). Other low-starch legumes include lentils, green peas, black-eyed peas, and mung beans. Here is a tip to make your beans more easily digestible. Cook them with kombu (a type of dried seaweed), since it contains alpha-galactosidase, the enzyme that breaks down the oligosaccharides in your legumes. This will result in less abdominal discomfort and flatulence.

Soy

Soy is one of the few plant foods that can be considered a complete protein, since it provides all nine essential amino acids.[296] Therefore, soy is frequently promoted as a valid alternative to meat. However, soy is surrounded by much controversy and discussion. Historically, soy traditionally has been consumed by Asian cultures, but what you probably don't know is that ancient writings from China suggest the soybean was initially considered unfit for human consumption.[297] This ended up changing with the discovery of the fermentation process, which allowed people to substantially reduce soybeans' antinutrient content.[298] So, most Asian traditional soy foods, such as tempeh, natto, miso, and tamari sauce, are fermented. Furthermore, these fermented foods, even though they were consumed often, were eaten in small amounts.

In contrast, nowadays, the most commonly consumed form of soy in the Western world is nonfermented tofu. To make matters worse, because of the growth of the vegan movement, the food industry is pumping into the market highly processed soy products like soy bacon, soy burgers, soy hotdogs, soy nuggets, soy milk, soy cheese, soy ice cream, etc. None of these are fermented to reduce antinutrients, and they're made even worse because of all the chemical food flavorings and vegetable oils added to them. And, by the way, as much as 94 percent of American soy and about 79 percent of soy worldwide may be GMO.[299]

Soy contains problematic lectins called soybean agglutinins, which have been found to cause inflammation and increased intestinal permeability.[300] Soy is also rich in phytates that, as you know, inhibit the absorption of nutrients in the intestine, which can depress your metabolism.[301] Soy also contains goitrogens that block iodine absorption and impair thyroid function.[302] Finally, soy contains saponins, which have been linked to an increase in intestinal permeability and even hemolysis (rupture) of red blood cells.[303,304]

If you choose to eat soy, please stay away from soybean oil, soy protein isolates, soy processed foods, and any unfermented soy products. Opt for non-GMO, organic, traditionally prepared and fermented soy foods like tempeh, miso, natto, and tamari.

Neo Note: Vegan Progression

I understand that this was a lot of information to take in, especially for my vegan readers. Some of you might realize that there are many things you should do to improve your health, including adding animal products. If you are not yet ready to adopt an omnivorous diet and add some meat to your plate, here are some of my recommendations in order to optimize your chances of healing:

• **First**, remove all the fake, processed foods from your diet. This is the most important step for everyone, vegan or not.

• **Second**, I challenge you to at least consider transitioning into a vegetarian diet with some animal-derived foods. Eggs and dairy will help you fill some of the typical nutritional gaps vegans have. Eggs are high in protein, fats, choline, vitamin B_{12}, and retinol (the usable form of vitamin A). Fermented dairy products are a great source of protein, probiotics, and vitamins, especially vitamin K_2, which is essential for proper calcium distribution and for a healthy heart.

• **Third**, compensate for your taurine, creatine, and carnosine deficiencies by supplementing. As we discussed before, these micronutrients are found only in meat and other animal foods and have many health benefits. Since you are not eating meat, get these important compounds in supplement form.

• **Fourth**, eat algae. A variety of algae in your diet will offset two common problems stemming from a vegan diet: low omega-3s and low iodine. Algae like spirulina and chlorella provide the marine omega-3s EPA and DHA, while nori, kelp, kombu, and dulse will take care of your iodine needs. Since we're talking about algae, I have to quickly highlight the amazing superfood spirulina (my absolute favorite). Besides packing a bunch of nutrients, spirulina has been shown to protect the intestinal wall from LPSs, promote stem cell production, boost mood, stimulate brain development in children, and protect the brain from degeneration in seniors.[305-307]

• **Fifth**, and finally, supplement with vitamin B_{12}. As demonstrated before, vegans can be substantially deficient in this vitamin. You can easily find several good and affordable vitamin B_{12} supplements, so don't think twice.

NEO SUMMARY

• Protein is an important nutrient since its amino acids are the building blocks for most tissues in the body.

• A recommendation of 70-120 grams of protein a day seems to be appropriate for most people.

• Both the carnivore and the vegan diets have pros and cons, but share the fact they are elimination diets.

• Following an elimination diet long term is not the best choice to achieve antifragility.

• Most individuals following a vegan diet end up developing substantial nutritional deficits.

• Pasture-raised meat consumption has been associated with better health outcomes.

• Industrial agriculture causes more death than animal farming.

• CAFOs and industrial agriculture are destroying the planet and both should be abolished.

• Regenerative agriculture can help us save the planet.

• Milk processing has made many dairy products "toxic."

• Best sources of protein are grazing animals, eggs and raw fermented dairy.

NEO ACTION

• Favor organic pasture-raised meats from grazing animals and pastured eggs.

• If consuming dairy, opt for raw fermented dairy products (if available) from A2 cows, goats or sheep, from small local farms.

• If you are intolerant to dairy, select unsweetened coconut milk as the alternative.

• Avoid processed meats, processed milk and fat-free milk products, yogurts sweetened with sugar, and animal products from CAFOs or industrial fishing.

• If vegan, please follow the recommendations given to minimize nutrient deficiencies.

NEO RECOMMENDATIONS

- *Carnivore Cure* by Judy Cho
- *Drawdown* by Paul Hawken
- *Eat Stop Eat: How Much Protein* by Brad Pilon
- *Food Fix* by Dr. Mark Hyman
- *It Takes Guts* by Ashleigh VanHouten
- *Nutrition and Physical Degeneration* by Dr. Weston A. Price
- *Protein Power* by Drs. Michael & Mary Dan Eades
- *Sacred Cow* by Diana Rodgers & Robb Wolf
- *The Bulletproof Diet* by Dave Asprey
- *The Carnivore Code* by Dr. Paul Saladino
- *The Carnivore Diet* by Dr. Shawn Baker
- *The Pegan Diet* by Dr. Mark Hyman
- *The Vegetarian Myth* by Lierre Keith

my.neodiet.co/neorecommendations

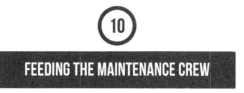

FEEDING THE MAINTENANCE CREW

The Evolution of Fiber from Poop to Gold

"The future of our nation depends on our ability to produce food and fiber to sustain the world."
Phil Bredesen

THE MISUNDERSTOOD NUTRIENT

Fiber is not sexy. You don't see it advertised in fitness magazines or as the basis of a new diet. But if we really understood what fiber can do for us, you would most definitely feel a little turned on. Okay, let's not go that far. The point is, fiber is like a sleeper secret agent. We pay little attention to it, but it might save the world, or in this case, our health! Although fiber is the "fourth macronutrient," it's clearly the most misunderstood of the bunch. Protein, fat, and carbs get all the love, while fiber is put to the side. After you read this chapter, you will understand that fiber is as important as any of the other three.

Historically, we used to eat a lot of fiber. It's believed that the diets of our hunter-gatherer ancestors share similarities to what present-day hunter-gatherer tribes like the Hadza eat. Their diets contain an average of 150 grams of fiber a day.[1] In contrast, the average Western diet contains only about 20 to 25 grams of fiber.[2] That is an enormous difference. Some people doing keto or carnivore diets don't even get to 20 grams a day. This is concerning, since research has shown that the less fiber we eat, the sicker we get.[2] As a society, we are overweight, and yet we are completely starving for fiber!

FIBER 101

When we were talking about carbohydrates, I mentioned that fiber would remain undigested throughout most of your digestive system. Therefore, some people think fiber just bulks our feces and makes us poop. But it doesn't work exactly like that. Although we cannot digest fiber, our bugs can. In fact, they thrive on fiber—but more on that shortly.

To begin with, we can split dietary fiber into soluble and insoluble. Want to tell them apart? It's simple. Add fiber to a cup of water. If it dissolves, it's soluble. If it doesn't, it's insoluble. Ta-daaa! To be fair, in nature, you tend to find fiber with a mix of both, so in truth, the example I just gave you will not be very accurate, but you get the idea. Another way to think about soluble and insoluble is to consider the concept of "flush and scrub." Soluble fiber will dissolve in water and move through the digestive tract, flushing it. Insoluble fiber, because it does not dissolve, will scrub your digestive walls, stimulating elimination of toxins and promoting epic bowel movements.

As humans, we lack the enzymes to digest fiber, but our microbiome may contain up to 60,000 digestive enzymes, capable of digesting most things we throw at them.[3] This is why we outsource many digestive processes to our bugs. Together, they work as a team to break down the different compounds in the foods we eat, and in the process they produce the incredibly health-promoting postbiotics. By consuming plenty of fiber, you provide abundant food for your digestive maintenance crew (your microbiome), and they pay you back by taking good care of you and releasing the highly anti-inflammatory SCFAs. On the other hand, if you don't feed your gut, your good bugs will start dying. Without your maintenance crew, all hell breaks loose. You may develop digestive issues, constipation, skin problems, allergies, low immunity, systemic inflammation, poor physical performance, and brain fog.[4]

BENEFITS OF FIBER

A 2016 study published in *Journals of Gerontology* followed a group of 1,600 adults for 10 years.[5] The researchers concluded that the individuals who ate the most fiber were 80 percent more likely to be free of hypertension, diabetes, dementia, depression, and overall disability. Additionally, the authors stated that fiber consumption was the most determinant variable for healthy aging.

When you eat prebiotics such as fiber, your microbiome produces SCFAs. These SCFAs, in turn, promote the production of satiety hormones like PYY and glucagon-like peptide-1 (GLP-1).[6] This is one reason fiber is associated with weight loss. In a five-year study with 1,114 participants, researchers found out that each 10-gram increase in daily soluble fiber consumption led to an additional 3.7 percent reduction in visceral fat accumulation.[7] In this study, soluble fiber showed a stronger link to weight management than smoking, sugar consumption, and even physical activity. Another reason behind fiber's weight management benefits is its effect on your metabolism. As we saw in chapter 6, when processed foods have their fiber stripped away, your body, in particular your mitochondria, might become overwhelmed. Without fiber, the digestion of your "multi-macronutrient" foods creates an energy "rush hour" in which your mitochondria get hit with all the fuels at the same time. This is one mechanism that can eventually lead to metabolic dysfunction and thus weight gain.

Another benefit of fiber is its ability to assist with detoxification and removal of metabolic waste from the body.[8] Not only does fiber help escort old bile acids and dissolved toxins, but it has also been shown to remove excess estrogen from the organism.[9,10] It seems that fiber may play an important role in clearing out recirculating estrogens from the body, preventing the accumulation of this hormone whose excess has been linked to many health issues, including weight gain and cancer.[11,12]

Fiber will also improve our immunity in many ways. For starters, by being food for our bugs, fiber causes them to produce SCFAs like butyrate that increase the synthesis and development of regulatory T cells (immune cells) in the colon, which mediate our inflammatory response.[13] Fiber intake has also been shown to reduce inflammatory markers like C-reactive protein, interleukin-6, and tumor necrosis factor.[14] Dietary fiber also promotes the growth of commensal bacteria, which in turn help decrease LPS formation and the consequent inflammatory response.[15,16]

I could cite a lot more studies on fiber and its amazing effects, but by understanding how dietary fiber is directly connected with metabolic health and inflammation in the body, we can easily see how fiber consumption (or the lack of) can be connected with risk of developing most diseases a human being can experience.

As a final note, it is important to point out that there are several contradictory studies on fiber consumption. One can find studies suggesting that dietary fiber is protective against heart disease and several cancers.[17-25] But there are also numerous studies that show no effect of fiber in those same pathologies.[26-34] This does not mean that fiber intake is not beneficial, but that we have to understand why some people had good results while others did not share the same success. Study participants may have different gut health profiles, and even the type of fiber might influence the results. Getting fiber from GMO grains obviously will not produce the same results as deriving it from organic vegetables, for example. Shortly, we'll discuss how to properly introduce fiber into your diet and what are the best sources of fiber for you.

Neo Note: Flatulence Is Good?

Some people are afraid of adding more fiber to their diet because they fear that it will cause too much gas. In fiber's defense, some people who suffer from gas and bloating are actually unconscious air swallowers. Yes, they swallow air while talking and breathing, and it eventually has to leave from one end or another. However, bacterial fermentation in the intestines also generates some gases, and a dysfunctional gut will indeed produce more gas. This is why we definitely do not want to radically increase dietary fiber in that situation.

The main gases our bacteria produce are carbon dioxide, hydrogen, methane, nitric oxide, and hydrogen sulfide. What I recently found out is that these gases are actually gasotransmitters.[35] Gasotransmitters are gaseous signaling molecules that are used to transmit chemical signals that induce certain physiological or biochemical changes in the organism, tissue, or cell. In a nutshell, these gases have been shown to influence mitochondria, alter blood flow, modulate inflammation, act as antioxidants, activate detoxification processes, improve learning and memory, and potentially protect from neurodegenerative diseases like Parkinson's.[36-44]

Research has shown that if you do not produce enough of these gasotransmitters (due to not properly feeding your microbiome), your body will downregulate your mitochondrial activity, slow your cellular processes, and potentially create metabolic dysfunction.[45-47]

This does not mean the more gas, the better. Large buildups of some of these gasotransmitters can be absolutely toxic. Once again, we have to follow the Goldilocks principle. They need to be just right for optimum results. One reason this is important is because it further reinforces the idea that your microbiome controls many aspects of your health. We already knew about SCFAs; now we know about gas.

Moral of the story: Some gas is actually a wonderful thing!

THE DIFFERENT TYPES OF FIBER

For the longest time, when I thought about fiber, I thought about grains and cereal. Let's face it, most of us have been brainwashed by TV ads to believe that grains and especially breakfast cereals are the only sources of fiber. While grains are indeed a rich source of fiber, they are probably not the best option for most people with damaged guts. Instead, we should consume more fiber from plant leaves, stems, tubers, and roots. A variety of these fibers is guaranteed to please the different gut bugs and consequently elevate your health. So, without further ado, let's look at some of your options.[48-50]

Cellulose

This is an insoluble fiber that comes primarily from plant cell walls of many vegetables (e.g., broccoli, cabbage, cauliflower, and kale), but also from legumes, nuts, and whole grains. Generally, cellulose is poorly fermented by gut microbes, but it increases gut transit and thus reduces the chances of bacterial overgrowths. This type of fiber also helps lower the risk of diverticulitis and can help with weight loss. It's considered "nature's laxative."

Lignin

Here we have another insoluble type of fiber. Some of the best sources of lignin are avocados, beans, cauliflower, flaxseed, green bananas, green beans, nuts, peas, rye, whole wheat, and zucchini. Lignin is also a great transit promoter that may even have positive effects on heart health and immune function.

Fructan

A fructan is a polymer of fructose molecules. When it has a short chain length, it is known as a fructooligosaccharide (FOS), whereas a longer-chain fructan is called an inulin.

Inulins are soluble fibers present in many foods such as agave, artichokes, asparagus, bananas, barley, garlic, jicama, onions, rye, and wild yams. As a supplement, inulins are usually extracted from chicory. They're known for promoting the growth of beneficial bacteria and improving GI and systemic health. Because they're highly fermentable, too much of this fiber can cause excessive bloating and flatulence.

A FOS, also called oligofructose or oligofructan, usually results from the degradation of inulins and is commonly used as an alternative sweetener. Its food sources and benefits are similar to those of inulins.

> **Neo Note: Galacto-oligosaccharides**
> Galacto-oligosaccharides (GOSs), a.k.a. oligogalactoses or oligolactoses, are not fructans, but they are structurally very similar to FOSs and are also excellent prebiotic sources. These are the prebiotics in milk that help children in particular develop their microbiomes. GOSs have been shown to stimulate the growth of good bacteria, improve intestinal transit, and boost the immune system.

Beta-glucans

These are a soluble, viscous type of fiber that your bugs adore. Beta-glucans are naturally found in algae, barley, beans, oat bran, oats, peas, yeast, and mushrooms such as reishi, lingzhi, shiitake, chaga, and maitake. This type of fiber has been shown to balance cholesterol, support the immune system, quell inflammation, and lower the risk of coronary heart disease and type 2 diabetes.

Pectin

Similarly to beta-glucans, a pectin is also a soluble and viscous type of fiber, and another one your bugs love to munch on. Pectins can be found in significant quantity in foods like apples, carrots, citrus fruits, guavas, potatoes, and strawberries. Industrially, they're also extracted very often from apples and citrus peel to create supplements. Pectins are associated with balancing cholesterol, combating diarrhea, supporting weight loss, and reducing the risk of type 2 diabetes.

Psyllium

Extracted from the husks of a plant called *Plantago ovata*, traditionally grown in India, a psyllium husk is part soluble and part insoluble, which makes it a great fiber choice. Because of its low fermentability, psyllium is well tolerated, but it still packs plenty of benefits. It has been linked to balancing cholesterol, softening stools and promoting intestinal transit, managing blood sugar, supporting weight loss, and improving heart health and blood pressure.

Wheat Dextrin

A wheat dextrin is a common soluble fiber found in many fiber supplements and as a bulking agent in processed foods, such as soups, stews, and baby foods. Though they're most commonly extracted from wheat starch, dextrins can also be extracted from corn, potatoes, rice, and tapioca. Since wheat dextrins and other dextrins are industrially processed, they probably should not be your first choice of fiber. However, they have been shown to help manage cholesterol, reduce blood sugar, and lower the risk of heart disease.

Polydextrose, Polyols, Maltodextrins, and Plant Gums

These types of soluble fiber are industrially processed (although plant gums can be minimally processed) and are highly fermentable. They're commonly added to processed foods as a bulking agent, gluten substitute (plant gums), or sweetener (polyols). I am not a big fan of polydextrose and polyols, but I think that supplementing with plant gums might be a fine way to increase your fiber options.

> **Neo Note: Soluble Fibers**
> Since the soluble fibers "attract" water, it is essential to make sure you are getting enough water while increasing your fiber consumption. This will ensure that your digestive tract is optimally hydrated. Sometimes taking in too much fiber without enough water can cause digestive discomfort.

Resistant Starches

Same authors include resistant starches as part of the fiber family, while some don't, since fiber is usually seen as a non-starch compound. I clearly am not one to get stuck in these little details, so to keep things simple, I'm just going to say resistant starches are part of the fiber family.

As the name suggests, these are starches that resist digestion. They pass through our GI tract intact and serve as food for our microbiome. They are naturally found in unripened bananas, raw potatoes (highly toxic, so please don't eat), oatmeal, and legumes. You can also "produce" resistant starches by cooking and then cooling certain starchy foods, like potatoes and rice. The cooling of these foods after they've been cooked converts some of their starches into resistant starches. Some authors claim that the more times the starches are heated and cooled, the more resistant they become. They have been found to lower blood sugar, help manage weight by increasing satiety, fight dysbiosis by promoting good bacteria, decrease inflammation, increase insulin sensitivity, and possibly reduce the risk of diabetes and some cancers.

> **Neo Note: Magic Beans**
> Undercooked beans have caused several outbreaks of food poisoning due to their high content of antinutrients.[51,52] But, as you already know, if properly prepared, beans can be a rich source of prebiotics for your bugs. Studies have shown that beans assist with promoting weight loss, managing cholesterol, lowering blood sugar (even to the point that many people have had complete remission of their diabetes), reducing inflammation, increasing numbers of beneficial SCFA-producing bacteria, reinforcing colonic barrier integrity, reducing bacterial endotoxin levels, and lowering the risk of heart disease and cancer.[53-58] Not bad at all!

FEEDING PATHOGENIC BACTERIA

Won't prebiotics also feed pathogenic bacteria? There are "test-tube" studies that show prebiotics increasing pathogenic bacteria, but this does not seem to happen in "real-life" (in vivo) scenarios, presumably because the growth of the good guys keeps the bad guys in check.[59,60]

While eating prebiotics is safe, this doesn't mean we have to take in ridiculous amounts of fiber. Despite the recent prebiotic hype, we have seen time and time again that taking things to the extreme doesn't work that well. Yes, more fiber is great, but drowning in fiber is just as bad as not getting any. If you have an excess of bacteria, as in SIBO, the last thing you want to do is give more food to that overcrowded population. Even people with IBS should be cautious, since SIBO may be the underlying cause, and eating more fiber might make everything worse.[61] Studies have shown that sudden increases in prebiotics in patients with Crohn's disease and ulcerative colitis caused their symptoms to double.[62]

The key in many of these conditions is to heal the underlying causes and then slowly, I repeat, slowly introduce prebiotics like fiber and resistant starches. One thing we do in the Neo Diet is not only go through a short elimination period to reduce overgrowths but also take advantage of ketone bodies to "feed" the cells of the colon, which will lower inflammation and improve intestinal wall integrity.[63,64] As the gut heals, we then introduce prebiotics.

THE FODMAP CONCEPT

If you have read a little about nutrition, you've probably heard about FODMAPs. This is an acronym for *fermentable oligosaccharides, disaccharides, monosaccharides, and polyols*, which basically are prebiotic compounds that are fermented by our microbiome. As you can guess, too much or improper fermentation can lead to issues such as excessive gas, bloating, discomfort, and diarrhea.

FODMAPs are mainly divided into the six categories below.

• *Lactose*: The sugar in dairy.
• *Galacto-oligosaccharides*: Prebiotic derived from lactose. Commonly found in dairy but also in legumes.
• *Fructose*: Sugar in fruits and some vegetables.
• *Fructans*: As we just saw, these are the prebiotics in some grains, fruits, and vegetables.
• *Maltodextrin*: Highly processed sugar primarily used in foods and beverages as a thickener, sweetener, and stabilizer. Said to be low carb, but it produces a substantial insulin spike.
• *Polyols*: Sugar alcohols like mannitol, sorbitol, xylitol, lactitol, and erythritol. These are often found in artificial sweeteners and some fruits and vegetables.

Considering that FODMAPs can cause digestive symptoms, we should eliminate them from our diets, right? Several authors believe we should. But after reading all that I've written so far, you already know better, *don'tcha*?

When the initial low-FODMAP-diet studies were presented, the authors clearly explained that this was a temporary elimination diet, not a permanent one. Unfortunately, many just ignored the temporary part and went all in with it, causing the misunderstanding we have today.

Research has shown that long-term FODMAP restriction can cause a substantial drop in beneficial bacteria and even lead to significant micronutrient deficits (for example, of calcium, retinol, riboflavin, and thiamin,).[65–68] FODMAPS like fructans and galacto-oligosaccharides are phenomenal prebiotics that should be part of a healthy diet. Yes, a temporary low-FODMAP diet is incredibly effective for many conditions like dysbiosis, SIBO, and IBS.[69–72] But after healing the gut, we should reintroduce the healthy prebiotic FODMAPs to keep our bacteria happy and get their awesome postbiotics. This controlled food reintroduction also helps us assess our potential food sensitivities and see which food groups we need to be more careful in reintroducing.

TAKING YOUR BUGS TO THE GYM

If you are reading this book, chances are your gut is not at its best right now. As you know, if the gut is struggling, eating fiber and other prebiotics might cause issues. And, it's not just prebiotics. If you have IBS, for example, you have a high probability of experiencing (or perceiving) significant food intolerances.[73] Some people right now might even be at a point where most things they eat cause them to have adverse reactions. How can I ask them to eat fiber? Well, in truth, these are the people who need it the most. We just need to do it in the right way.

After completing an elimination period, we need to be consistent with the reintroduction of these foods. It's not like you can eat some artichokes today and then only try again next week. You need to eat a particular food in small doses, but frequently. As you train your microbiome, not only will your bugs be able to consume higher doses of fiber, but they will also become better at processing that fiber. With practice, they can process prebiotics in a more efficient way, producing more postbiotics like vitamins and SCFAs for you, without provoking the GI distress they once caused.

When you go to the gym, you shouldn't just focus on one exercise only. Let's say you do only arm curls. You might develop biceps like Popeye's, but the rest of your body will be weak. The same applies to the microbiome. You have different bugs that thrive on different foods and that produce different postbiotics. If you eat only a single type of prebiotics, you feed only a certain group of bugs. While that group will thrive, the entire intestinal ecosystem will be fragile. To get the maximum benefits, you should feed your microbiome an ample range of the foods they love, so your entire microbiome can grow stronger and you can obtain all possible postbiotics. Variety is the key. The goal is to eventually reach the point where you can mix several types of prebiotics into your weekly diet. Now, it might seem impossible, but I promise, I'll get you there!

I should add, there aren't many studies that recommend clear fiber consumption limits, but according to anecdotal reports, more than 150 to 200 grams of prebiotics a day might be too much for most people. So don't overdo it.

Neo Note: Prebiotic Supplements

I am not a fan of relying only on supplements to address gaps that could easily be remedied through diet. Nevertheless, I can definitely see a place for fiber supplements. They can be a great tool, especially during the initial reintroduction stages, when you are slowly increasing your intake of different prebiotics. It's essential, however, to be selective about these supplements. For example, it's pretty common to see beta-glucan or dextrin supplements being extracted from grains. Even though we are talking about important prebiotics, we have to consider that if the grains used were exposed to glyphosate and other toxins, we might be depositing those toxins into our intestinal ecosystem. As another example, let's say that you suffer from celiac disease. Consuming beta-glucans from wheat, barley, and rye is obviously contraindicated, but if you choose beta-glucan extracts from mushrooms and seaweed extracts, this is perfectly safe.

Some of the best (and gentlest) choices to start with are psyllium and plant gums like guar and acacia. In the resources section of the book, I share some of my favorite prebiotic supplements.

NEO SUMMARY
• Fiber is commonly misunderstood, but it is essential for optimal health.
• Most people are fiber deficient.
• There are different fiber types and all are important for a healthy body.
• Fiber improves detoxification, lowers inflammation, and boosts metabolic health.
• Excessive fiber might exacerbate symptoms and its increase should be gradual.

NEO ACTION
• If you commonly experience GI distress symptoms, it might be a good idea to adopt a low FODMAP diet.
• If you currently do not have GI distress symptoms, start slowly expanding your prebiotic variety.

NEO RECOMMENDATIONS
• *Fiber Fueled* by Dr. Will Bulsiewicz
• *Healthy Gut, Healthy You* by Dr. Michael Ruscio
• *The Energy Paradox* by Dr. Steven Gundry
• *The Longevity Paradox* by Dr. Steven Gundry

my.neodiet.co/neorecommendations

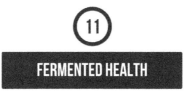

FERMENTED HEALTH

The Traditional Foods That Made Us Stronger

"Fermentation may have been a better invention than fire."
David Wallace

FERMENTATION AND PROBIOTICS

Go to any store today and you will find dozens, if not hundreds, of products infused with probiotics. The probiotic movement boomed in the '90s with probiotic-rich yogurt, but since then this craze has expanded to other foods like kefir and kombucha. These foods look like a recent phenomenon, but in reality, we have been fermenting foods and "growing" probiotics for millennia. In fact, scientists have found in Jordan fermented bread that was estimated to be 14,000 years old.[1] In Israel, archeologists found a 13,000-year-old wheat-and-barley-based beer mixture.[2] Other findings of the use of fermentation with more than 8,000 years have been found in Sweden and China, for example.[3,4] It's a fact! We have been using fermentation for a long time and all over the world.

Before the time of preservatives, fridges, freezers, and canning, fermentation was one of the best strategies we had to preserve food. Fermentation allowed people to eat foods like meat, fish, dairy, grains, vegetables, and fruits that usually would be scarcer during the winter. This is why, still to this day, you can find fermented traditional foods in most cultures. We have kimchi from Korea, tempeh from Indonesia, natto and miso from Japan, injera from Ethiopia, kvass from Russia, sauerkraut from Germany, and a whole lot of other traditional foods made with yogurt, fermented meat, and fermented fish in various countries.

With the industrialization of food production and the new methods of food conservation, humans stopped relying on these traditional foods. With the spread of the Western diet, only a select few fermented foods, such as wine, beer, bread, yogurt, cheese, chocolate, pickles, and ketchup, continued to thrive. Yes, these are all foods created through fermentation. Or at least, they used to be. Luckily, because of all the studies on probiotics that started in the 1990s, fermented foods are in an upward spiral, and even culture-specific foods are starting to spread all over the world.

FERMENTATION 101

One common mistake is to confuse decomposition (spoilage or rotting) with fermentation. Technically, decomposition is a form of fermentation, because it results from the transformation of organic matter by microorganisms. But we attribute completely different meanings to these two. We use the term *decomposition* when the transformation process makes the organic compound go bad (like rotten meat or spoiled fruit). Conversely, we use the term *fermentation* when the transformation process makes the organic compound "go good"—meaning, the foods convert into something better than before. They become easier to digest and more nutritious.

By tweaking the environment of this transformation, we can determine whether the food will decompose or ferment in a positive way. Let's look at sauerkraut, for example. When you put the cabbage under water, this "tweaks the environment" for the anaerobic bacteria (those that can live without oxygen). These bacteria ferment the cabbage and transform some carbs and fiber into different acids (such as SCFAs). As acids accumulate, the pH of the solution drops and creates a toxic environment for most microorganisms. Only a few good bugs (probiotics) can thrive in such an acidic environment, so your sauerkraut does not decompose. Instead, it continues to build up more probiotics and amazing postbiotics that result from the fermentation.

BENEFITS OF FERMENTATION

Think of the fermentation that occurs in a jar of kimchi the same way you think about your microbiome breaking down hard-to-digest foods in your intestines. In a way, what is happening in the jar is similar to what's going on in your gut. The microorganisms break down the food into simpler substances that you can absorb, and in the process, the bugs create postbiotics that enhance the food's nutritional value.

As we've seen, fermentation of certain foods can eliminate several of their antinutrients, such as gluten, phytic acid, and lectins.[5] Fermentation has even been shown to help us degrade pesticides in our foods, making them less harmful.[6] These two facts may explain why people with IBS generally tolerate sourdough bread but suffer when they eat traditional wheat bread.

Fermentation can ramp up the nutrient value of the food. For example, researchers found out that the fermentation of sourdough creates 25 different antioxidant peptides that help you fight oxidative stress and inflammation.[7] Studies also uncovered that fermentation of soy milk with certain bacteria may activate isoflavones and increase bone volume and thickness, which is essential to reducing the risk of osteoporosis.[8] In South Korea, a clinical trial concluded that the fermentation of red ginseng increases the number of bioactive saponins in it and helps control blood sugar.[9] And other studies have shown that fermentation can use nonvitamin precursors (compounds that do not contain vitamins) to produce B vitamins and vitamin K.[10,11] This list could go on and on. The point is that fermentation makes food safer and more digestible, and increases its micronutrient profile.

MICRONUTRITION

So far, I've dedicated entire chapters to macronutrients but made only a few brief mentions of micronutrients. My bad. I guess size does matter! According to its definition in the *Merriam-Webster Dictionary*, a micronutrient is "a chemical element or substance that is essential in minute amounts to the growth and health of a living organism." It's because of the minute quantities needed that we call them *micro*nutrients. But needing something in small quantities differs from not needing it at all. In fact, according to the CDC, micronutrients are vital to healthy development, disease prevention, and overall well-being.[12] Micronutrients are essential for many bodily functions. Scratch that! Micronutrients are essential for all bodily functions. As we've discussed before, at a fundamental level, everything we are is expressed by our cells. To operate, our cells need energy, which comes from the macronutrients we take in. But in order to use that potential energy, guess what cells need. You got it. Micronutrients! Micronutrients such as B vitamins, magnesium, and sulfur are required for your mitochondria to power your cells and make them function properly. Without them, your cells would not last long.

When we think about micronutrients, we think about vitamins and minerals, but there are hundreds of different compounds that belong to the micronutrient family (for example, antioxidants, carotenoids, enzymes, polyphenols, trace minerals, and so on). Heck, scientists are still discovering new micronutrients every year. What is important to know is that these substances are important and that by eating nutrient-dense "real" food, we will get different combinations of them that, together, potentiate our human health experience.

Unfortunately, that is not what happens with most people. Our separation from authentic food is not allowing us to obtain all the micronutrients that we need in order to thrive. We were brainwashed to worry about calories when, in fact, we do not have a calorie issue. We have a micronutrient issue. As I've said before, we are overfed but undernourished. If you want to stop food cravings, boost your vitality, and feel at the top of your game, eat micronutrient-dense foods!

Neo Note: Micronutrient Deficits and Behavior

I know that by now you have no questions about the importance of proper micronutrient intake for your overall health. But I still have one more study I would like to present to you.[13] A group of researchers studied a possible connection between nutrition and violent behavior of young male prison inmates in the UK. To do so, the researchers performed a double-blind, randomized trial in which one group of inmates was provided a multivitamin and essential fatty acid supplement, while the other group received a placebo. During the 4½ months of the study, violent incidents involving the inmates receiving nutritional support dropped by 37 percent. That's right! By getting better nutrition, the inmates were more emotionally stable than before. Something to really think about!

Some people try to adopt the convenient approach and just take a daily multivitamin. While I understand the thought process, I have to reinforce that synthetic supplements cannot be compared to real food. Real food has all the right micronutrients with the right combination of cofactors to create the balanced nutrition your body needs. Synthetic supplements don't. Some good brands try to source supplements from actual food and avoid overisolating compounds in order to create properly balanced supplements, but unfortunately, these represent less than 1 percent of the products out there.

The supplements most people take are the ones with high quantities of isolated compounds like vitamins or minerals. These high doses of a single micronutrient can end up causing serious deficiencies of its antagonist micronutrient. For example, many people have been supplementing with zinc lately in an effort to boost their immunity. A great natural source of zinc is oysters. But one of the differences between supplements and actual oysters is that this shellfish also contains the mineral antagonist copper. So, when we eat oysters, there is no risk of creating deficiencies by "overdosing" on the "opposing mineral." But most people supplementing with zinc are becoming copper deficient.[14] People are getting their zinc to support the immune system, but the copper deficiency they're creating is causing anemia, fatigue, weakness, connective tissue disorders, osteoporosis, ataxia, and, ironically, increased risk of infection.[15–17]

Then we have the entire issue of synthetic supplements being made out of crude oil, petroleum, coal, and formaldehyde. I kindly invite you to google this. It's not surprising, then, that studies have shown that synthetic supplements are absorbed differently and are unlikely to be used by the body in the same way as their natural counterparts.[18–20] There are even studies showing that synthetic supplement intake was associated with a higher risk of cancer and death.[21–24]

My goal was just to make a quick comment on micronutrients, since fermented foods are a great natural source of them. I guess I got a little carried away. The point here is that one of your main goals should be to focus on micronutrient-rich foods like animal foods, some fruits and vegetables, and of course, the amazing fermented foods. Not only are they nutrition bombs, but they are also the best way to optimize your probiotic intake.

BENEFITS OF EATING FERMENTED FOODS

Since fermented foods combine probiotics and prebiotics, you get the benefits of both. Actually, their combined benefits may even be superior to their sum. How can you not love these superfoods?

In one study, individuals with diabetes who ate probiotic yogurt showed a whopping 30-point reduction in blood glucose compared with the placebo group.[25] These glucose-lowering effects of probiotics were further supported by several meta-analyses of placebo-controlled trials.[26,27] Furthermore, the metabolic effects of these fermented foods don't stop here. Their probiotics have also been shown to promote weight loss in obese men and women.[28] Previously, we also saw how probiotics were linked to substantial improvements in mental health. It seems they are also great at boosting mental performance. Using magnetic resonance imaging (MRI) scans, researchers were able to see that women who regularly ate yogurt containing probiotics had improved connectivity within the prefrontal cortex.[29] This may indicate superior planning, organizing, and self-regulation abilities. Other studies also support the possibility of these probiotics working to promote memory and cognitive health.[30,31]

Some benefits from probiotics in fermented foods also have to do with their ability to synthesize postbiotics. In fact, fermented foods are rich in SCFA postbiotics.[32] The main SCFAs in your body are butyrate, acetate, and propionate, all of which have been linked to health promotion and longevity. As you have probably noticed by the number of times I've already mentioned it, butyrate is by far the most-studied SCFA. In earlier chapters, we've already seen that butyrate is critical to control mitochondrial oxidative stress, boost cellular metabolism and health, soothe inflammation, and regulate the immune response. Other studies also show that a deficiency in SCFAs (especially butyrate) has been connected with the development of obesity, metabolic syndrome, inflammatory bowel disease, and certain types of cancer.[33,34]

We can theorize that the metabolic benefits of SCFAs may be connected with their ability to promote ketone production.[35] Also, for cancer in particular, SCFAs have been shown to regulate cell growth and differentiation, which is the fundamental premise for carcinogenic growth.[36] Malignant cells need histone deacetylases (HDACs) in order to copy themselves and multiply. Butyrate is well known for being able to inhibit HDACs, thus inhibiting cancerous cell replication.[37-40] On top of that, SCFAs have been shown to promote apoptosis (cell death), which eliminates the mutated cells that cause cancer.[41-44]

Finally, since SCFAs seem to cross the BBB, they can have a direct effect on brain cells.[45,46] Not only may fermented foods (with their prebiotics and SCFAs) be able to improve children's cognition (multitasking, working memory, and maintaining focus), but researchers believe they might also

262 THE NEO DIET – CHAPTER 11

protect the brains of adults from diseases like Parkinson's and Alzheimer's.[47-53] Some of these findings regarding the brain may be related to butyrate's ability to raise levels of BDNF, which, as you know, directly slows neurodegeneration and boosts neuroplasticity.[54] Considering all these benefits of fermented foods, it seems safe to say there is no other type of food with such health-promoting potential.

THE HISTAMINE ISSUE

Last chapter, as we discussed the increased consumption of prebiotics, we noted the need to train the body for FODMAP foods. We have a similar "problem" with fermented foods. The problem is called histamine. Histamines (and other amines) are compounds produced by the immune system to trigger a defense response against allergens (although they also work as neurotransmitters). You naturally produce histamines, but you can also get them from your diet. And, as I'm sure you've already guessed it, fermented foods are rich in them.

For most people, this is not a problem because they can break down histamine. But if you suddenly increase your histamine intake, your body might struggle to break them all down, and they might accumulate. This can stir up allergy symptoms like an itchy throat, a stuffy nose, skin reactions, digestive discomfort, joint pain, and even, in more severe cases, neurological symptoms.[55] As with FODMAPs, with "practice," the body becomes more efficient, and this stops being an issue. The same concept of slow introduction and increase also applies here.

It's important to note that there are people with genetic mutations that cause them to have a hard time producing diamine oxidase (DAO), which is the main enzyme that degrades histamines in the body.[56] These people are "histamine intolerant." The good news is that even someone with reduced histamine tolerance can supplement with DAO or eat plenty of pea sprouts or kidney meat, which are said to be great natural sources of this enzyme.

If, with the careful introduction of fermented foods, you still experience allergy symptoms, it is important to rule out food sensitivities. Try to change the type of fermented food and see whether it was the food or the histamines in it. Also, try to eliminate fermented foods completely and check if the symptoms persist. If they do, it's either another food that you are reacting to, or it might even be something environmental, like pollen. If that is the case, it means that your gut needs further healing in order to better modulate your autoimmunity issues.

Another thing you can do is to bump up your fiber consumption. Research shows that increased fiber intake can boost levels of DAO and help you break down histamines.[57,58] Another hack is to supplement with quercetin or eat foods rich in it, such as capers, lovage leaves, okra, or onions. Quercetin has been shown to be a great histamine blocker.[59]

Women may also notice that depending on their menstrual cycle, they can have higher or lower tolerance to histamines. Studies have uncovered that after ovulation, women have higher levels of DAO, which makes the breakdown of histamines in fermented foods a lot easier.[60]

Please keep in mind that you may also find out that you are actually genetically intolerant to histamines. In that case, you may have to always eat foods rich in DAO or take a DAO supplement. I say "may" because studies suggest that certain strains of bacteria, such as *Bifidobacterium infantis*, *Bifidobacterium adolescentis*, *Lactobacillus plantarum*, *Lactobacillus rhamnosus*, *Bacteroides thetaiotaomicron*, and *Bacteroides fragilis*, are able to degrade histamine or reduce the body's reactivity to it.[61–65] What this means is that the healthier your gut is, the more tolerant you become, despite your genetic mutation.

Finally, I just want to note that the histamine issue is not exclusive to fermented foods. You can find high histamine levels in many foods, like bone broth, canned foods, eggplant, mushrooms, nuts (especially cashews and walnuts), processed foods, shellfish, spinach, vinegar, and leftovers that are a few days old (the less fresh the food is, the more histamines it has).

KEEP THEM COMING

One of the great reasons to start eating fermented foods is because of their probiotic content. And one reason to continue eating them frequently is . . . because of their probiotic content. Confused? I'll explain. Apparently, most probiotics cannot colonize you. According to research, our microbiome is not very welcoming to newcomers and makes it almost impossible for new microbes to establish a home in the gut.[66] This is a defense mechanism so we do not get colonized by pathogenic bacteria. It's almost like when our parents would tell us not to open the door to strangers. Not allowing strangers into our guts is a good thing, but it also causes us to have increased difficulty in bolstering our good long-term residents. These findings are supported by other studies that demonstrate that a week after intake of probiotics stops, they largely disappear from the stool.[67]

Does this mean we should not eat probiotic-rich foods? Not at all! Even though most of them will be only temporary visitors, while they are there, they communicate with the locals and help digest food, maintain your intestinal walls, kick out the bad guys, and boost your immunity.[68,69] Free labor in exchange for a bed. A concept that never gets old.

These transient probiotics are so great that they still benefit you even if they're dead. Weird, right? According to several studies, probiotics that have been "heated to death" were somehow still able to produce beneficial results. Heat-killed probiotics have been shown to boost the immune system of seniors and also treat diarrhea, improve IBS symptoms, resolve skin allergies, and decrease the incidence of colds in the general population.[70–74] I honestly

264 THE NEO DIET – CHAPTER 11

am still scratching my head over this one. The only justification I can come up with is that pathogens get scared by seeing all the dead bodies passing through your GI tract and run away. And the good guys get a reality check and start performing better at their jobs. Too far-fetched?

> **Neo Note: Taking Probiotic Supplements**
> As you know, I always favor real foods. But probiotic supplements have their place in a healing protocol, since people's guts might be too fragile to handle natural sources of probiotics like fermented foods. By temporarily adding a good probiotic supplement, you may give your gut the boost it needs to crowd out some of the bad guys causing dysbiosis and lower the inflammation to a point where you can tolerate fermented foods.

RECOMMENDED FERMENTED FOODS

Before we go through my list of favorite fermented foods, it's important to remind you that not all foods are created equal. Fermented foods are no exception. For example, if you're choosing some sourdough bread from an artisanal bakery, you should opt for bread made with organic ancient grain flour. Or, if buying yogurt, grab the one made with "A2 milk" from pasture-raised cows. Also, another important tip is to make sure the probiotic foods you eat are not pasteurized, since the heat will kill the bacteria.

Sauerkraut

I'm sure we can agree that most people would not rate cabbage as a nutritional powerhouse. However, when fermented, it becomes a rich source of vitamins and minerals, like B vitamins, vitamins C and K, and iron. Sauerkraut is also a significant source of fiber, probiotics, and SCFAs. Research has shown that just one serving of commercial sauerkraut can provide around 28 different strains of bacteria.[75] And let me emphasize that these results were in commercial preparations. Just imagine how much bacteria will be present in a homemade, raw sauerkraut.

Depending on where in the world you live, you might have a hard time finding raw sauerkraut in stores. If you find it, please make sure the ingredients are just cabbage (sometimes makers add more vegetables to it), water, and salt. Sauerkraut does not need any additives and preservatives, so please stay away from them. In case you can't find it, don't worry. It's actually extremely easy to make sauerkraut at home. In broad brushstrokes, you just add cabbage, water, and salt (and some love) to a jar and wait. Just type *sauerkraut* on YouTube and you'll find a ton of detailed tutorials.

Kimchi

Kimchi can be considered a more diverse sauerkraut. On top of the cabbage base, it can include different ingredients like ginger, garlic, daikon radishes, carrots, peppers, and scallions, just to name a few. Depending on who made the kimchi, it may pack too much of a kick for some, but you can also do it at home and make it less spicy. As mentioned earlier, kimchi is a traditional food from the Korean Peninsula. It's so beloved by their natives that it's estimated that the average South Korean person eats 48 pounds of kimchi a year. No wonder a 2017 study published in the prestigious journal the *Lancet* revealed that by 2030, South Korea will probably have the highest worldwide life expectancy.[76] Several studies have shown that eating kimchi lowers cholesterol, promotes weight loss, improves insulin sensitivity, soothes inflammation, boosts anticarcinogenic processes in the body, and may even confer antiaging benefits.[77-83]

Natto

When boiled soybeans are fermented, they form an enzyme called nattokinase, which causes the soybeans to transform into the traditional Japanese food natto. Natto is not one of those foods that is eaten in large quantities, being mostly enjoyed as a small dish for breakfast. Not everyone is a big fan of natto, since it has an ammonia-like smell and a gooey consistency similar to mucus. But don't let the smell or texture throw you off, because this fermented food is a tremendous health booster. The nattokinase in natto has been shown to destroy clots, lower blood pressure, and balance cholesterol, among other benefits that have been linked to a reduction in cardiovascular mortality.[84] Probiotic strains (*Bacillus subtilis*) in natto may also improve our immune function.[85] And natto is one of the best sources of vitamin K_2, which, as we've seen, has important roles not only in blood coagulation but also in bone metabolism.[86] Natto might be difficult to find beyond Asian markets, but it's definitely worth the work of looking for it.

Miso

Miso is a paste made by fermenting soybeans with a fungus called koji (*Aspergillus oryzae*). If you've ever been to a Japanese restaurant, I'm sure you have at least been offered some miso soup. If you ever try miso soup, please don't make the same mistake I did, of assuming that the white squares are the miso. That's actually tofu. The miso paste is diluted in the soup water. At least the waiter and I had a good laugh. Miso adds a lot of umami flavor to foods and is a great addition to soups, broths, marinades, and dressings. Just be careful not to cook the miso paste, so you don't kill the probiotics. Add it only after you turn off the heat.

A Japanese study concluded that miso eaten with a meal led to improved insulin function and a faster normalization of blood glucose levels after the meal.[87] So it's not a coincidence that they offer you miso soup before sushi. Miso is also rich in calcium, vitamin K, and isoflavones, all of which contribute to preventing osteoporosis.[88] Research has also shown that eating miso may help prevent several cancers.[89-91]

Tempeh

To end our soy fermentation sequence, let's talk about tempeh. Because of its high protein content and dense consistency, this is a commonly used meat alternative for many people adhering to a vegan diet. There aren't as many studies on tempeh as we have for the other fermented foods, but due to its prebiotic and probiotic content, we can imagine that some benefits might be in the same line as the others presented here. One study published in the journal *Pharmaceutical Biology* uncovered that tempeh has a good antioxidant capacity.[92] Even though I occasionally eat some tempeh, especially when I'm with some vegan friends (yes, it is okay to be friends with people who have different ideologies), I am not the biggest fan for two reasons. First, tempeh is usually cooked, which kills the probiotics. Second, even though fermenting soy removes most of its antinutrients, soy is not something we want to overconsume. While natto and miso are usually eaten in small quantities, tempeh is consumed in larger quantities, since it is a meat replacement. That being said, if you follow a vegan diet, tempeh is much better than any processed fake meat you can buy.

Yogurt

Thanks to all the research that started in the '90s, yogurt is probably the most famous source of probiotics in the world. As you know, yogurt is made from the fermentation of milk. We already discussed extensively the importance of the source of the milk and its treatment. Obviously, this will affect the quality of the yogurt. Keep in mind that most of the studies done on yogurt were performed with commercial, pasteurized yogurt. What this means is that if even commercial yogurt shows good results, just imagine what a good A2 raw yogurt from pasture-raised cows can accomplish.

Several studies have shown that yogurt consumption is associated with enhanced integrity of the gut lining, better regulation of intestinal transit, reduced inflammation, improved glucose metabolism, better weight management, lower blood pressure, and improved cardiovascular health.[93-99]

Besides the probiotics for which it's famous, yogurt is also rich in protein, healthy fats (in good yogurts, at least), and an array of micronutrients, in particular calcium, vitamins B_2 and B_{12}, magnesium, phosphorus, and potassium. A good-quality yogurt may even be suitable for some people with lactose intolerance. If it's fermented long enough, the bacteria can break down almost all the lactose for you.

Kefir

Kefir is a fermented drink similar to a liquid yogurt. It is said to be one of the oldest cultured milk products in existence, having originated in the Caucasus region but having become famous in Russia. Some say that the word *kefir* comes from the word *kefi*, which in some Caucasus languages meant "choice" or "best quality." Others claim that it comes from the Turkish *keyif*, meaning "which gives pleasure." No matter who's right, kefir is indeed a great choice, since its benefits give us pleasure. Too corny?

Kefir was originally made by adding kefir grains (which we know are actually cultures of bacteria and yeast) to goat's or cow's milk. Nowadays, we have more options, like coconut kefir and even water kefir.

Several recent studies have shown that regular consumption of kefir is associated with improved digestion and tolerance to lactose; antiallergic, antibacterial, antidiabetic, antihypertensive, and anti-inflammatory effects; better cholesterol metabolism; improved microbiota modulation; immunomodulation; higher antioxidant activity; and anticarcinogenic activity.[100-103] But many of the smaller studies supporting these findings were conducted in vitro or in animal models, so more human in vivo research is needed. Kefir is a good source of vitamin K_2 and also contains kefiran, a unique compound that can reduce inflammation and modulate the immune response.[104]

Kombucha

Kombucha is said to have originated in China or Japan about 2,000 years ago. It is produced through the fermentation of black or sometimes green tea with specific strains of bacteria. More recently, people started to make it more appealing to the masses by adding many different teas and fruits. Every day, you find new brands popping up in stores around the world. This phenomenon is probably spurred by kombucha's effervescence created by fermentation, which makes it a healthier soda substitute. It's definitely an acquired taste, and it might take you a couple of tries before you begin to like it. But once you start enjoying it, you might get hooked.

Although kombucha has many health benefits, it's important once again to reinforce that the production method is essential to its quality. Some commercial kombuchas are not fermented properly and still have too much sugar left in them. On the other hand, some batches of kombucha might have fermented too much, which can cause alcohol to form. In fact, some kombuchas in stores actually report an alcohol percentage of 3 percent, which is comparable to that of a light beer. Depending on the type and quantity of kombucha you drink, you might get drunk. So, as this beverage gains popularity, we might see a new slogan on highway advertisements: "Don't drink too much kombucha and drive."

Kombucha's acidity means that excessive consumption also may have the potential to erode tooth enamel. This is one of those examples of too much of a good thing being bad for you. Some people dilute their kombucha with water just to reduce the acidity a little. Others suggest drinking it out of a straw to decrease contact with the teeth. Either way, I don't think this is a huge concern as long as you're not drinking enormous quantities every day.

Because of its probiotics, kombucha has been shown to have antibacterial and antifungal effects, which may be important contributors in reducing pathogenic bacteria and reestablishing microbial balance.[105] Other studies suggest that beyond its probiotic effects, kombucha is also rich in antioxidants that seem to help heal the liver and boost detoxification.[106] On top of these benefits, a 2020 review adds that kombucha may help fight constipation, improve glucose metabolism, and offer anticarcinogenic effects.[107]

I personally haven't tried doing this yet, but I've heard that it is pretty cool to make your own kombucha at home. Give it a try. Let me know how it turns out.

Kvass

Kvass is still a somewhat unknown fermented beverage in most places except for Eastern European countries. This beverage was originally made from the fermentation of rye or barley, so it tasted almost like beer. Kvass is also made through the fermentation of beets (and other root vegetables), and some people add fruits, spices, and herbs to give it extra flavor. The fermentation of these grains or beets removes a significant portion of their antinutrients and boosts their nutritional profile. Not to mention that it adds a ton of awesome probiotics.[108]

There aren't many studies available on the benefits of kvass, but just by focusing on its probiotics, we can expect an overall boost in many areas of our health. Beet kvass might be the most beneficial one because of the amazing phytonutrients present in beets. Research on beet fermentation shows significant antioxidant and anti-inflammatory effects.[109] Other studies on the phytonutrients in beets also suggest strong immune-boosting properties (even help in fighting cancer) and powerful cardiovascular effects that improve athletic performance.[110-113]

Pickles

Pickling food has been a preservation technique used for millennia in different parts of the world. People have pickled vegetables, fruits, and even meat, fish, and eggs. Probably the most famous pickle is the cucumber with its many seasonings. But please keep in mind that the majority of pickles we find in stores are not fermented. They are produced in mass scale, which involves their pasteurization. The fermented taste comes from added vinegar.

Many times, these are also filled with additives and preservatives. Definitely not the fermented food we're looking for. However, you can still find some true "raw pickles." If you can't, it's definitely an easy fermented food to make at home.

A 2018 review found several studies highlighting the benefits of pickles.[114] Pickles have been shown to balance the microbiome, enhance digestion, improve cholesterol, help with headaches and fever, boost immunity, and enhance cellular health. Pickles and especially pickle juice have also become popular among athletes as an aid to recovering from exercise and reducing cramps, because of these foods' naturally occurring electrolytes and antioxidants.[115]

Apple Cider Vinegar

As the name indicates, apple cider vinegar (ACV) is made through the fermentation of apples. It has been used for centuries in cooking and especially as a health elixir. ACV seems to be a great metabolic stabilizer. Studies have shown that having just a tablespoon of ACV along with a starchy meal helps lower glucose and the insulin effect.[116] It may even improve blood sugar control in individuals with type 2 diabetes.[117] Other research has concluded that taking two tablespoons of ACV in the evening helps blood sugar levels the following morning.[118] Besides the glucose management effects, raw ACV has also been found to kill pathogenic bacteria, promote healthy weight loss, scavenge free radicals, and lower heart-disease risk factors.[119–124]

Obviously, there are more fermented foods, including some that I've probably never heard of. My goal here hasn't been to list them all, but to give my favorite recommendations. I just want to note that I am also a big fan of sourdough bread, but since I had already talked about it earlier, I didn't find the need to extoll its benefits again. The key is that you explore your options, find different fermented foods, and make them a consistent part of your diet.

NEO SUMMARY
• Fermentation has been used for thousands of years to preserve and revitalize food.
• Fermented foods combine the benefits of their prebiotics, probiotics and postbiotics.
• Fermentation improves the nutritional profile of foods.
• Histamines are present in fermented foods. They may cause allergy symptoms.
• Your histamine tolerance improves as your gut heals and it can be increased with practice.
• Even with increased histamine tolerance, it's advisable not to overconsume fermented foods. Besides too much histamine buildup, they may cause SIBO.
• There are many fermented foods around the world with amazing health benefits.

NEO ACTION
• Explore different fermented foods and slowly add them to your diet.
• Enjoy these foods but don't overconsume them.

NEO RECOMMENDATIONS
• *Deep Nutrition* by Dr. Catherine Shanahan
• *Eat Dirt* by Dr. Josh Axe
• *Eat Smarter* by Shawn Stevenson
• *Fiber Fueled* by Dr. Will Bulsiewicz
• *Gut and Psychology Syndrome* by Dr. Natasha Campbell-Mcbride
• *Paleo Principles* by Sarah Ballantyne
• *The Big Book of Kombucha* by Hannah Crum & Alex LaGory
• *The Kimchi Diet* by Dr. Susanne Bennett
• *Wild Fermentation* by Sandor Ellix Katz

— my.neodiet.co/neorecommendations

THE MISSING MACROS

What Many Consider the Elixirs of Life

"Everyone has limits. You just have to learn what your own limits are and deal with them accordingly."
Nolan Ryan

THE MISSING MACROS

Did you know that alcohol is a macronutrient? That's right. Alcohol is the fourth energy-yielding macronutrient, after carbs, protein, and fat. (Fiber does not directly yield energy.) I'm not big on calories, but just for reference, carbs and protein each contain four calories per gram, fats have nine calories per gram, and alcohol contains seven calories per gram.

I'm not finished, though. I still have another macronutrient for you. *Whaaaat?* I know, I just keep on giving. The secret macronutrient we still have to cover is water. Water can be considered a macronutrient because, similarly to fiber, it's also needed on a macro scale and can provide energy, but indirectly. More on that shortly, but to keep things simple, let's just focus on alcohol (a.k.a. the "fun macro") for now.

Obviously, we do not drink alcohol with the goal of meeting our energy requirements. If you use that excuse, you might have a problem. We consume alcohol because it is part of our tradition and because it's a symbol of connection and community. Some even say that it is the soul's elixir. Unfortunately, alcohol is also considered a toxin and a promoter of disease. Thus, I feel it is important to briefly touch on how alcohol has been part of our lives and what effects, good or bad, it may have on us.

ALCOHOL: FRIEND OR FOE?

There isn't an exact notion of where alcoholic drinks were first consumed, but their "invention" is believed to have occurred during the Neolithic era, possibly around 8500 BC.[1] This is another reason for the title of this book. *Just kidding!* Archaeological findings suggest that alcohol use might have started in the Caucasus and then spread west. But it seems humans were brewing alcohol in northern China around 7000 to 6600 BC, based on residues found in pottery jars.[2] This is to say, we might have had different geniuses around the world coming up with this idea. Regardless of where it was first used, alcoholic drinks have been part of most traditions across the globe for a long time. Alcohol consumption has been used for ceremonial reasons but also as a symbol of community and celebration.

Wine and beer in particular were initially seen as sources of health, vitality, and longevity, but slowly this narrative changed as humans discovered the deleterious effects of excessive alcohol consumption. The shift in perspective was so dramatic that many countries even banned alcohol during different periods (the most known being Prohibition in the United States). To this day, there are still several countries in the world where alcohol consumption is forbidden for religious and political reasons.

According to the WHO, the harmful use of alcohol is a causal factor in more than 200 diseases and injury conditions. In fact, 5.3 percent of all deaths worldwide might result from harmful use of alcohol.[3] Short-term liberal alcohol consumption is linked to several issues, including motor vehicle accidents.[4] But most of the negative health effects of alcohol seem to be associated with more long-term use. Some of these negative consequences are alcohol dependency, alcoholic liver diseases, pancreatitis, neurological diseases, psychiatric illnesses, hormonal disorders, cardiovascular diseases, and cancer.[5] Studies show that alcohol creates inflammation and induces gut permeability, which possibly explains why chronic alcohol consumption damages the liver and other organs.[6] Even a single night of excessive drinking of vodka has been linked to increases in inflammatory cytokines and endotoxins in the blood.[7]

Common belief is that having a "nightcap" is a great way to unwind and sleep better. But according to research, this is not true.[8] Yes, you might fall asleep faster, but alcohol does not promote the rejuvenating sleep you need, which occurs during the rapid eye movement (REM) stage. Besides making it harder for you to achieve the REM stage, as the alcohol wears off, it ends up disrupting your sleep even further. It might even lead to sleepwalking, sleep talking, and memory problems.[9]

Be that as it may, alcohol consumption is not all bad. As the German doctor Paracelsus once wrote, "whether wine is a nourishment, medicine, or poison is a matter of dosage." This is further supported by studies showing that over time, alcohol consumption seems to have a classic hormetic curve, in which some is good and too much is bad.[10] In one study that followed 9,000 men in US for 16 years, the authors concluded that those who drank an average of two small servings of alcohol a day had lower rates of heart disease and lived longer than those who abstained, rarely consumed alcohol, or overindulged.[11] In France, another study showed that moderate wine consumption was associated with a 33 percent reduction in all-cause mortality.[12] Yet another study, this time in China, also reported a 19 percent reduction in risk of death in people who drank rice wine in moderation.[13] Lastly, research from the

Netherlands that followed subjects for over 40 years uncovered that compared with abstinence, drinking about half a glass of alcohol per day might extend life by five years.[14]

Let's not get carried away, though. It's important to note that even studies that show these positive effects of moderate alcohol consumption also report that excessive alcohol intake was found to be dangerous in both young (due to higher risk of violent deaths and accidents) and older adults (because of the development of metabolic diseases).[15,16]

But research shows that in low doses, alcohol stimulates the blood vessels' endothelial cells to produce fibrinolytic (clot-busting) proteins that have the power to dissolve clots and prevent deep vein thrombosis (DVT), heart attacks, and strokes.[17] Additionally, low concentrations of alcohol induce increased release of nitric oxide (NO) from the endothelium, which promotes dilation of the vessels and improves blood flow.[18] This same study also reports that high intakes of alcohol will reverse the effect and cause reduced NO bioavailability. And, guys, the authors also state that chronic excessive alcohol intake also impairs penile erectile function. Remember the maxim "a little makes you bigger, a lot makes you lose your shot."

Red wine is also famous for having a phytonutrient called resveratrol. Resveratrol in wine has been shown to fight oxidation, help heart cells regenerate, and promote heart resilience against ischemic (oxygen deprivation) injuries.[19-21] There is even one study showing that people drinking between one and two glasses of red wine daily for 20 days may actually boost the health of their microbiome, augmenting their friendly bacteria and lowering their levels of pathogenic bugs.[22]

PICK YOUR POISON

Thus far in this chapter, I have been talking about alcohol without distinguishing much between the different beverages. It's easy to guess that different beverages will have different effects on the body. Let's briefly look at the main ones.

Wine

Most research on alcohol has analyzed the effects of wine consumption. Wine, especially red wine, seems to be the beverage with the most benefits, thanks to phytonutrients from the grapes, which are behind many of the health benefits attributed to moderate wine intake. Unfortunately, not all wine is made the same. Studies report that about 50 percent of wines contain mold toxins (although most are within a range that's considered safe).[23] As we have seen before, mold content has a lot to do with production and storage methods. With wine, it seems that many producers may not be adopting the best possible practices, especially in the US, since American wines are said to have higher toxin levels than wines from Europe (where there are stricter

274 THE NEO DIET – CHAPTER 12

regulations).[24] Also, research shows that occurrence of mold toxins is higher in red and sweet than in white and dry wines.[25]

Another concern, especially for US wines, is the worrisome levels of arsenic, pesticides, and added sulfites. There is very poor regulation of the wine industry (and many other industries) in the US, which causes many producers to attempt to game the system and cut corners to bring down the cost of their wines. This issue is so concerning that in 2015, a class-action lawsuit was filed in California against 28 top winemakers over the high levels of arsenic in their wines.[26] It was alleged that some wines had up to four to five times the maximum amount the Environmental Protection Agency allows for drinking water.

The key is to choose high-quality wine that is made with conscientiousness and care. This does not mean that you have to drink only the most expensive wines you can find. Not at all. Some of these expensive wines might have inflated prices because of marketing and reputation but still have high toxin levels. You can find affordable wines produced without pesticides, chemical additives, or added sugars, and with proper filtration methods and agricultural practices to reduce mold and other toxins. You just need to do your research. If you suffer from an increased mold sensitivity, a better option for you would be a dry wine or dry (brut) champagne.

Beer

Though it pains me to say it, I have to confess that this is not the best choice of alcoholic beverages. For starters, most beers have a high carb content. Then, they are made from grains, which may be highly contaminated with chemical toxins. Beer also tends to have more mold toxins than wine. Finally, we have all the issues that result from the lectins in the grains. As much as I love beer, I've felt significantly better since I started opting for wine instead.

Vodka, Gin, Tequila, Whiskey, and Moonshine

Distilled spirits, even those derived from grains, are a decent option. Because of the way these types of liquor are processed, lectins are eliminated and sugar levels drop. Overall, distilled spirits are good choices, but they will get you intoxicated faster. While you can safely drink one to two small glasses of wine, you have to shrink that glass to a shot for these alcoholic beverages. They are commonly used for cocktails, but adding juices or sugary liquors will wipe out the benefits. Either drink it pure or add some sparkling water and lime if you're feeling more exotic.

FINAL RECOMMENDATION ON ALCOHOL

Drinking some alcohol can have hormetic effects and can promote health, but do not feel that you need to drink to become healthier. There are several other things you can do to become more antifragile. My point with this chapter is to let you know that there is nothing wrong with low alcohol consumption and you shouldn't blame yourself if you enjoy a glass of wine with some friends and family. I know I do. The important thing is to understand the hormetic curve and to know that drinking one to two glasses three or four days a week is different from chugging a box of wine every day. If you feel you have a problem limiting yourself, you are better off just staying completely away from alcohol.

Focus on quality and make it a treat for yourself. I don't drink much now, but when I do, I make sure it is a good-quality wine. And I do my best to find out as much as I can about the producer.

If you like wine, it's difficult to go wrong with a good-quality Portuguese wine. (I'm not biased at all. Pinky swear!) Otherwise, nothing wrong with a shot of a nice moonshine.

Neo Note: Hangover Killer

I am not advising that you get hammered, but once in a blue moon, there might be a special occasion when some excesses might be committed. For those rare situations, there are ways to hack your body to process that excess of alcohol in a friendlier way.

During

Among its many effects, alcohol dehydrates you. So, while you are drinking, a good hack is to always have two glasses: one with the alcoholic beverage of your choice and another with water. That way, you will offset some of that dehydration with the water you consume along with the alcohol.

Before Bed

Once you're ready to call it a night, it's time to fight some of the damage you've caused. It's important to replenish some lost minerals, get rid of some toxins, take in plenty of antioxidants, and set yourself up for a good night's sleep. To achieve these goals, 30 to 45 minutes before you sleep (so you have enough time to pee):

• Fill a big glass with water, add the juice of one lime or lemon, and mix in ½ teaspoon of salt (e.g., Himalayan). Alternatively, use "unsweetened" coconut water. This is to help with the dehydration.

• (Optional) If you're brave enough, set a shot of raw fermented pickle juice on the side. Add a pinch of powdered ginger for flavor and to soothe your stomach.

Before-Bed Supplements
• Take 300 to 400 milligrams of magnesium. This helps replenish the magnesium levels depleted by alcohol and helps your gut move things along.
• Take one gram of either liposomal vitamin C or vitamin E to help reduce oxidative stress.
• Take one to two grams of activated charcoal to bind to toxins, especially the endotoxins caused by the excess of alcohol.
• Take one serving of your favorite milk thistle and/or fenugreek supplement.
• Take 3 to 10 milligrams of melatonin. Not only is it a great antioxidant, but it will compensate for the melatonin deficit caused by alcohol, allowing you to have a better night's sleep.

The Following Day
Repeat the hydration strategy from last night:
• Fill a big glass of water, add the juice of one lime or lemon, mix in ½ teaspoon of a good salt, and add a pinch of powdered ginger.

If things are still rough, you might need the **Neo Potion**:
• Full glass of "unsweetened" coconut water
• ½ teaspoon salt;
• ½ teaspoon powdered ginger
• Juice of 1 lemon or lime
• 2 egg yolks
• 2 tablespoons broccoli sprouts
• 1 tablespoon ghee (or pasture-raised butter)

Add everything to the blender and chug it down. It's not tasty but it works. You're welcome!

WATER AS THE SOURCE OF LIFE

Saving the best for last. Water, the last macronutrient. It makes up two-thirds of the human body by weight and 99 percent of our molecules by number.[27] Water is a major component in all our tissue and is involved in most biological functions. It's so important that we consider it a basic requirement when searching for life on other planets. However, on our own planet and in our bodies, we neglect it and seem to consider it irrelevant.

Water is far more than just a filler or a transporter of nutrients. Water has an important role in every system. Thus, if you get enough "healthy" water, you will feel vibrant and full of vitality. On the other hand, if you don't get enough water (or drink polluted water), all systems will be compromised and you will feel far from your best. Remember the concept of fats and proteins being the building blocks of many other compounds and tissues in the body?

If you eat healthy proteins and fats, you build a healthy body. If you eat bad proteins and fats, you build a sick body. Water is no different. The quality of the water you put inside of you will either move you toward health or bring on disease. Water carries nutrients and oxygen in and out of every cell, regulates temperature, lubricates and protects joints and organs, is part of the detoxification system, facilitates all metabolic reactions, and helps in the transmission of electrical and chemical (hormone and neurotransmitter) signals, connecting your entire body.

DEHYDRATION

While humans can survive around two months without food (possibly even longer if they're obese), we can survive only a few days without water (8 to 21 days).[28] However, we do not seem to be too concerned about this, since it's believed that most people live in a state of dehydration[29]. A 2013 report from the CDC concluded that in their sample, only 22 percent of the people actually drank the recommended eight cups of water daily. And 7 percent even reported not drinking any water at all.[30] This is concerning, since we cannot accumulate water like we do with fat. This means that replenishing our supply daily is a must.

Even slight states of underhydration can lower tissue oxygen, impair healing, and increase wound infection.[31] Certainly our bodies are resilient enough to survive a state of mild dehydration, but are we reaching our full superhuman potential that way? Of course not. My goal with this book is not to help you survive; it's to help you thrive. And that is why water is so important!

The truth is that the early signs of underhydration are hard to notice. We may feel a bit tired, both physically and mentally, and even develop a light headache. But that's about it. Many people make little of these symptoms and just eat something or grab a cup of coffee to get that afternoon pick-me-up. Unfortunately, the snack or coffee doesn't do anything for your hydration. On the contrary, they might aggravate the underhydration state. If this happens once in a while, your body can get over it, but when it becomes chronic, you develop more serious issues like cellular dehydration. This can manifest in a myriad of different ways, since all your tissues and organs are ultimately made of cells.

In a 2020 review, the authors explained that insufficient hydration is directly linked to metabolic dysfunction.[32] Low water consumption causes the body to produce arginine vasopressin (AVP), which is a hormone that triggers water retention in the kidneys. Although this is a good protective mechanism, long-term high levels of AVP increase the risk of hyperglycemia, type 2 diabetes, and other cardiometabolic risk factors. The authors also concluded that all these findings could be reversed with proper water intake.

Remember histamines? Studies show that dehydration stimulates the production of histamines, which cause the exacerbation of allergy symptoms.[33] It can also trigger symptoms in people who rarely have allergies. These people, in fact, are not reacting to allergens in the environment but are having a reaction to the excess of histamines in their bodies. When they drink water, the symptoms improve.

As I briefly mentioned, underhydration can lead to fatigue and headaches. In a 2012 study performed with young female test subjects, researchers concluded that a mere 1.36 percent dehydration sufficed to cause poor mood, increased perception of task difficulty, lower concentration, and headaches.[34] Once they were properly hydrated, all the issues cleared up. This link between hydration and brain performance is further supported by other studies showing that these negative effects might be even more noticeable in vulnerable populations like children and the elderly.[35,36] Dehydration also increases our perception of pain.[37]

Water consumption can influence the risk of kidney stones; cancers of the breast, colon, and urinary tract; childhood and adolescent obesity; mitral valve prolapse; salivary gland function; and overall health in the elderly.[38] I could surely present a couple more studies, but I'm confident you get the idea. Water is essential for our bodies to function properly. Instead of grabbing a coffee when you're tired or reaching for the painkillers when you have a headache, drink two or three glasses of water. Chances are you are just dehydrated.

Neo Note: Thirst

Some people think it's enough to drink water once they're thirsty. After all, that is the body's dehydration alert system. While a dry mouth will accurately inform you that you need water, this signal comes when your cells have already been underhydrated for a while. As your water level becomes low, other organs relinquish their water so the brain can maintain its hydration. It's only when the brain actually starts needing more water that you experience a dry mouth and thirst. By this time, most of your systems are already underperforming.

The takeaway: thirst should not be seen as the first sign of needing water but as a sign that we could have done a better job staying hydrated. For optimal health and performance, try to stay ahead of thirst.

WATER QUALITY MATTERS

Water is described as an inorganic, transparent, tasteless, odorless, and nearly colorless chemical substance. However, you certainly have experienced smelly water or have drunk different-tasting waters. This is because water is not just pure H_2O. Water has many other compounds in it. In fact, water is known as the universal solvent because of its ability to dissolve more substances than any other liquid on earth. Depending on what is dissolved in it, water can promote health or make you dehydrated and sick. Water, dehydrate you? Sure! Drink some ocean water and then let me know. (On second thought, don't.) Ocean water is still H_2O but with a lot of salt dissolved in it. And that excess of salt can pull water out of your cells and dehydrate you.

Water can also have lots of dangerous chemical pollutants, heavy metals, organic substances, medications (from antidepressants to pain relievers to hormone replacement medications) dissolved in it. According to the Environmental Working Group (EWG), heavy metals, fertilizers, herbicides, and many other chemicals are commonly found in concerning levels in US tap water.[39] The EWG has even detected radioactive substances and known carcinogens in the water supplies of 170 to 232 million Americans.[40,41] Sadly, this is not a problem exclusive to the United States. Go online and type "tap water contamination" and you will find literally thousands of studies reporting concerning levels of known toxins all over the world. When I did this, the US, France, Spain, Pakistan, South Korea, and China were just some of the countries listed on the first page of results alone.[42–47] This is scary because many of the contaminants found in our tap waters around the world have been linked to several chronic health problems, including cancer, autoimmune diseases, thyroid problems, and brain diseases, among many others.[48–50]

How do these contaminants get into the water in the first place? Easy! Big industries dump chemicals in our rivers, oceans, and sewer systems; fertilizers and herbicides we use in agriculture also end up going into our water; even just flushing some ibuprofen—or even cocaine—down the toilet will send these drugs into our water supply.[51] Drugs in our natural bodies of water are such a problem that there was even an article published in the *Independent* titled "Record Cocaine Levels in Thames Probably Not Making Fish High, Experts Say."[52] Hilarious, but also sad because it's true.

Our cities process and "recycle" water, but they don't filter most of this crap out of the water. We have the technology to make water safe, but since it would be more expensive to adopt it, most places just do some basic filtration and add a bunch of fluoride to prevent bacteria from growing. And there you go.

If you drink tap water, please stop. That is probably one of the best and simplest changes you can make for your health.

CHOOSING YOUR WATER

Considering that we should stay away from tap water, one might turn to bottled water. But not all bottled water is the same. Not only do plastic bottles and containers cause environmental issues, but compounds in the plastic may disrupt the human endocrine system and even lead to cancer.[53,54] A better alternative would be water bottled in glass. With glass, you are not increasing your risk of exposure to toxins in plastic, nor are you exacerbating our current environmental issues. Most glass-bottled water comes from springs that naturally filter the water. Yet most brands do quality control and check the water frequently for environmental contaminants.

I do drink glass-bottled water, especially when traveling, but my number one choice is water filtrated at home. I have a water filtration system that gives me confidence that my water does not have any pollutants and has the minerals I need to thrive. And even when I'm not at home, I just carry my stainless-steel bottle with water from home.

There are many water filtration systems on the market. Although I can't guide you in what system to choose because there are so many, I can at least give you some recommendations on what to look for.

First thing to know is that filtering pitchers like you commonly see in stores are not sufficient. They still let several toxins through and are not nearly as efficient as a water filtration system. There are several under-the-counter or over-the-counter filtration systems, but look for at least a four-stage reverse-osmosis system. This usually comprises a prefilter and a carbon filter to remove sand, dust, rust, other debris, and volatile organic compounds (VOCs). The third stage is the reverse-osmosis membrane, which removes even more chemical compounds and converts the water to 85 to 90 percent pure H_2O. The fourth stage is usually a mix of carbon filtration plus remineralization and alkalization to add flavor and minerals. Some more expensive (five-stage) systems also have a deionization filter that basically puts the water through electrically charged resin beads after the reverse-osmosis membrane to capture even more impurities. If you can afford it, go for it, but a four-stage filtration system produces great results.

Please be aware that some systems do not possess a remineralization stage. If yours doesn't, you would need to buy ionic mineral drops to add to the water, or mix a pinch of salt in a full glass of water. Remember, we also need minerals in our water for proper water balance and cellular health.

SPORTS DRINKS

It's impossible to talk about hydration without talking about sports drinks. While sports drinks contain electrolytes and can be useful to replenish mineral needs after intense exercise, we also have to keep in mind that most of them are also full of sugars and synthetic additives that are not doing you any favors. Furthermore, a 2012 study concluded that out of the 431 claims made in 104 different sports drink advertisements, most had no hard scientific evidence supporting them.[55] Finally, we also have to consider that excessive sports drink consumption can lead to mineral imbalances and cause serious issues. In a case study, it was found that a football player who was ingesting five grams of potassium a day from sports drinks suffered potassium-induced complex ventricular arrhythmia.[56]

Neo Note: Homemade Sports Drink—"Neo-Ade"
Do you have an intensive physical activity planned and have a concern about replenishing your electrolytes? Not to worry. Neo-Ade to the rescue.

Neo-Ade **Recipe**
- 1 full glass water or coconut water
- ½ teaspoon salt
- Juice of ½ lime or lemon
- 1 teaspoon basil seeds (more about this shortly)
- 1 teaspoon honey or maple syrup OR 1 serving of an essential amino supplement **PLUS** 1 tablespoon MCT oil (if you're accustomed to it).

My favorite version of this recipe is the one with honey or maple syrup, but the second option is ideal for individuals who are aiming to stay in ketosis longer.

PHASES OF WATER

Most of us learned in school that water has three phases: solid, liquid, and gas. Recently, scientists have uncovered a fourth phase. In this form, water is almost like a gel and is slightly more viscous than in the liquid state. Some names given to water in this fourth phase are structured water, gel water, EZ water, liquid crystalline, ordered water, or coherent water. Throughout this book I'll call it EZ water, because that is the term I'm most familiar with since reading Dr. Gerald Pollack's book *The Fourth Phase of Water*. He calls it EZ water, with *EZ* standing for "Exclusion Zone" because the water excludes impurities, as ice does.[57] In this state, water is not your typical H_2O but is in a slightly different configuration, H_3O_2.

While liquid water has a neutral charge, EZ water has a negative charge. Having a negative charge is actually a very positive thing. According to Dr. Pollack, this makes EZ water work as an antioxidant (since it has electrons to give to free radicals), causes it to hydrate more efficiently (high dipole moment makes it enter the cell with ease), gives battery-like properties to the water, and boosts electrical conduction in our bodies.

As Dr. Pollack explains, EZ water can be created through the sun's radiant energy. Water absorbs light energy freely from the environment and uses that energy to build EZ water by naturally splitting positive and negative moieties and originating H_3O_2. Beyond light energy, research from Dr. Pollack and a separate study done in 2020 have shown in a lab setting that certain fats (such as ghee, coconut oil, and lard) also promote the conversion of water into EZ water.[58] The authors even theorize that the "EZ-water-promoting" abilities of these fats are one of the reasons these foods lead to good health outcomes. Because of this, healthy fats facilitate hydration. This is probably why camels' humps are made of fat, as Dr. Dana Cohen cleverly observes in her book *Quench*.[59]

When reading Cohen's book, I was pointed toward Chris McDougall's book *Born to Run*, in which he shares the story of the Tarahumara tribe in the desert canyons of the Sierra Madre in Mexico.[60] The Tarahumara are famous for being excellent long-distance runners even in the harsh conditions of the Mexican desert. It seems their hack to deal with dehydration is to drink a mixture of fermented corn beer and chia seeds when they run. When mixed with liquid, the chia seeds create gel-like water that hydrates more slowly and effectively than regular water. This may suggest that the soluble fiber in the chia seeds (and other seeds) might also assist in structuring water.

Unfortunately, there is no scientific data on this, but I definitely would love to see some studies testing this theory. Besides soluble fiber, chia seeds are also rich in omega-3s. These have been found to help increase the cell membrane surface area so that more water and nutrients can pass through, promoting their hydration.[61,62] This is another reason chia seeds may be so efficient with hydration. I personally prefer basil seeds because they do not have lectins, which is why I suggested adding them to my Neo-Ade.

Finally, some authors suggest that water found in nature—in fruits and vegetables, springs, mountain streams, and rain—is mostly structured water. This is further supported by a Harvard study that showed that water inside cellular proteins forms an ordered hexagonal shape that comes in many sheets or layers, just like EZ water.[63]

One thing we know for certain is that water is more complex than most people think, and these complexities may mean better energy levels, faster hydration, and overall better health.

HACKING HYDRATION

Instead of focusing on getting your eight eight-ounce glasses (about two liters) a day, why not take advantage of the knowledge about EZ water, healthy fats, and fiber to hydrate more with less water? It's commonly said that if you eat one apple and drink one bottle of water, you will be more hydrated than if you just drank two bottles of water. Although I haven't found any evidence supporting this, I understand the logic, since the fiber in the apple will help retain the water and might even help add "structure" to it.

Have you ever seen in spas, cucumber slices inside the water jars? It's the same concept being used here. The plant fiber and even phytonutrients may help add structure to the water and make it more easily absorbable by your cells. In fact, research has shown that phytonutrients like lutein and zeaxanthin can help increase hydration.[64]

At the end of the day, hydration is the water that your cells receive and not the water that passes through you. I used to get dry skin and dry lips all the time, even when drinking two to four liters of water a day. Unfortunately, I was not really retaining any of that water. It would go in and out in less than 20 minutes. That is not hydration. As soon as I started focusing on healthy fats, fiber, and even getting water from raw plants, my skin and lips got much better, while I consumed half the water I did before.

My favorite strategy to hack my hydration is to get healthy fats, fiber, and phytonutrients from smoothies, soups, and broths. I highly recommend that you do the same. For the smoothies, just keep in mind not to add too much fruit so you don't end up inadvertently creating a fructose bomb. Focus on berries, some low-antinutrient vegetables (listed later in the book), some good fats like avocado and ghee, and some fiber using hydrated basil seeds and psyllium husk, for example. Same concept applies to soups. Please avoid starchy vegetables.

Neo Note: Hydrogen Water

One of the things being marketed a lot lately is hydrogen water. Some say it is the next big thing, others say it's snake oil. Hydrogen water is regular water with hydrogen molecules added to it. The idea behind it is that the extra hydrogen molecules could scavenge free radicals and help decrease inflammation.[65] Even though logically it makes sense, our body is complex, so it's important to see what science has to say.

Current research into the effects of hydrogen water is limited, but some studies show promising results. Recent human studies suggest that hydrogen water may have antioxidant effects, lower inflammation, enhance endurance, relieve fatigue, boost physical performance, enhance mood, reduce symptoms of anxiety, improve autonomic nerve function, lessen risk factors of metabolic syndrome, and even help decrease radiotherapy side effects and improve symptoms of Parkinson's disease.[66-74]

Hydrogen molecules have been shown in several studies to improve health outcomes in several diseases, especially Parkinson's, since Parkinson's patients have been found to have fewer hydrogen-producing bacteria species than normal.[75-77]

But please note that there are also studies showing that hydrogen water had no effect compared with a placebo.[78]

I personally have never tried hydrogen water, but I am inclined to believe that it might indeed be beneficial. Nevertheless, since its cost is still relatively high at the moment, I prefer to recommend other, more affordable strategies to naturally boost the production of hydrogen molecules in the body, like eating fiber and letting your microbiome create the hydrogen for you.

WATER RECOMMENDATION

Hydration is important, but let's not go with the hype of having to drink two gallons of water a day or needing sports drinks any time you do some exercise. As we've just discussed, there are strategies to be more efficient in hydrating the body. I believe that a safe range for most people is to drink between 70 and 100 fluid ounces (two to three liters) of water a day. Obviously, the more you sweat, the more you should drink. Similarly, the elderly should also drink more water because of their commonly less-optimal kidney function.[79,80]

Please remember that water quantity is not necessarily quality. It's all about absorption. Drinking too much water can actually deplete your body of vital nutrients and electrolytes, which will then affect your performance and overall health. Drink a properly filtered water or a good-quality spring water in glass bottles. Also favor vegetables and some fruits (even unsweetened coconut water), and consume plenty of smoothies, broths, and soups, with fat and soluble fiber.

Start your day with one to two big glasses of water. This is how I have started my days for the past few years. With my two glasses of water, I also take a pinch of salt to "charge" my adrenals for a new day. Another recommendation is to have a medium-size or large stainless-steel bottle you fill at home and drink from throughout the day. Usually, by having the bottle by my side, I end up reminding myself to drink it. Not to mention that I don't have to constantly purchase glass-bottled water throughout the day, which can become expensive long term. Final recommendation comes from Dr. Cohen's *Quench*, in which she explains that immobility slows down water delivery into the cells, as well as compromising the outflow of waste particles.[81] What this means is that by moving and doing some light stretches throughout the day, you will improve your hydration status.

COFFEE WORLD

Coffee is one of the world's most popular beverages. Some even call it the "elixir of life."[82] No one knows exactly how coffee was discovered, but legend has it that a goatherd on the Ethiopian plateau noticed his goats getting hyper and not being able to sleep after eating the berries from a certain tree. He shared his discovery with the local monastery, and the monks made a "tea" with the berries. They noticed that this "tea" energized them, so they started to use it. Coffee was born!

Regardless of the veracity of this story, we know that eventually coffee reached the Arabian peninsula, since several historians believe that toward the end of the 14th century or the beginning of the 15th century, coffee was being cultivated and brewed in the Sufi monasteries of Yemen. By the 16th century, its use had spread to Persia, Egypt, Syria, and Turkey. From Turkey, because of the strong trade routes the Ottoman Empire controlled, eventually it reached Europe. The Europeans took it all over the world. The rest is history.

ELIXIR OR POISON

The number one reason people drink coffee is not because it's the most delicious thing out there, but because coffee's caffeine content gives them an energy boost. Caffeine is also well known for being addictive, which is probably why people keep getting their coffee day after day.[83] In fact, caffeine is the most popular psychoactive substance in the world.[84]

There is more to this coffee story than caffeine, though. Coffee contains many other compounds. Research has discovered more than 1,000 antioxidant compounds in coffee, which is even more than in green tea and cocoa.[85] Some of them, such as polyphenols, chlorogenic acid, trigonelline, and diterpene alcohols, are known for having antioxidant, anti-inflammatory, neuroprotective, hypolipidemic, and hypoglycemic effects.[86,87]

Moderate coffee intake (two to four cups of coffee a day) is compatible with a healthy diet and an active lifestyle.[88] In fact, coffee is not only compatible with but might even promote performance and health. Moderate coffee consumption has been associated with lowering the risk of developing type 2 diabetes, cardiovascular disease, and cancer, and preventing premature death from these diseases.[89-94]

Where coffee seems to shine even brighter is with regard to brain health. Research also shows that coffee may block inflammation in the brain, slowing cognitive decline and lowering the risk of developing Parkinson's, Alzheimer's, and other neurodegenerative disorders.[95] Coffee also influences serotonin and dopamine activity in the brain, which possibly justifies why studies have found potential effects in improving mood and reducing anxiety, depression, and even suicidal ideation.[96-98]

Although there is no question that coffee can be a true health elixir, high doses of coffee (or any other central nervous system stimulant) can spur resistance to neurotransmitters and not only cause addiction but also create a constant need to increase the dosage to derive the same effects. One of most studied neurotransmitter deregulation phenomena occurs with adenosine.[99-101] Adenosine induces a state of tiredness and facilitates sleep. But because caffeine is molecularly similar to adenosine, caffeine links up with the brain's adenosine receptors and doesn't let adenosine work its magic. This is why coffee blocks the feeling of tiredness. To balance this, your brain is forced to create more adenosine receptors over time in order to open a few slots for real adenosine. With more receptors available, now you need to drink more coffee to produce the same effects. And as you ratchet up your coffee consumption, this problem only gets worse.

This means it's important to take regular breaks from caffeine so your brain can balance its receptors and so you stay sensitive to coffee and don't suffer from withdrawal syndrome. Sudden interruption of coffee intake can lead to withdrawal symptoms such as fatigue, brain fog, anxiety, headaches, and tremors.[102–106] I've seen this not only in myself when I did a caffeine detox a few years ago but also in my mother after a surgery she had. Because of the medical procedure, she was not allowed to have coffee for about 24 hours. As the withdrawal effects kicked in, she was nauseated and had headaches. Once she was authorized to get her "hit" of caffeine, the symptoms miraculously disappeared.

Research also shows that caffeine addiction (and its consequent caffeine resistance) is associated with chronic depression and anxiety, and its withdrawal is also not pleasurable.[107–109] High coffee consumption may also cause increased urination and loss of important minerals such as sodium, chloride, and calcium.[110,111] That being said, heavy coffee drinkers benefit from upping their salt consumption in order to balance some of these losses. The calcium loss is particularly concerning in the elderly, since it can lead to osteoporosis.

In some countries it's traditional to add a pinch of salt to coffee to enhance its flavor.[112] This might be a great way to kill two birds with one stone.

TOXINS IN COFFEE

Even the highest-quality coffee beans may contain several toxins with deleterious health effects. One of those substances is acrylamide. Acrylamide is recognized as a potential carcinogen, having been linked to multiple types of cancer.[113–115] This toxin is also commonly ingested through baked and fried foods (nuts, crackers, bread, breakfast cereals, french fries, potato chips, etc.), but depending on the roasting method, coffee may have especially high levels of it.[116,117] Roasting at high temperatures seems to eradicate acrylamide, but it also produces more PAHs, which you already know about.[118] Luckily, there are other roasting methods, like "smokeless roasting," which reduce both acrylamide and PAHs. Although these methods are rare, you should prioritize companies that process their beans in this way.

Another concern is that coffee crops are highly sprayed with pesticides like glyphosate. So, choosing organic coffee or brands that regularly test their beans for pesticides and other chemicals is a priority.

Finally, we also have the mold issue. Coffee beans are regularly stored for long periods and many times not under the right conditions. This can lead to mold development. Research shows that coffee is often contaminated with mycotoxins such as ochratoxins A and B, penicillic acid, citrinin, fumonisins, and aflatoxins.[119–121] Once again, purchase coffee that's been tested for mycotoxin content.

FINAL RECOMMENDATION ON COFFEE

Coffee has amazing benefits but also has its dark side. As long as you can maintain a healthy relationship with it and keep from overdoing it, you can take advantage of its benefits without suffering the consequences of excessive consumption or addiction.

How do you know if you're going too heavy on the coffee? For most people, consuming more than four cups a day seems to be excessive. But we all process caffeine differently. The best approach is to pay attention to your body. If you feel you need coffee every day to wake up, you are probably overconsuming. Similarly to what we discussed with regard to wine, you should enjoy it, not need it. When you depend on a substance just to function, your relationship with it is no longer a healthy one.

Enjoy your coffee, but make sure you take a few breaks in order to balance your brain's biochemistry. As Ben Greenfield suggests, avoid caffeine for 7 to 10 days every other month.[122] Finally, make sure you are getting great-quality coffee beans. The brand you choose should have strict quality standards, roasting the beans with lower toxin-producing techniques and regularly testing their batches for mold, pesticides, and other chemicals. Remember, depending on its use, coffee can be considered a nutrient or a drug of abuse. You choose how it works for you!

TEA TIME

Despite coffee's popularity, tea is purportedly still the most-consumed beverage in the world (other than plain water).[123] Tea has been part of many traditional cultures for thousands of years because of its health benefits and supposed longevity-promoting compounds. Scholars believe that tea was first used as a medicinal elixir in the Yunnan region of China during the Shang dynasty.[124] For centuries, tea drinking spread throughout China, and with the arrival of Portuguese traders during the early 16th century, tea was brought to the Western world.[125]

I know this may catch some readers by surprise, since the British are probably the European culture best known for their love of tea, but it's believed that the marriage of King Charles II in 1662 to the Portuguese princess Catarina de Bragança (Catherine of Braganza)—who brought her tea from Portugal—popularized the tea-drinking habit in the UK.[126] Between its natural expansion in the East and the influence of the Portuguese and British in the West, tea eventually reached all parts of the world and became the symbol it is today.

Tea is typically prepared through the infusion of *Camellia sinensis* leaves. From this plant we get the white, green, oolong, pu-erh, and black tea varieties. Yes, they all come from the same plant and differ only in the method and duration of processing.

BENEFITS OF TEA

Tea contains more than 4,000 chemical compounds that may affect the human body in many different ways.[127] Many of these compounds, such as flavonoids, theanine, theophylline, epigallocatechin gallate (EGCG), and other catechins, have been studied extensively.[128,129]

In traditional Chinese medicine, tea is often recommended as a natural remedy for high blood pressure. Several modern studies confirm the validity of these claims, as shown by a 2020 meta-analysis.[130] The flavonoids in tea have been found to promote healthy artery walls, prevent blood clots, and decreasing heart-disease risk.[131,132] In fact, in a large Dutch observational study that followed 37,514 individuals for over 13 years, it was concluded that drinking tea was linked to decreased risk of developing heart disease.[133] Other recent studies have also supported the heart-health-promoting benefits of tea, in particular green and black varieties.[134-136]

Tea, especially green tea, has also been shown to be a great metabolic health promoter. Research has linked tea consumption with reduction of insulin resistance, oxidative stress, and inflammation.[137] Other studies suggest that the catechins (EGCG in particular) and other phytonutrients obtained by drinking tea may decrease levels of the hunger hormone, ghrelin; boost basal metabolic rate; improve muscle glucose metabolism; facilitate fat burning; and lower the risk of type 2 diabetes and metabolic syndrome.[138-147] Many authors defend the anticarcinogenic properties of tea, and several recent studies, including a 2020 literature review, suggest protective effects of tea against various cancers.[148-154] At the same time, there are some inconsistent results, and more quality long-term studies are needed.

Neo Note: Tea Can Be Toxic

The pattern keeps repeating in each chapter. All foods can be good or bad, depending on quantity and quality. This also applies to tea, since some varieties have been found to contain substantial doses of fluoride, heavy metals, pesticides, and other environmental toxins.[155] Most tea production occurs in China and India, countries known for their high use of pesticides and other toxic chemicals, and also known for not having the best standards for quality control and testing.[156,157] So it's best to opt for organic teas, which will ensure that you're getting fewer toxins. The quality of the water you use to brew your tea is also essential. You can buy the most expensive organic tea out there, but if you use unfiltered tap water, you're still getting a big toxic load.

PS. Tea bags may be convenient but they have been found to release microplastics into our organism.[158] Your best choice is to brew your tea using a stainless steel infuser.

CHOOSING YOUR CUP OF TEA

This is not a tea encyclopedia, so I have to keep this last section as brief as possible. I'll present some benefits of the main teas we just discussed, and I'll also give you some suggestions of other teas you can choose depending on your health goal. If you want to explore more about tea, at the end of this chapter you'll find excellent book recommendations.

• *White tea*: Known for its light flavor. Since white tea goes through the least processing, it contains the least amount of caffeine but still has most of its antioxidant content. Great choice for later in the day.

• *Green tea*: Currently the most famous of them all, and for good reason. Green tea has some of the highest levels of catechins, in particular the super-powerful EGCG. Research suggests that EGCG may improve skin health, lower cardiovascular disease risk, fight metabolic dysfunction, reduce inflammation, promote brain health, decrease cancer proliferation, and even promote longevity.[159]

Neo Note: Matcha

Matcha has become very popular in the past few years, but it has been consumed for centuries in Asia, especially in Japan. Matcha is a green powder made from a specific type of green tea leaf. This variety is grown in the shade for several weeks before harvest in order to bump up its chlorophyll levels. Then the leaves are dried and ground into powder. Among green teas, matcha has one of the highest concentrations of EGCG, the catechin responsible for most of the positive effects of these teas,[160] and also has plenty of chlorophyll. Research shows that chlorophyll may improve detoxification, block lipopolysaccharides and mold toxins, lower inflammation, and help fight cancer.[161–165]

• *Oolong tea*: From this list, this is the tea people tend to care the least about. But oolong has very interesting effects, especially for weight management. Studies show that regularly drinking oolong revs up fat metabolism and suppresses the creation of new fat cells, helping reduce weight.[166,167] Oolong is also said to be easier on the stomach than green tea.

• *Pu-erh tea*: The decision to drink this tea usually has to do with its health benefits, since its taste is definitely an acquired one. Research suggests that this is also an excellent tea for weight loss because it boosts hormone-sensitive lipase (HSL), promoting fat metabolism.[168] Pu-erh might also be the perfect companion for fasting, as it not only promotes fat metabolism but also has been shown to help preserve muscle mass, scavenge free radicals, and detox the body from cellular waste products.[169,170]

• *Black tea:* The old-school tea and the undisputed popularity champion. Because of its caffeine content, it is a splendid choice for the morning or for an afternoon boost. Black tea is rich in theaflavins, which are known to have significant antioxidant effects.[171]

• *Teas to relieve anxiety and stress:* Some of the best teas to help you relax are chamomile, kava, passionflower, and tulsi (a.k.a. holy basil).[172–175]

• *Teas for insulin regulation:* Some teas that are especially good at helping balance sugar levels and promote a healthy metabolism are bilberry, hibiscus, and lemon balm.[176–178]

• *Teas for detoxification:* Some standouts to help you flush toxins out of your body are burdock (*Arctium lappa*) root, dandelion, milk thistle, and red clover.[179–182]

• *Teas to heal the gut:* For help in repairing a damaged gut lining and promoting gut health, try licorice, peppermint, marshmallow root, and slippery elm.[183–185]

• *Teas to fight inflammation:* Some of the best teas to bring down inflammation in the body are nettle leaf, ginger, rose hips, and yerba maté.[186–189]

• *Teas to boost immunity:* Teas skilled at fighting off bacteria and viruses are Indian echinacea (*Andrographis paniculata*, or andrographolide), astragalus, echinacea, elderberry, and hibiscus.[190–194]

NEO SUMMARY
• Alcohol can have a hormetic effect in low-to-moderate consumption.
• The quality of the alcoholic beverage is essential in order to decrease exposure to toxins.
• Proper hydration is vital for mental and physical performance.
• Most people are underhydrated.
• Hydration is deeply connected with metabolic health.
• Tap water is contaminated and needs to be filtered.
• Consuming healthy fats and soluble fiber can increase your hydration efficiency.
• It doesn't matter how much water you drink. What matters is how much water actually reaches your cells.
• Coffee and tea present anti-inflammatory and metabolic-boosting properties.
• Caffeine in coffee and tea can cause addiction.

NEO ACTION
• Stay away from water packaged in plastic bottles.
• Opt for filtering water at home or purchasing glass bottled spring water.
• Consume soups, broths, and smoothies for optimum hydration.
• Either refrain from alcohol, or keep its consumption to 1-2 glasses, 2-4 times a week.
• Prioritize good quality wine or plain distilled beverages.
• Cycle your coffee consumption to prevent addition and resistance.
• Try pu-erh tea during your fasts.

NEO RECOMMENDATIONS
• *20,000 Secrets of Tea* by Victoria Zak
• *Eat Smarter* by Shawn Stevenson
• *Intuitive Fasting* by Dr. Will Cole
• *Quench* by Dr. Dana Cohen & Gina Bria
• *Regenerate* by Sayer Ji
• *SuperLife* by Darin Olien
• *The Bulletproof Diet* by Dave Asprey
• *The Fourth Phase of Water* by Gerald H. Pollack
• *The Longevity Solution* by Dr. James DiNicolantonio & Dr. Jason Fung
• *Your Body's Many Cries for Water* by Dr. Fereydoon Batmanghelidj

SCAN ME

my.neodiet.co/neorecommendations

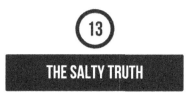

THE SALTY TRUTH

More Than a Source of Flavor

"Be salt, and a little bit of salt keeps the whole society from going rancid."
Philip Yancey

SALT LIFE

We've all had it drummed into us that salt is bad. So bad that the Center for Science in the Public Interest has even called it "the single most harmful substance in the food supply."[1] The guidelines are clear. We need to drastically cut down on salt. After all, salt causes high blood pressure and heart disease. That's what I learned in school, and that is what most doctors still recommend.

Not surprisingly, once again, we have not heard the full story. Sadly, our health authorities are still holding on to outdated and disproven theories about salt. Because of this, common knowledge still recognizes these concepts as facts and contributes to the health crisis we're experiencing. Fortunately, as with fat and meat, the truth is finally coming out. Several researchers have made substantial contributions to expose these lies. My goal with this chapter is to share their work, so you finally understand the importance of salt for a healthy body. It's no coincidence that humans are genetically wired to crave salt. We crave it because we need it.

SALT THROUGH HISTORY

Salt has been actively sought after by humans since the Neolithic era.[2] While there is no evidence that our Paleo ancestors engaged in salt extraction or took an interest in inland salt deposits, this doesn't mean you can "be Paleo" and skip salt altogether. Hunter-gatherers may have dipped food in seawater, or gotten salt through seafood or the blood of the animals they ate.[3,4] Either way, even accepting the possibility that our earliest ancestors consumed less salt than most humans throughout history did, we also have to recognize that because of their unique lifestyle and diet, prehistoric people probably did not need as much salt as we do now.

THE SALTY TRUTH   293

Some believe that formal salt mining or extraction started about 8,000 years ago in the northern province of Shanxi in China, but there is evidence of its spread shortly thereafter to different regions around the world, such as Egypt, Greece, Italy, Spain, and the Celtic territories.[5,6]

Researchers estimate that the average Roman consumed 25 grams of salt—equivalent to 10 grams of sodium per day, which is more than 2.5 times what we consume today, on average. By the 16th century, people in most European cultures took in about 40 grams of salt per day. And by the 18th century, this had risen to about 70 grams of salt daily.[7] Even with all this salt, there are no historical findings of an epidemic of heart disease in Europe during those times. Heck, even nowadays, three of the countries with the lowest rates of death because of coronary heart disease (Japan, France, and South Korea) are notorious for their high salt consumption.[8]

Salt is our biggest source of dietary sodium, which is an essential nutrient for our health. Without sodium, our cells would not hold water, we wouldn't have proper fluid balance in our tissues and organs, our muscles couldn't contract, and our nerves would not be able to properly send electric signals. Why have we been told all our lives that salt is bad? Let's find out.

THE SALT PARADOX

For the past 50 years, the theory has been that salt consumption increases water intake and retention. This raises blood volume and, consequently, blood pressure. Although this seems straightforward and logical, our body is pretty complex, and things are not processed linearly—so much so that we never really had any good scientific evidence to support this theory. Even in 1977, when salt restriction guidelines were already in place, a report from the US Surgeon General admitted there was no scientific data proving that a low-salt diet would stave off increases in blood pressure.[9] Despite the lack of evidence, these recommendations somehow prevailed up to this day. As I write this, the CDC and WHO websites still include recommendations for low salt intake.[10,11] I was also surprised to find out that there is a Salt Awareness Week.[12] In 2021 its slogan was "More Flavor, Less Salt!" *Let's agree to disagree.* It seems we are really making an effort to vilify salt, yet we still lack the evidence for it.

Research suggests that about 80 percent of people with normal blood pressure are not sensitive to the "blood-pressure-raising effects" of salt. In individuals with prehypertension (slightly high blood pressure), approximately 75 percent are also not sensitive to salt. And finally, even among those with hypertension (high blood pressure), roughly 55 percent are not sensitive to salt's effects on blood pressure.[13] Ironically, later studies have actually demonstrated that higher salt intakes decrease vascular resistance and cause blood vessel relaxation, while lower salt intakes lead to an increase in vascular resistance and blood pressure.[14]

Salt homeostasis in the body is essential for proper cell performance. We worry about getting the salt concentration too high, but as we're going to find out, we have mechanisms to expel excess salt. However, we do not have mechanisms to get more salt, other than eating it.

Did you know that several deaths suffered by runners during marathons have occurred as a result of drinking too much water and thus losing too much salt? It has been noted that excessive water intake can cause a state of hyponatremia (low sodium), which can cause symptoms such as vomiting, loss of appetite, headache, abnormal mental status (hallucinations, confusion, change in personality), muscle weakness, convulsions, and, in some cases, even death.[15,16]

Some scientists have suggested that chronic low salt intake may cause a state endocrinologists call "internal starvation." When the body detects low sodium levels, it reacts by causing insulin to "tell" the kidneys to retain as much sodium as possible (through the hormone aldosterone, as we saw in chapter 6). Metabolically, this shifts the body into "carb mode," which can then trigger sugar cravings, promote weight gain, and eventually cause insulin resistance and metabolic disorders.[17] Low-salt diets have also been shown to cause an increase in the levels of the hunger hormone, ghrelin, further aggravating the metabolic dysfunction.[18,19] On the other hand, optimal salt intake will have an inverse effect on insulin, optimizing the levels of leptin, adrenaline, and thyroid hormones, and even allowing glucagon's fat-burning activity, as seen in chapter 6.

A 2012 review of 23 observational studies and 9 randomized trials concluded that restricting sodium to less than 2,500 milligrams per day not only causes aldosterone deregulation and consequent hypertension but also makes plasma renin activity go up, which substantially increases the risk of heart disease.[20,21] Yet somehow our official guidelines recommend sodium intake to be lower than 2,300 milligrams.[22] Who is coming up with these RDAs? This does not make any sense! Although there is some evidence that short-term sodium restriction can slightly lower blood pressure, this effect is reversed and turns into hypertension with the continuation of the low-salt diet.[23]

One reason we need more salt than our Paleo ancestors did has to do with our stress levels. Even though they had an incredibly higher chance of being eaten by a wild animal, they were pretty chill about it. In contrast, we stress about everything. Chronic stress spurs overproduction of cortisol, which in turn can lead to aldosterone deregulation and imbalances of sodium and potassium levels.

Low salt intake reduces libido, causes women not to become fertile until later in life, decreases the chances of getting pregnant, reduces the weight of infants, and increases erectile dysfunction, fatigue, and sleep issues.[24-26] Salt is also important for the immune system, in that it has antimicrobial properties that help us get rid of pathogens in the skin, increases T cell function, and boosts macrophage-driven immune response, which fights off infections.[27–29]

SALT RECOMMENDATIONS

We are all unique and have different nutritional requirements, but, as in the protein situation, scientists believe there is a salt consumption range in which most people will thrive. Researchers such as Dr. DiNicolantonio suggest that the optimal range for sodium intake is 3 to 6 grams per day, which represents roughly 1½ to 3 teaspoons of salt.[30]

Some people might require even more. You should consider increasing your salt consumption if you

• just started a low-carb diet;
• suffer from a chronic disease such as hypothyroidism, adrenal insufficiency, or congestive heart failure (commonly associated with low sodium, or hyponatremia);
• take medications such as diuretics, antidepressants, or antipsychotics (these meds can cause sodium depletion);
• are exposed to intense mental stress;
• frequently do high-intensity exercise; or
• drink too much coffee.

Then we have people who have medical conditions that compromise sodium balance in the body. These conditions have very specific medical guidelines that should be followed in detail. The conditions are hyperaldosteronism, Cushing's disease, and Liddle syndrome.

Another point I want to touch on is salt quality. When most people think about salt, they think of table salt (refined salt). Unfortunately, table salt is a dangerous mix of chemically extracted pure sodium and toxic aluminum anticaking agents. Table salt is what's been giving salt a bad rap. Although these aluminum anticaking agents are considered safe by the FDA, I have my reservations, since aluminum can accumulate in the body and potentially cause several issues.[31] A good salt will not contain fillers but will provide you with more than just sodium. Good salts contain several precious trace minerals. Some of my favorite options are Celtic salt, pink Himalayan salt, black or red Hawaiian salt, Redmond Real Salt, and any other salt that is mined from old seabeds (no toxins back then).

By the way, most commercial kosher salt is just larger grains of table salt. Still bad for you!

NEO SUMMARY
• Your body needs salt.
• We used to consume a lot more salt and didn't have an epidemic of heart disease.
• Low salt causes high blood pressure and metabolic dysfunction.
• Higher salt consumption is important for cellular, metabolic, hormonal, and immune health.
• Table salt is bad for you because it is pure sodium mixed with aluminum anticaking agents.
• Choose salt from ancient sea beds.

NEO ACTION
• Stay away from table salt.
• Eat more "good" salt.

NEO RECOMMENDATIONS
• Salt by Mark Kurlansky
• SuperLife by Darin Olien
• The Salt Fix by by Dr. James DiNicolantonio

my.neodiet.co/neorecommendations

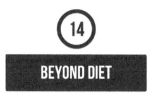

BEYOND DIET

Lifestyle Is the Other Half of the Equation

"To insure good health: eat lightly, breathe deeply, live moderately, cultivate cheerfulness, and maintain an interest in life."
William Londen

THE HEALTH EQUATION

For the longest time, I didn't pay any attention to what I ate because I felt that as long as I was active and exercised regularly, I would stay healthy. But here's the thing. Staying fit and being healthy are two different things. You can be "fit" on the outside while being "rotten" on the inside. There is no point in looking good when your diet is giving you cancer. Is there?

The opposite situation is also true. You can follow the most perfect diet in the world, but if your lifestyle is toxic, diet alone won't save you. This is how it stacks up for the thousands of individuals who thoroughly follow a diet but don't see any results. The diet is not failing; the lifestyle is blocking their progress.

Fortunately, improving your lifestyle is easy, and a couple of simple changes can go a long way. In this chapter I'll show you how to improve your health in an efficient and holistic way. After all, health can only be achieved when you consider the two variables of the health equation: diet and lifestyle.

$$Health = Diet + Lifestyle$$

Even if math is not your thing, together we will crush this equation, so let's do this!

EXERCISE IS ENCODED IN OUR GENES

It doesn't take a genetic scientist to realize that humans were designed to be active creatures. We have all the physical attributes that allow us to walk, pick up heavy objects, jump, climb, run, or even fight. That's how we made it through the toughest times in our evolution. Many authors talk about the Paleolithic times when our ancestors used to run after wild animals and roam the land for several miles daily. But we don't need to go to that extreme.

From the Neolithic era up to the Industrial Revolution, our ancestors were incredibly active. Everything was manual labor, and, for most folks, if they needed something, they had to get up and make it. Nowadays, though, we don't move nearly as much as our bodies need. The average person in the Western world drives to work and then sits in front of their desk the whole day—or, increasingly, works from home, plunked in front of a computer. Even manufacturing jobs are being replaced by machines, and the few workers left are mostly sitting while operating these machines. If these eight to nine hours of sitting during the day weren't enough, after being done with work, the average person goes home and sits on the couch watching TV until it's time to hit the sack. Some individuals are so lazy, or in such terrible shape, they even sleep in their reclining chairs. Don't even get me started on how common it is to see individuals, especially here in the US, using electric scooters to shop for food because they're so fat they can't walk. The irony!

Research has linked chronic sitting with increased risk of all-cause mortality.[1] The good news is that research also shows that when we just add a tiny bit of movement during the day, this association becomes weaker. Studies have concluded that simply getting up and walking about two minutes every hour is enough to reduce the early death risk by 33 percent, while one hour of moderate-intensity exercise daily completely clears the early death risk.[2,3] As you can see, we don't need to be ultramarathoners or gym rats to respect our genes. In fact, those examples are harmful for us, as you are going to find out. You just have to fight the lazy voice in your head and add some movement during the day, especially on weekends (or whatever are your days off), since there is nothing forcing you to stay put. Unless you are in jail. In that case, future Kevin really did a great job with marketing.

I know this might sound like I am lecturing you from my high horse, but that's not what I'm doing. I, too, still enjoy a weekend of movie bingeing. But I also know that I feel much better physically and mentally when these are the planned exceptions and not the every-weekend rule. Knowing and feeling the difference is what I want for you. I would love for you to get in touch with your physical self and improve your human experience.

Physical activity and exercise should not be seen as grunt work or a chore. Make it fun. I personally cannot run 15 minutes on a treadmill, but I can spend two hours running after a ball, playing soccer with friends. The key is to find something you like to do. You don't have to hit the gym. Go outside and play with your kids. If you don't have kids, play with someone else's kids. Whoops, I just noticed how that sounded. Forget that second option. The important thing is that you add movement to your day-to-day so you can respect your biology and become healthier.

THE BENEFITS OF EXERCISE

I think we all know that exercise is good for us, but we tend not to know exactly how it makes us healthier. This is what we are going to find out in this section.

Exercise is the perfect example of hormesis. It creates some stress in the body, and the body reacts by becoming stronger. That's why we commonly hear the cliché "no pain, no gain." You indeed need a certain level of "pain" in order to induce the wanted change. But, like all hormetic stressors, too much exercise can be bad for you. When you are in the gym, you are intentionally increasing your heart rate and damaging your muscle tissue, creating micro muscle tears and generating free radicals and inflammation. Your body reacts by producing hormones, enzymes, and antioxidants that trigger a cascade of anti-inflammatory processes that will put you in "healing mode."[4-6] During this healing process, not only does your body reverse the acute oxidative and inflammatory damage caused by exercise, but it also increases its resilience in order to tolerate a higher dose of stress next time.[7,8] This overcompensation is what makes you stronger and healthier.

At the microscopic level, one thing we can see is the metabolic improvement created by exercise. During exercise, the enzyme AMPK (the "metabolic master switch") gets activated and promotes improved mitochondrial activity. For several years, we've believed that AMPK's primary function was to regulate glucose uptake and fat oxidation during exercise. But some authors have recently suggested that these metabolic improvements may have a higher association with other regulators, such as nitric oxide, Rac1, and ROS, also produced during exercise.[9] Nonetheless, as seen before, AMPK will stimulate the elimination of cellular metabolites, promote the recycling of damaged mitochondria (mitophagy), and create more mitochondria (mitochondrial fission).[10,11] This, in turn, will boost your muscular metabolic efficiency and increase your insulin sensitivity at a systemic level.

Another important thing to mention is that the uptick in mitochondria seems to go beyond the muscle tissue, in what's known as cross-adaptation. Studies show that AMPK has been associated with an increase in mitochondria in fat cells (a process known as browning) and even in the brain.[12-15] Besides improving your brain's metabolic health through AMPK signaling, exercise will also increase the blood flow to this organ, ramping up the delivery of nutrients and oxygen.[16] Another way your brain is improved is by the effects of BDNF. Exercise promotes the increase of BDNF, which, as you already know, protects the brain and facilitates neuroplasticity.[17,18] Studies have shown that introducing an exercise plan in sedentary individuals leads to learning and memory improvements, even in cases of mild cognitive impairment.[19-22] Other studies also show that exercise can improve mood, reduce anxiety, decrease symptoms of depression, and boost psychological resilience against stress.[23–26]

Exercise is also essential for detoxification, since muscle contraction is the main pump for the lymphatic system.[27–29] According to paleoanthropologist Daniel Lieberman, the sedentary lifestyle of the modern human does not include enough physical activity to support the lymphatic system for optimal health.[30] This is the perfect example of diet alone not being enough. You can eat incredibly healthy, but if you don't add some exercise to your life, you will have a congested lymphatic system and increased difficulty getting rid of toxins.

Recent studies show that a sedentary lifestyle is associated with dysbiosis, while physical activity increases microbial diversity and overall health of the microbiome.[31] Moreover, exercise has also been found to help preserve intestinal wall mucus thickness, lower bacterial translocation, diminish intestinal permeability, and decrease autoimmunity by modulating TLR signaling.[32,33]

Finally, exercise, in particular weight training, can make you live longer. Studies show that strength training is directly linked to a reduction of all-cause mortality risk.[34] That's right. While real guns kill, "biceps guns" make you live longer!

Neo Note: Overtraining

Some exercise is fantastic; too much can be problematic. Overtraining is a serious problem that can lead to chronically high cortisol levels, which can cause weight gain, muscle loss, hormonal imbalance, and burnout. Don't be fooled, thinking this occurs only in older or sedentary people. There are studies suggesting the development of overtraining syndrome (OTS) even in young athletes.[35] This is concerning not only because of the increased risk of injuries but especially due to the development of serious hormonal, immunological, neurological, and psychological disturbances.[36,37]

Extreme forms of cardio like marathons, ultra-trails, Ironman triathlons, and so on, without proper recovery, can stress the heart muscle beyond recovery and eventually trigger cardiovascular disease and even deadly heart attacks.[38–41]

Studies also show that excessive exercise may damage the gut and cause leaky gut syndrome.[42] This is probably because too much exercise can cause immune suppression. Other studies have shown that while moderate exercise may reduce the risk of colon cancer, excessive exercise may damage your gut.[43–45]

HACKING EXERCISE
Walking

Going to the gym and hitting the weight room is not the only form of exercise. In fact, the concept of the nonathlete going to the gym only developed in late '60s and early '70s. Until then, people found other ways to work their bodies, like running, swimming, practicing sports, or walking. In fact, walking might be the most important form of exercise one can do—so important that I even recommend it to high-performance athletes.

Remember the first chapter, when we spoke about killer genes? Well, since walking has been such an important part of our human experience, one can theorize that our genes are programmed to recognize it as something healthy individuals do. Think about it; back in the day, if an individual couldn't walk, that person would not keep up with the group and would have more difficulties surviving. That being said, it would only make sense that if your genes notice you are not "keeping up with the group" (not walking enough throughout the day), the autodestruct mode might be turned on. On the other hand, if you can "keep up," your genes feel you are important to the species and keep you healthy. So much so that research shows that simply walking and moving during the day have been linked to decreased risk of infections, inflammatory diseases, metabolic syndrome, cardiovascular disease, brain disease, and some cancers.[46-53]

Trying to build up to a minimum of 10,000 steps a day is a great place to start. Obviously, this varies for everyone depending on pace and stride length, but we can average it out to around 90 minutes of walking. Considering that you are awake for about 16 to 18 hours a day, it's not a lot of walking at all. As you get used to walking more, slowly keep on working toward increasing those numbers.

Heavy Lifting

Another form of exercise our ancestors often did was carrying heavy things. Back then, the only way to bring game, tubers, water, or even firewood back to the camp was by using the body. People could not afford to go back and forth several times. They had to be efficient and carry all they could in the least number of trips possible. Kinda like I do when bringing in the groceries from the car. If I have to do more than one trip, I feel that I have dishonored my family. I'm sure I'm not the only one. The point is, both men and women were used to lifting and carrying heavy things, and this kept them muscular and healthier. Nowadays, because most of us don't have physical jobs, we have to turn to gyms to practice this same function—lifting or pushing heavy stuff.

I know some people are afraid of or feel uncomfortable with the idea of weight training (a.k.a. resistance training). Some women, in particular, avoid it at all costs for fear of getting too muscular or bulky. If this is a concern you share, don't worry. You have nothing to worry about. I wish it were that easy to gain muscle mass. Unfortunately (or fortunately, depending on how you look at it), years of high-intensity weight training are necessary in order to become bulky, especially for my female readers.

Adding weight training to your routine is essential not only to become stronger but also to improve your health. Not to mention that it is *waaay* better than cardio for losing those extra pounds. Research shows that while aerobic training—that is, your typical cardio (running, using a treadmill, cycling, etc.)—will increase your metabolic rate during the exercise, resistance training will keep your metabolic rate elevated for almost two days.[54] In other words, not only will you burn calories while doing resistance training, but you'll continue burning them at a higher rate even while resting during the next one to two days.

In another study, researchers divided test subjects into two groups.[55] Both groups consumed a similar diet with the same number of calories (only 800 calories per day), but one group did one hour of cardio four times a week, while the other group performed resistance training (10 resistance exercises) three days per week. After 12 weeks, both groups lost weight; but the participants who did the resistance training lost more fat, preserved their muscle mass (even at 800 calories), and increased their metabolisms. The cardio group lost muscle mass and slowed their metabolisms. Not the way one should lose weight, for sure.

Resistance training will also help you pack much-needed muscle, increase insulin sensitivity, enhance cardiovascular health, prevent bone loss, boost testosterone and GH levels, improve self-esteem, and possibly even improve cognitive and memory skills in older adults.[56-61]

Unless your goal is to become a bodybuilder, 15 to 30 minutes of weight training two or three times a week is all most people need to get these benefits. The trick is to perform the exercises to failure within the 8-to-12-repetition range. If you can go over 12 repetitions, the weight you're using is not heavy enough. Time to level up. Another form of progression is to increase the contraction time: instead of taking one second to do a chest press, try to do this movement in slow motion, taking about four seconds in each direction. Trust me, you will feel the burn even with less weight than you usually do.

What about the number of sets? Well, there are several theories, but I don't find the need to get too technical. As long as you are doing your exercises to failure, one set of each is all you need. Additionally, since we are doing sets to failure, I recommend using machines, because the chance of injuries is much higher with free weights. Since you are going to work out until muscle failure, do a two-minute dynamic warm-up to get your blood flowing. Some of my favorite warm-up exercises are kettlebell swings and burpees. Pick your poison. Please note, you don't need to do fancy workouts. Focus on the foundational moves. My top five are: chest press, overhead press, pulldown, seated row, and leg press. Squats and deadlifts are also great exercises but if done incorrectly can easily result in injuries.

You can easily find detailed videos on each of these exercises on YouTube. Most gyms also have personal trainers providing help. They will gladly show you how to perform these safely.

High-Intensity Interval Training

Genetically speaking, running for hours on end is wasting energy, and there is no direct benefit from this activity. But when we talk about short, high-intensity sprints, the story changes. Most animals benefit from being able to sprint in order to hunt or to avoid being hunted. For the survival of the species, this makes perfect sense, thus it is encoded in the animals' DNA. As you can figure out, humans are no different.

Humans were designed to be great walkers and to occasionally sprint. Yet we have been challenging our own biology for millennia—not out of necessity but out of competition and pride. It's said that the concept of the marathon came from the battle of Marathon, between the Greeks and Persians around 490 BC.[62] Common belief is that there was a man named Pheidippides who ran from Marathon to Athens (about 25 miles, or 40 kilometers) to bring the news of the Greeks' victory. If I had to guess, I would say that our ancestors started running "marathons" just to prove they could do it faster than Pheidippides. You know, the typical "big ego syndrome."

Even though we've been doing extreme cardio (like running marathons) for ages, our genetic code still does not see the advantage of doing it, and our killer genes penalize us for going against our biology. As we've seen, extreme forms of cardio, without proper recovery, can cause heart disease and even death.

I'm not suggesting that if you enjoy this type of physical activity, you should stop. Heck, as I'm writing this, I have an obstacle course half-marathon waiting for me in about a month. What I am suggesting is to be aware that this type of stress puts you on the bad side of the hormetic curve. Meaning, it's more stress than the body can handle. So, you should really prioritize proper nutrition and recovery to reverse some of the damage you're doing to yourself.

Chronic cardio like running for long periods of time has not only been shown to promote heart disease, but research also reveals that it leads to significant muscle-mass loss, increased intestinal permeability, a drop in immune function, greater risk of injuries, and decreases in testosterone levels.[63-69] To all my guy friends who are always bragging about how long they last running, let me ask you, how long do you last in bed, though? Just busting your balls. Although it seems like you're already doing a great job at that yourselves. *Haa-haaa.*

Alternatively, what I recommend is adding some form of high-intensity interval training (HIIT) to your routine, because this is something "recognized" by our biology and that consequently gives us several health benefits. Think of HIIT like running away from a lion in the savanna. Actually, let me give you another example, since you would definitely get eaten by the lion. Imagine running away from a pissed-off goose in the park (much better). You will sprint for a couple of seconds. Stop to check where the goose is. Run again because he is still trying to attack you. And stop, because you've finally gotten to your car. HIIT is basically short bursts of intense exercise with a few brief breaks.

One of great things about HIIT is that it gives you the benefits of longer-duration exercise in a fraction of the time.[70,71] In fact, one study shows that as few as three 10-minute HIIT sessions per week, in people with cardiometabolic disorders and even in healthy individuals, was enough to improve aerobic capacity, skeletal muscle oxidative capacity, exercise tolerance, and markers of disease risk.[72]

If your goal is to lose weight, HIIT has to be part of your exercise routine. A 2015 study concluded that HIIT outperformed other forms of exercise in calorie burning by an average of 25 percent to 30 percent.[73] Additionally, HIIT has been shown to increase metabolic rate not only during exercise but also hours after the workout stops.[74,75] HIIT is so powerful that in one study it was even discovered that only 2 minutes of sprint-interval exercises were enough to bump up metabolism for 24 hours, "burning" as much calories as much as 30 minutes of running.[76] I don't know about you, but I'll take the 2 minutes of sprints over 30 minutes on the treadmill.

In addition to weight loss, research also suggests that HIIT may help you increase muscle mass, elevate human growth hormone levels, improve insulin sensitivity, reduce blood pressure, boost overall cardiometabolic health, and even facilitate neuroplasticity and improve cognitive function.[77-88]

For people just starting, I recommend doing your HIIT session using a stationary bike or rowing machine, or just performing body-weight exercises like burpees, for example. These will allow you to put in your maximum effort while still keeping your risk of injury relatively low. There are many variations, but the one I suggest is the 30/90 combo. Let's say you decide to do your HIIT session in a stationary bike. Before getting on the bike, start by doing a 2-minute active warm-up, walking and moving your main joints. When you feel ready, jump on the bike and go all in for 30 seconds. Actively rest by pedaling at a light speed for 90 seconds. Repeat this sequence until you complete a total of 10 to 15 minutes. Not trying to discourage you, but I am expecting most first-timers to last only two or three rounds. And that is perfectly fine. The goal is to slowly build your condition so you can tolerate the whole 15 or even 20 minutes.

Alternatively, especially after the whole COVID-19 situation, there are plenty of 20-minute HIIT programs on YouTube. Most of them rely on body-weight exercises, so you don't need to buy fancy equipment. Go online and find a trainer you like.

As you get more conditioned, there is another method of training that's popular with "biohackers" because of its time efficiency. It is called the Tabata protocol. This exercise protocol was created by Izumi Tabata of Japan and basically is HIIT 2.0.[89] You pick one exercise and do eight rounds of 20 seconds of "all you got" exercise, following each round with 10 seconds of rest. One set of Tabata will take you only four minutes to complete, but because it is one of the most energetically effective HIIT training methods, you'll still get incredible results. But I recommend this only for people already used to HIIT. If you are in good shape and really want to challenge yourself, you can try to do three to five four-minute sets of Tabata with one-minute breaks between sets. This is guaranteed to make you sweat.

CREATING AN EXERCISE ROUTINE

I believe in following guiding principles. But one should understand that each person is unique, and so should be their exercise routine. There is no "one size fits all." Some might already be in good physical condition and able to do more, while others might be trying to take that first step toward a healthier life. Obviously, their exercises should be different. We need to respect each person's situation.

If you are already in good shape, these concepts you just read are probably not new to you. My main recommendation to you is that more is not always better. Please make sure you don't overtrain and especially that you get proper rest and nutrition.

And for my readers who are now starting their fitness journey, please don't be too hard on yourselves. Things take time, and if you put too much pressure on your shoulders, you will burn out and have difficulty achieving any results. Start slowly! Anything you introduce will already be much better than what you are doing right now.

As suggested in the beginning of this section, the first step should be to be more active during the day. Park a little farther away to force yourself to walk more. Take the stairs, not the elevator. Every hour, try to stand up and walk for a minute or two. And whenever you go to the bathroom, do a couple of squats. Although these random activities throughout the day don't seem like much, they add up. In fact, research suggests that three 10-minute sessions of exercise spread throughout the day provide at least the same benefit as, if not more than, a single 30-minute workout.[90,91]

What about the type of exercise you choose when you do workout? What is the best form of exercise? I know this is cliché, but it's true: the best form of exercise is the one you'll actually do. If walking is all you can do right now, I'll take it. The important thing is that you develop the habit of being more active. Then you will want to do more because you'll feel the difference. In my opinion, the best exercise routine most people should follow combines all the principles mentioned above. Ideally, you would hit your 10,000 steps every day, and do two or three resistance training days and one HIIT day per week. If this is your very first week working out in a long time, probably aim to walk every day but do only one weight-lifting workout, since you might be sore for the rest of the week. Then, the following week, you can add the HIIT and a second weight-lifting day.

Most importantly, don't stress too much about it. Do your workouts with no other expectation beyond becoming healthier. When a person gets obsessed with weight loss and the exact amount of muscle mass gained, stress hormones like cortisol become elevated and compromise progress. If you take a relaxed approach and try to enjoy the process, results will naturally occur, I guarantee.

THE CIRCADIAN RHYTHM

By now, you're already familiar with the concept of the circadian rhythm. As shown before, when we are in sync with our circadian rhythm, our bodies function as they were programmed to, and thus we achieve better health outcomes. Being in tune with our internal clock not only allows us to live better, but researchers believe it might even allow us to live longer.[92]

In chapter 8, we learned that the "circadian sensors" in our digestive system use periods of eating and fasting to regulate our circadian clock. Another important circadian regulator is light. Our eyes and the cells in our skin detect light (or its absence) and use this stimulus to sync up the entire body.[93,94] When light is strong, it's time to be active, and the body should be firing on all cylinders. When the light fades, it's time to recover and sleep. Pretty simple, right?

The problem here is that our current lifestyle is messing up these light signals. Nowadays, most of us are not outside much and don't have the privilege of being exposed to natural light. Most people spend their days in enclosed workplaces with artificial lights. To make matters worse, their eyes are being blasted with blue light coming from electronic devices like computer screens, TVs, and smartphones. While exposure to natural sources of blue-spectrum light is important to activate our bodies, promote alertness, and boost cognitive performance during the day, chronic exposure to blue light later in the day will wreck your circadian rhythm and disturb your ability to sleep and recover.[95] In fact, research shows that narrow-bandwidth blue LED light has a potent effect in suppressing melatonin in the body.[96] And, as you know, melatonin is the main circadian rhythm regulator and sleep inducer.

This disconnection from natural light patterns is part of what researchers call Paleo-deficit disorder—the way our lifestyle has made us diverge from our genetic programming.[97]

Other forms of circadian rhythm disruptors are chronic emotional stress, travel between time zones (jet lag), late-night eating, and night-shift work, for example. Research suggests that the disruption of the circadian rhythm may trigger weight gain, metabolic dysregulation, low energy, inflammation, autoimmunity, and even cancer.[98–101]

TIME TO UNDERSTAND YOUR INTERNAL CLOCK

When we know what is supposed to happen at a certain time, we can make better lifestyle decisions. This is what we are going to discuss here. We will review your circadian timeline and what happens in your body. This section won't be a detailed 24-hour guide, but we will cover what I consider the most important aspects. Please understand that this is just an average timeline. The exact hours vary with the time of year and even with the specific chronotype (natural inclination of the body to sleep) of each individual.

That being said, generally around 6 a.m., your body starts to activate. Cortisol levels rise, which makes you wake up. When you're in a fasted state, cortisol also promotes fat burning to power the body—one reason we should skip breakfast. At this time, your body also starts producing higher levels of vasoactive intestinal polypeptide (VIP), which spurs vasodilation, more circulation of nutrients, and increased muscle activity to get you ready for the day. The best way to anchor these physiological responses is by exposing yourself to sunlight in the early morning. Ideally, try to expose your skin and eyes to the red light from the sunrise, if you have that opportunity. Exposure to sunlight in the morning will optimize cortisol's effect in the body and will charge your body with energy for the day ahead of you. Since morning light serves as a circadian anchor, it will also promote relaxation and better sleep. Early mornings are the perfect time for a fasted walk outside while listening to your favorite podcast or audiobook.

Throughout the morning, your body continues to energize so you can be productive. Around 2:30 p.m., your muscle coordination peaks, and around 5 p.m., it's time for your muscle contraction to reach its full potential.

Sunset marks the end of your "active day." The red light from the fading sun tells your body to start shutting down. From this point on, being exposed to blue light will throw off your circadian rhythm. Thus, you should avoid exposure to smartphones, tables, TVs, and so on after dusk, or at the very least, use blue-light-blocking glasses. If you don't confuse your circadian sensors with blue light or late meals, after the sunset is also the period when your body increases its levels of leptin and adiponectin to burn fat while you sleep. Around 10 p.m., your body wants you in bed. Melatonin production steps up to make you feel tired and sets your body for a healing night of sleep.

Most authors talk about dimming the lights at home, using red or orange lightbulbs, installing apps to reduce blue light in electronic devices, and wearing blue-light-blocking glasses. But even though I agree with these tips,

I don't believe most writers on sleep reinforce how important the timing of your last meal can be. That late-night snack will cause insulin levels to be higher than they should before you sleep. This takes you out of catabolic mode (fat burning and protein recycling) and puts you in anabolic mode (mostly accumulation of fat, unfortunately). Also, because of the inverse relationship that insulin has with the satiety hormone leptin, chronically high levels of insulin may trigger low levels of leptin. Because you don't feel satiated, you will want to snack more and more, creating a vicious circle. Finally, this peak in insulin can also thwart your glymphatic system, as we saw before. You definitely do not want to stop "deep-cleaning" your brain, because it then can accumulate toxins and other metabolites that will lead to inflammation and disease.

From 11 p.m. to about 2 a.m., your body slows most systems down so it can start doing its work of repair. Not only do you have high levels of melatonin at this point, but you also have an increase in growth hormone to facilitate the daily muscle repair. Then, until 6 a.m., your body tends to increase the activation of immune cells to take care of any ongoing immune issues and to bring down levels of inflammation. With this, body temperature also drops, which allows neural repair and plasticity.

Beep, beep, beep. The alarm rings. And the cycle repeats itself again.

As you can see in this overly simplified version of events, your body knows what to do and when to do it. You just have to stop confusing it. Set the proper circadian anchors. Get natural sunlight in the morning. Skip breakfast. Get a good meal anywhere from noon to 2 p.m. Be an Instagrammer and chase all the sunsets. Finally, avoid blue light after sunset and don't have late dinners. That's it!

Caveat: I believe it is important to have a social life and go for dinner with friends. Most times, these dinners are later than your usual routine. This is perfectly fine as long as you understand that this should be the exception and not the rule. This is the typical example of the Neo Diet's 90/10 principle. But more on that later.

HACKING THE CIRCADIAN RHYTHM

Following an eating schedule that matches your biology is easy to implement. So is getting blue-light-blocking glasses to use at night. But what about people with stressful jobs or people who cross time zones often? You should actively find strategies to reduce your levels of stress. Later in this chapter, we are going to discuss several methods, like being outdoors, socializing, meditating, and other things. However, I understand that sometimes one might have to travel or have a particularly difficult day. For these exceptions, we can hack our internal clocks through supplementation.

Three of the most studied adaptogenic herbs that have been used by Ayurvedic practitioners for hundreds of years are ashwagandha (*Withania somnifera*), *Rhodiola rosea* (golden root), and *Bacopa monnieri* (water hyssop). Overall, researchers have found that these herbs are efficient at fighting stress because of their strong antioxidative and neuroprotective effects.[102-117] While fighting the stress in the body, they may also assist you in keeping your circadian rhythm in order.

For my readers who are often jet-lagged after travel, there are also some hacks to help you sync your clock with the local time zone. One of the best things you can do is what researchers call grounding or earthing. This basically entails having your bare feet in direct contact with the ground to connect with the earth's electromagnetic field. If this is the first time you are reading about this, I know how it sounds, but there is plenty of high-quality research supporting this concept. I won't explore more than this, since it goes beyond the scope of this book. Just remember that taking off your shoes and walking in sand, grass, dirt, rocks, and natural bodies of water will help you "sync up."

Another hack is to supplement with melatonin.[118] By taking a melatonin supplement around the time when your melatonin levels would naturally spike (around 10 p.m.), you give your body a strong circadian anchor that will help you correct the circadian phase shift.

> **Neo Note: Seasonal Foods**
>
> Circadian rhythms are present everywhere in nature. Here, we discussed the rhythm around the day according to its traditional definition, but there are many other, larger rhythms in nature. Our planet has different seasons, animals have mating periods, plants flourish and produce fruits at different times of the year, and women go through different physiological changes during their menstrual cycle, just to name a few examples. The point is that we should understand and respect these cycles of life. One of these cycles, and one that we have been neglecting, is seasonal nutrition. Nowadays, because of the advances in transportation and refrigeration systems, we can eat vegetables and fruits year round that used to be exclusive to a short season or even to parts of the world far from where we live. While you won't become seriously ill by doing so, you are also not doing your body any favors if you skip seasonal local foods.
>
> In his book *The Forest Unseen*, biologist David George Haskell observes that cows eating out-of-season foods could become sick, and deer doing the same may even die.[119] While our physiology is different, I believe these examples should be taken as a warning sign about what can happen to us long term.
>
> By favoring local seasonal foods, you get the most nutrition out of them. Not only that, but you benefit from the right seasonal microbes that will help you digest and absorb these foods. Research shows that as part of these seasonal cycles, plants create symbiotic relationships with the microbes from

the soil.[120] And, as seasons change, the plants' needs change and the microbes on them also change. When eating seasonal plants, you get the right microbes that will help your microbiome stay healthy during that season. In fact, seasonal change in microbiomes has been seen not only in animals but also in tribes still eating seasonally, like the Hadza.[121,122] In contrast, people living in an urban setting where seasonal nutrition is not common did not show that variability.[123]

When you eat seasonally, you are getting fresher foods with more nutrition, and you're also obtaining all the good microbes your body needs to be more resilient in that particular season and place in the world.

SLEEP AS THE MAIN CIRCADIAN EVENT

It's estimated that most humans sleep for about eight hours a day, which translates into spending one-third of their day in shut-eye. Nowadays, being in la-la land for so long is not a big problem, since you do it in the safety of your home. However, as biohacking master Dave Asprey notes, for our ancestors, sleep put them in great danger, because while they slept, they were completely defenseless against wild animals.[124] If we are genetically programmed to sleep, it's because it must be really necessary. So necessary that it outweighs the risk our Paleo grandfathers had of being attacked during the night.

Recent studies have confirmed this evolutionary theory.[125] Sleep is really important if we want to be healthy, happy, top-performing, long-living human beings. Even though I am going to present some research to support my claims, I'm sure this is not a new concept for you. Certainly, you've already had at least a couple of bad nights' sleep that made you feel like crap the following day. Am I right?

Sleep deprivation is so bad for you that it is considered torture. In fact, it violates the third Geneva Convention (1949).[126] Keeping someone awake for a prolonged period has such an effect on the body that researchers believe it can cause death—possibly by the accumulation of too many free radicals in the body.[127] For obvious reasons, there are no studies with human subjects to support this theory, but there are animal studies with dogs and rats in which this fatality theory was confirmed.[128,129]

Probably one of the best human experiments I can reference is one from 1964 in which a San Diego high school student named Randy Gardner stayed awake for 11 days and 24 minutes as part of his science fair competition.[130] By day three, he became irritable, and his speech began to slur. As time passed, his cognitive abilities declined, and he developed not only memory and concentration problems but even paranoia and hallucinations. According to reports from that time, Randy took it like a champ and, although clearly affected by such a challenging experiment, at the end, he even held a press conference. Now, this makes me understand the comments some of my older clients make about younger generations not following through. Randy really showed some incredible commitment. I hope he won the fair, at least.

All right, if you're wondering what happened to him, he ended up making a full recovery after a couple of long nights of sleep.

BENEFITS OF SLEEPING

Your brain may be the organ that suffers the most from inadequate sleep. As you already know, the glymphatic system is activated while you sleep. If you're not sleeping well, this process is not as efficient. This is supported by research showing that poor sleep is associated with more amyloid plaque in the brain.[131]

According to a 2020 study by UC Berkeley researchers, sleep disruption is a recognized feature of all anxiety disorders.[132] In other words, poor sleep can cause anxiety. To make this worse, anxiety in turn aggravates sleep issues, which can then create a vicious circle.[133,134]

Researchers believe that poor sleep impairs the activity of the prefrontal cortex, and this is what causes anxiety.[135] But the prefrontal cortex is also believed to be responsible for self-control, reasoning, decision making, and planning, and indirectly involved in learning and memory. It's no surprise, then, that studies also show that sleep deprivation causes deficits in all these cognitive functions.[136–139]

Proper sleep removes toxins, boosts neuroplasticity, and helps the brain repair itself.[140] This allows humans to improve their cognitive performance and emotional health.[141,142]

Many authors comment on how a sleep-deprived brain leads to weak self-control and bad diet decisions, which then can lead to metabolic consequences. Although this is true, it is important to note that sleep deprivation can mess up your metabolism even if you can preserve your better judgment. Studies show that just one bad night of sleep is enough to cause temporary insulin resistance and an increase in the hunger hormone, ghrelin.[143,144] Having less self-control, more hunger, and reduced capacity to process the sugar in the blood is definitely not the best combo if you are trying to lose weight. In fact, sleeping less has been shown to increase people's intake of sugary foods.[145,146] Chronic sleep disturbances have also been associated with increased obesity, intestinal dysbiosis, IBD, and higher risk of type 2 diabetes and metabolic syndrome.[147–150]

Not sleeping enough is also bad for the heart. Studies show that moderate sleep restriction may cause arterial endothelial dysfunction and increase the risk of cardiovascular disease (including heart attacks) and death.[151–154]

Your time in bed is also essential for your immune system. Researchers have found that you can increase your risk of autoimmune disorders if you are not sleeping enough.[155,156] This seems to occur because of a decrease in a phenomenon called immunological memory. This biological process is the ability of our immune cells, in particular T cells, to recall pathogenic bacteria and viruses they've fought in the past. If our immune cells remember how to fight these aggressors, they will be much more efficient in their job of keeping us healthy. The same way sleep is important for our mental memory, research shows it is also essential for our immunological memory.[157] Additionally, sleep deprivation studies have also shown that when people don't sleep enough, their levels of pro-inflammatory markers like C-reactive protein, IL-6, and TNF-alpha increase.[158,159]

Remember epigenetics? Sleep also seems to be an important regulator of your epigenome. Since this is such a new field of investigation, more research is called for. But there is already plenty of evidence suggesting that epigenetic alterations occur following sleep deprivation.[160] Researchers believe that quality sleep helps regulate DNA methylation.

Many people are sleep deprived and don't know it. They think that feeling like a zombie is normal and that they just need one more cup of coffee. In part, this is the fault of the current "social media entrepreneur" mentality. Our culture rewards sleep deprivation. The less you sleep and the more you grind, the cooler you are. But what's the point of bragging about the few hours you sleep, if you're not productive and can't perform at your best? You take double the time to get the same work done, and you put your health at risk. Not worth it. As some of my mentors say, don't work harder, work smarter!

So how much should one sleep? That's another million-dollar question. There is no right answer because we are all different. Not to mention that quantity does not mean quality. You can be in bed tossing and turning for 12 hours and feel terrible the following day. But let's not complicate this even further. Systematic reviews with meta-analyses published in 2009 and 2010 suggest that sleeping less than 7 hours or more than 9 hours per night puts you at a higher risk of disease and even death.[161,162] Another systematic review, this one from 2015, puts the ideal sleep duration range between 7 and 8 hours.[163] I'm sure this is no surprise, since this is what most of us have heard all our lives. However, a 2021 study contends that sleeping more than 6.5 hours a night increases the chances of cognitive decline and dementia.[164] As you can see, science gets confusing.

My take on this is that we are all different and each one of us has a different biology and lifestyle, which makes our sleeping requirements vary. While a high-performance athlete might benefit from 10 or even 12 hours a night, others might feel amazing with just 6.5 (a number that's been trending in biohacking forums). But don't follow trends. See what works best for you. As much as I have tried to follow that social media grind mentality of sleeping only 5 or 6 hours a night, I simply cannot do it. I need my 7 hours to function properly. You might need more or less. Just know that less than 6 is most likely bad and more than 9 might be a bit much unless you really exert yourself regularly.[165,166] Within that 6-to-9-hour range, find your sweet spot, and be consistent with it.

HACKING YOUR SLEEP NATURALLY

Diet plays a major role in the quality of your sleep. As we discussed earlier, getting some good carbs at night may help you increase your brain tryptophan and serotonin synthesis, which will relax you and promote better sleep. But eating these carbs too late, or in excess, may cause your insulin levels to remain high and block the action of your glymphatic system, which cleans your brain while you sleep. That's why it's recommended that your last meal of the day should be at the very least 3 hours before you go to sleep.[167]

Beyond diet, there are several things you can do to boost your chances of having a great night's sleep. Here are my top 10 suggestions.

1. Get direct sun exposure in the morning within 15 minutes of waking up, if possible.
2. Give yourself at least 8 hours between your last coffee and your bedtime.
3. You may have one glass of wine at dinner, but don't drink after that, since it will affect the quality of your sleep.
4. After sunset, use blue-light blockers
5. Don't exercise right before going to sleep. Give yourself at least 2 hours.
6. Take a warm shower or bath before bed to drop your body temperature.
7. Meditate for 5 to 10 minutes to relax your mind before sleeping.
8. The bedroom is your sleep and sex sanctuary. This is not the place to watch TV, scroll social media, or work on your laptop. Keep technology outside the bedroom.
9. Your room should be pitch black. You should be able to wave your hand in front of your face and not see a thing. Even the slightest bit of light can affect sleep quality.
10. If possible, keep the room temperature on the cool side.

HACKING YOUR SLEEP WITH SUPPLEMENTS

Supplements are not supposed to replace a healthy diet and lifestyle, but in the beginning of your quest for better sleep, they might give you the push you need. There are literally dozens of supplements said to improve sleep quality, but I am a fan of keeping things simple. That's why I'll only mention my favorites. These are the ones that have produced the best results for me and my friends and clients.

Magnesium

Magnesium makes the top of my list because not only can it help you sleep better, but it is one mineral our population is generally deficient in.[168,169] Magnesium is essential for maintaining normal cellular and organ function, and its deficiency is associated with skeletal deformities, cardiovascular diseases, and metabolic syndrome.[170] Regarding sleep, magnesium helps convert serotonin into melatonin, which you already know is essential for sleep. There are numerous forms of magnesium supplements, and various authors have different opinions about them. Overall, the most absorbable and beneficial forms seem to be magnesium aspartate, chelate, citrate, glycinate (or bisglycinate), malate, orotate, and taurate. The best type to improve your sleep is said to be magnesium glycinate, but if you can get a supplement containing multiple forms, you're probably better served. In the book's resources, I recommend some of my favorite brands. Additionally, you can also use topical forms of magnesium. A nice Epsom salt bath before you go to bed is a great way to relax and get sleepy.

Glycine

Glycine is another multifunctional supplement. When you take it before going to bed, it helps lower your body temperature, which is essential to inducing sleep.[171] Glycine may also reduce the risk of atherosclerosis, heart failure, inflammation-driven syndromes, metabolic syndrome, and some cancers.[172] Since glycine competes with glyphosate for binding sites in tissues, it may help lower the accumulation of this toxin in the body.[173] You don't necessarily need to supplement with this amino acid, because it's present in organ meats, ligaments, poultry drumsticks and skin, and bone broths. But as a sleep aid, the supplement form is more convenient. You can add it to your before-bed tea (possibly valerian or chamomile), since it also works as a light sweetener.

Reishi

Reishi and other medicinal mushrooms have been increasing exponentially in popularity in the supplement world. And for good reason. They are fantastic not only for sleep but also to boost many other physiological processes. Reishi mushrooms have been shown to make people fall asleep faster and increase sleep time and quality.[174] On top of that, reishi mushrooms have been recognized as a potent cancer-fighting food and have been associated with improved mood, immunity, blood sugar control, and heart health.[175-183] Want to sleep like a baby? Forty-five minutes before bedtime, make some reishi tea, add some glycine to sweeten it, and take your magnesium supplement. Lights out!

L-theanine

L-theanine is an amino acid found in tea leaves. It has been shown to modulate neurotransmitter activity, increasing serotonin, dopamine, and GABA levels in the brain, which in turn counteracts stress and promotes sedation and sleep.[184–188] If you want to make L-theanine even more powerful, take it with a GABA supplement. Research shows that the sleep-promoting effect becomes much stronger.[189]

Chamomile

Chamomile is an ancient herbal remedy that has been used to promote relaxation and sleep for hundreds of years. A 2019 systematic review of literature concluded that chamomile intake causes significant improvement in sleep quality.[190] Similarly to reishi, there are extracts in pill form, but I usually prefer to drink chamomile tea.

Melatonin

First things first: I do not recommend taking melatonin as a frequent sleep supplement. You don't want to be constantly taking substances your body is supposed to produce naturally. If you keep feeding your body things it knows how to create, it becomes lazy and stops producing them. This applies not only to melatonin but to any other hormone or enzyme. That being said, the occasional use of melatonin might be a powerful tool, especially when your circadian rhythm is off balance. I take about three milligrams of melatonin (I mention the dosage because most melatonin supplements are too strong) when I travel between the US and Europe, to help anchor my circadian rhythm.

TIME TO GET DIRTY

Most people in the Western world have become hygiene freaks. There is the idea that if you get dirty, you will get deadly bacteria, puke your guts out, and die. While this scene from a sci-fi movie can happen if you are "lucky" enough to be in contact with deadly bacteria, and you have an incredibly weak immune system, the chances of this occurring are infinitesimally small. You actually have a better chance of getting sick because of your choice to be immaculately clean, as we saw in chapter 5.

We have to realize that human beings evolved in the wild. For millennia, we lived outdoors, and being exposed to the elements made us strong and resilient. Only recently did our technology promote the lifestyle change we see nowadays. Now, we are indoors all the time, and we are obsessed with keeping a sanitized bubble around us. Think I'm exaggerating? I challenge you to drop some food on the floor, then pick it up and eat it. Here is one condition, though. You have to let it sit on the floor longer than five seconds. *What? You're asking me to break the five-second rule?* I sure am! #YOLO

So, were you able to do it? Don't feel bad if you weren't. You have been conditioned to act this way. But if you could do it, let me welcome you to the 1 percent. The dirty rebels. Should we get some matching jackets, or am I getting carried away here? Jokes aside, it is important for you to realize how disconnected you may have become from nature, because this not only has implications for your immunity and physical health but also has a powerful effect on your ability to thrive emotionally.[191] Your genes are still programmed to enjoy the outdoors, and they will make you healthier and happier if you give them what they want.

There is a concept that is very famous in Japan called *shinrin-yoku*. In English, this translates to "forest bathing."[192] And it is what it sounds like: total immersion in nature. According to a 2019 review of literature, forest bathing was associated with improvements in the immune function and reduction in blood pressure, heart rate, and stress hormones such as adrenaline, noradrenaline, and cortisol.[193] The same article also linked this practice with decreased fatigue, confusion, anxiety, anger, and depression.

Knowing what we've learned thus far, we can argue that many of these benefits may come from exposure to the microorganisms in the forest, which can boost our microbiome even if only through their transient influence. As you know, a healthy microbiome is linked to all the benefits just mentioned. But studies show that volatile organic chemical compounds called phytoncides, released by plants and trees, are directly involved in triggering all these health benefits.[194,195]

What is even more fascinating is that the simple act of observing nature produces significant health benefits. A 2021 review suggests that being exposed to nature through virtual reality may contribute to psychological and physiological relaxation.[196] Obviously, the genuine experience is much more beneficial, but with this example, one can see how deeply ingrained the outdoors is in our programming. Research shows that the closer one lives to a green space, the less likely that individual is to experience stress.[197] Furthermore, several studies have concluded that separation from nature because of our Western style of living is detrimental not only to our well-being but to human development and health.[198,199]

If you are lucky enough to live in a place with plenty of nature around you, connect with it and to expose yourself to some green and some dirt. If your outdoors is all asphalt, concrete, and glass, find your nearest park and spend a couple of minutes there daily. When possible, try to go out of the city and immerse yourself in the wild. Go for a hike, roll in the dirt, run in the park, lie on the grass while listening to your favorite podcast, or even play in the ocean. In fact, the minerals in salt water may reduce inflammatory diseases like rheumatoid arthritis and psoriasis.[200] On top of that, salt water is rich in bacteriophages, which essentially are "good" viruses that attack pathogenic bacteria and can help us fight infections.[201] You should use any excuse possible to be in contact with nature. You need to get dirty. No excuses, please. Like Shia LaBeouf yelled, "*Just dooooo iiiit!*"

GET YOURSELF SOME D

One of the indirect benefits of spending time outdoors is being exposed to the sunlight. While I clearly state this as a benefit, I know that some will cringe at the idea of letting the sun shine on their skin. *After all, that's how you get skin cancer, right?* For decades, we've been hearing that sun exposure will make us develop skin cancer and that we should avoid sunlight at all costs. Once again, we haven't heard the full story. I promise I will get to it shortly, but what is important for now is for you to know that sun exposure is good, and it is an essential circadian anchor. Letting your eyes and skin get sunlight will help you sync your circadian rhythm daily and will also enable you to produce the indispensable vitamin D. In fact, vitamin D is so important that one of its active forms, calcitriol (1,25-dihydroxycholecalciferol), is considered a true steroid hormone.[202]

For the longest time, we never really appreciated vitamin D to its fullest. Although, particularly in the past two decades, many articles and even entire books on vitamin D have been written, this message was not spreading within the medical community. Most health professionals knew vitamin D only for its role in boosting calcium absorption. That was about it. Functional medicine doctors and antiaging specialists were the only ones really trying to show the world how essential this vitamin is. Fortunately, I think the mainstream medical community is finally waking up. Especially during the COVID-19 pandemic, vitamin D finally got the recognition it deserves because of its important role in the immune system.

Vitamin D may be one of the most important compounds in our bodies because it regulates at least 1,000 different genes, which in turn control virtually every tissue in the human body.[203] The influence of vitamin D over your epigenome is best known for regulating muscle and immune function, bone mineralization, and cellular metabolism.[204] Proper vitamin D levels have therefore been associated with prevention of osteoporosis, sarcopenia, metabolic conditions, autoimmune diseases, and even cancer.[205–207]

Have you ever heard of telomeres? They are basically the end caps of our chromosomes, and they protect our genetic material. Although this is controversial, some researchers believe long telomeres are related to greater longevity, while shorter lengths are associated with aging and higher risk of death.[208] The reason I'm mentioning this is that studies show the individuals with the highest levels of vitamin D in their blood have the longest telomeres.[209] In other words, having the right levels of vitamin D in your body may let you live longer.

Considering all this information, I have no question in my mind that our decreasing sun exposure is one reason we have been getting sicker and more fragile. Biologically, we need to get that energy from the sun in order to, among other things, produce the incredibly powerful vitamin D. So, don't be scared. Go get yourself some D. Some vitamin D, that is.

SUN EXPOSURE AND VITAMIN D

There are a ton of vitamin D supplements on the market, but I believe these may not be necessary for a significant part of the year, as long as you make an effort to get some sun on your skin. Why spend money on a supplement when you can produce the real deal for free just by spending time outdoors?

Before I continue, let me address your possible concerns about the relationship between sun exposure and cancer risk. This relationship was first introduced within the dermatology community in the late 19th century, but it didn't start reaching the general public until the 1930s, especially once the US Public Health Service began issuing statements about sun-related health risks. In the following decades, this subject was continually studied, and researchers eventually linked excessive ultraviolet (UV) radiation from the sun with the development of skin cancer, in particular melanoma, basal cell carcinoma, and squamous cell carcinoma. As you can imagine, even at that time, the results of these studies were controversial, since, up to that point, skin cancers were incredibly rare. And people were actually exposing themselves less and less to the sun because of the new industrialized lifestyle.

In the 1970s, scientists finally believed they had an answer for this skin cancer paradox. They attributed the uptick in skin cancer cases to the destruction of the stratospheric ozone layer and the consequent increase in UV radiation reaching us. Because this theory, at first glance, makes sense, it has been widely accepted by health officials since. But if you spend just two minutes doing some research, you can easily learn that this theory is caca. NASA scientists have analyzed 30 years of satellite data and found that the amount of UV radiation reaching Earth's surface has indeed increased, especially the closer you get to the poles, with the Patagonia region showing an increase of about 20 percent.[210] They attribute this in part to ozone depletion.

Wait, is Kevin actually supporting the theory? Not so fast! In that same study, NASA also concluded that these increases in UV radiation have stabilized since the mid-1990s. But skin cancer cases have not slowed down since the '90s. On the contrary. I guess we can say this is red flag number one.

One can still say that the 20 percent increase was enough to put us over the tipping point and trigger this epidemic of skin cancers. But what most of us don't realize is that a 20 percent increase in UV radiation is incredibly insignificant for our health. Here is an example so you can better comprehend this. Let's say that you live in Belgium and you decide to move to Hawaii because you're tired of the cold winters. That latitude change during the winter would increase your UV radiation exposure from around 0.4 MED (minimal erythema dose) to 14 MED.[211] That is a whopping 3,400 percent increase. Certainly, this insane increase in UV radiation has to show in the number of skin cancer cases, right? *Wrooooong!* At the time of this writing, according to data from the World Cancer Research Fund, Belgium, even with its lower UV radiation levels, ranks 9th in the world for the most cases of skin cancer, while the US sits at 17th.[212] One can still argue that the US is a big country and that Hawaii's cases are diluted in the nation's average. Correct, but that is not the case. According to data from a major US health insurance company, Hawaii is actually the state with the fewest skin cancer cases in all of the United States.[213] In other words, sunny Hawaii presents significantly fewer skin cancer cases than cloudy Belgium, despite the insane difference in UV radiation.

While there are studies associating excessive UV radiation exposure with skin cancers, there are also plenty of studies showing the exact opposite. In fact, a 2010 article from the University of Texas MD Anderson Cancer Center contended that the animal study most referenced to associate UV radiation with the development of melanoma should be questioned, and that UVA (ultraviolet A) exposure is unlikely to have contributed to the rise in the incidence of melanoma.[214] In addition, most melanomas occur on the least sun-exposed areas of the body, and exposure to sunlight actually reduces the risk of developing melanoma.[215,216]

So, if sun exposure is not the primary cause of the higher prevalence of skin cancers, what is? That is a complex question, but the answer lies in the diet and lifestyle changes that occurred with the Industrial Revolution—the same changes that led to obesity, autoimmunity, and all the metabolic diseases we explored in the previous chapters. And some of these dietary changes also may have contributed to a decreased ability to use sunlight to produce the anticarcinogenic vitamin D. Additionally, our exposure to toxic chemicals has been increasing at a concerning rate since the 1930s, which could also be a significant contributing factor.

You should not fear sun exposure. At the same time, please don't assume you can go outside and tan for 5 hours straight and suffer no consequences. Besides turning into a lobster, you may develop serious issues from that sunburn. Think of sunlight as an amazing tool to keep you healthy. But, as with any other tool, you need to know how to use it properly so you can get the most out of it without injuring yourself.

THE BEST SUNSCREEN

The best way to get all the benefits from the sun is to expose as much bare skin as possible. Note that I specify bare skin. If you add a sunscreen, you are blocking the UV ration necessary to produce vitamin D. I know we've been told that sunscreen allows us to have all the benefits of the sun while filtering the bad stuff. Unfortunately, those are nothing more than hyped marketing claims. If sunscreens are so good, why do our rates of skin cancer continue to grow?

Some authors even argue that there is a direct correlation between the use of sunscreen and the increase in skin cancer. They claim that many sunscreens alter the way UV radiation interacts with our skin, triggering skin inflammation and even the same cancer they're supposed to prevent. Although I did not find enough evidence to support these claims, what I can definitely say is that many sunscreens on the market, even "organic" ones, have dangerous toxic compounds in them that may be affecting your overall health.[217-219] In fact, research suggests that ingredients commonly used in sunscreens may compromise GI function, disrupt your endocrine system, and cause neurological problems.[220] And don't forget the effects most sunscreens have on coral bleaching and contamination of other marine life.[221,222]

A better option, in my opinion, is to eat your sunscreen. Hold on. I'm not suggesting you eat *sunscreen*, okay? I'm saying to use your diet to improve your body's ability to process sunlight, like a sunscreen is supposed to do. Our skin is not as fragile as we're told. Our epidermis (the most superficial layer of the skin) can block at least 95 percent of UV radiation, and the collagen beneath the epidermis can absorb the rest.[223] If you have a good diet, your body can regenerate the epidermis at a fast pace and have enough collagen to keep you safe. A poor diet, on the other hand, will not give you the right raw materials and may cause inflammation that in turn can progress into sunburn, age spots, wrinkles, and other skin issues.[224]

With the Neo Diet, we'll be removing all the highly inflammatory vegetable oils, grains, and processed foods and introducing collagen-rich foods like slow-cooked stews and bone broth, for example. We'll also eat plenty of healthy fats, which are essential for cell rebuilding. Besides that, another hack to consider is getting plenty of vitamin C, which is essential to skin repair and collagen production.[225] So, by making sure you have good vitamin C levels, you are promoting proper skin regeneration. My preferred way to do it is to add some camu camu (one of the best sources of vitamin C in the world) or acerola to my smoothies.

BUILDING UP YOUR UV TOLERANCE

Once your body gets enough UV radiation to produce the needed vitamin D, then it has to protect itself from overexposure. One way it does this is by synthesizing melanin, the predominant pigment responsible for skin color.[226] Melanin converts ultraviolet radiation into heat. That's why when people are exposed to sunlight, they tan. Your skin produces more melanin to combat the excessive UV exposure, and as a side effect, your skin gets darker. Melanin may also have other physiological roles, such as free radical scavenging and toxin chelation.[227]

If you haven't exposed yourself to sunlight for some time and decide to go out and tan for six hours, this will not work out well for you. Your body won't have enough melanin produced in your skin to protect you from the excessive UV radiation. This is when you can cook your cells and develop issues like skin cancer. The trick here is to have regular, moderate exposure so you can build up your tolerance and be protected. Let's say you live somewhere where it's really cloudy, and for three or four months of the year, it is impossible for you to get sunlight on your skin. The first few times you do get some sun on you, do it after 3 or even 4 p.m. so the UV index is not as strong. Until then, stay in the shade or cover up. Even if you are on vacation and really want to go for a swim at 1 p.m., there are plenty of UV-protectant swim shirts you can use. After a couple of sun exposures, you can get sun even in the "stronger" hours. Just see how your skin reacts and use common sense.

Once you build up that tolerance, the goal is to be outside for about 1 hour a day, with as much skin showing as possible. Please note that by following the Neo Diet, you will have a body to be proud of. Still, don't go to extremes with the "showing as much skin as possible" part, since there are laws against public indecency in most countries.

OTHER BENEFITS OF SUNLIGHT

Sunlight is exceptional in allowing the body to produce vitamin D, which, as you already know, is essential for optimum health. And, by producing it naturally, you don't incur the risk of overdosing on vitamin D as can occur with supplements.[228] However, being in the sun has more benefits than just the natural production of vitamin D. As discussed before, sunlight is a great circadian anchor. It helps regulate levels of serotonin and melatonin, which will promote improved mood and better sleep. Research also suggests that sunlight triggers the skin to release nitrogen oxide, which then causes arteries to dilate, lowering blood pressure and the risk of cardiovascular disease.[229]

In a very interesting 2005 study, researchers analyzed 89 postoperative patients who'd had cervical or lumbar spinal surgery.[230] Some of these patients were in bright rooms with lots of sun exposure, while the others were in rooms with less sunlight. Researchers noticed that the patients on the bright side of the hospital consistently used less analgesic medication and experienced less perceived stress.

If you still have doubts, please know that several studies have also associated sunlight exposure with reduced risk of all-cause mortality.[231–233]

Neo Note: Light as a Source of Energy

Plants can use sunlight for energy. The process in which this occurs is called photosynthesis. Photosynthesis is possible because of a compound named chlorophyll, which is present in algae and plants.[234] While I'm sure this is not breaking news for you, what you might not know is that by eating these plants and then being exposed to sunlight, you might also produce energy. Researchers who performed a 2014 study proposed that chlorophyll pigments from these ingested plant foods enable mitochondria in mammals to capture photonic (sunlight) energy and produce ATP.[235] In another study, researchers suggested that the skin pigment melanin can convert light into chemical energy through the hydrolysis (breakdown) of water molecules in the body.[236] In other words, the human body may be able to harness the energy of the sun as well.

STRESS AS A CAUSE OF DISEASE

In the Western world, we see stress as just a normal part of life, something we simply have to deal with. In the East, however, it is seen as something to be cautious about. According to Chinese traditional medicine and Ayurvedic medicine, stress is a contributing factor in most diseases and should be put on the same level of importance as diet in order to achieve a healthy life. Several authors even mention that between 75 percent and 90 percent of all doctor's office visits are for stress-related ailments and complaints.[237] Although these numbers seem to come from outdated studies, I think most of us can agree that our lives have become more stressful in the past 50 years and that these numbers may be more accurate now than ever before.

Stress can have important effects on the body that can trigger diverse pathological responses. For example, studies show that chronic stress can alter the structure of the brain, leading to insomnia, dementia, and other mental health issues.[238-240] Other studies have concluded that chronic stress is directly linked with chronic inflammation and GI diseases like GERD, IBS, and ulcers.[241,242] While the specific mechanisms by which stress triggers or exacerbates these conditions may be different, we must note its importance as a cause of disease.

When you are under stress, your body produces cortisol and adrenaline. Among many things, these hormones put you in fight-or-flight mode and get you ready for war. Although this may seem exaggerated, your genes do not comprehend modern-day stress. They are still programmed to see stress as you being under attack by a predator. They don't understand that you now stress about traffic, your asshole boss, your sports team that never wins, or that neighbor who doesn't let you sleep. And, even though you are just stressed about minor things, your body goes all in and puts you in attack-or-run mode. Your heart rate and blood pressure rise, blood sugar is released from your liver, and muscle activity is prioritized by temporarily turning all other cells insulin resistant. Simultaneously, your body suppresses your digestive and immune systems, since they are not needed while you are "fighting this predator." While this was a great response back in the day, it's simply too much for the stress we are dealing with now. Chronic stress is causing poor digestion, leaky gut, metabolic disorders, and even increased risk of infections and disease.[243-251]

> **Neo Note: Long-term Consequences of Traumatic Stress**
> Acute traumatic stressful events can also cause long-term consequences beyond the obvious mental health issues. Research has shown that individuals who experience early adverse life events (traumatic stress) have a greater risk of developing GI symptoms and even IBS.[252] This finding might be justified by the microbiome-gut-brain (MGB) axis. As discovered by UCLA researchers, traumatic experiences can dramatically change our microbiomes.[253] This change can then result in the GI issues mentioned in other studies.
> A 2019 literature review concluded that traumatic childhood experiences are also linked to a higher risk of developing cancer.[254] Chronic stress is dangerous, but acute traumatic stress should also be addressed with the help of a skilled professional to avoid negative long-term consequences.

There are many authors stating that stress can cause cancer. While this is still a debated topic that needs more research, I feel we have enough evidence to point out that stress can at the very least amplify cancer's progression. Studies show that the adrenaline released during stress induces resistance to chemotherapy drugs, thus protecting cancer cells from the effects of most conventional treatments.[255] Stress is linked to increased activity in the mitogen-activated protein kinase (MAPK) pathway, which ultimately leads to chemotherapy resistance and cancer propagation.[256]

We should all model the ancient Chinese and Ayurvedic practices and learn how to manage stress in order to live happier and healthier lives.

MANAGING STRESS

I purposely wrote "managing" stress because stress will always be present. Even monks get stressed and argue about who is meditating better. At least that's what I imagine. The point is that stress will show up uninvited, and when that happens, you need to find strategies to get rid of it as soon as possible.

Please put this in your head. Stress comes from our perception of things. For example, if I see a strange Doberman running toward me, I might piss myself, but if the Doberman is my pet, I would most likely be happy because "my boy" is excited to see me. Things will happen to you, but the meaning you put into these things and how you react to them is what is going to produce stress or not.

Let me tell you a secret. All of us have the demon and the angel voices in our ears, just like in the cartoons. For many of us, the demon voice is louder and is always shouting. At the slightest thing, it makes you snap and go overboard. But you can learn to invite the "angel voice" into the conversation more often and react differently to events you'd usually see as stressful. There are many ways to do this, and my goal is not to explore them all. I'll just focus on the main strategies supported by science and the ones that have worked the best for me and my clients.

PNS Toning through Breath Work

As you know, stress creates the fight-or-flight response, which is nothing more than the activation of the sympathetic nervous system (SNS). The "opposing" system, and the one we want to keep activated most of the time, is the parasympathetic nervous system (PNS). The PNS brings down cortisol levels, normalizes heart rate and blood pressure, facilitates healing, awakens your digestion, and boosts your immunity. In this state, you are more relaxed and happier. There are many ways to tone your PNS, but one of the best ways is through your breathing.

Research shows that deep abdominal breathing (inhaling while expanding your belly) can increase activity of the vagus nerve and tone the PNS.[257,258] Studies show that a weekly practice of deep breathing is enough to improve mood and reduce levels of stress in the body.[259] And of course this tactic can be used when stressful situations arise. Something as simple as breathing deeply a couple of times is enough to override the temporary SNS activation from stress, keeping you cool and under control.

There are many breathing techniques. The one I usually recommend is box breathing. This technique is really simple. You inhale, expanding your belly, for four seconds, hold your breath for four seconds, exhale for 4 seconds, hold for once again 4 seconds, and then repeat the sequence for a few minutes. I like to do this before important meetings or even when I'm having difficulty falling asleep.

Other ways to tone your PNS include cold exposure, fasting, physical contact (like hugging or massages), laughter, singing or chanting, yoga, and meditation.[260–270]

Meditation and Mindfulness

Growing up, I used to think of meditation as something monks did to achieve enlightenment. Somehow, I associated this practice only with seeking connection with a higher self, the divine, the matrix, or whatever you want to call it. Only about 10 years ago did I notice that people from all walks of life were using it to control their emotions and stay grounded.

Please keep in mind that meditation can be a lot more than just sitting with eyes closed focusing on your breath. Meditation can be anything that helps quiet the mind and relax the body. Yoga, Pilates, singing, playing an instrument, and listening to music all can be forms of meditation. Instead of focusing on being the perfect meditator, as I did for so long, try just to be more mindful and to take 10 to 20 minutes every day to quiet your mind with some breath work or any of the other activities mentioned. By taking these moments to pause and breathe, you train your body to bring down that overactivation of the SNS.

Another strategy is to be more mindful of what happens around you and how you react to it during the day. Instead of automatically reacting to situations, make a conscious effort to stop, breathe in deeply, and then analyze the situation with a fresh mind. If, even after pausing, you're still too triggered, don't engage with the situation; if possible, return to it the following day. Sometimes the best way to solve a problem is to leave it for the following day, when you can see it with different eyes.

Gratitude, Affirmations, and Visualization

I know, I know, this nutrition and lifestyle book is now looking like the new version of *The Secret*. While this "hippie stuff" might throw some people off, I would not be spending the time writing this if it weren't important.

Although I would love to see more high-quality studies on this topic, several researchers maintain that something as simple as expressing gratitude is enough to improve sleep quality, overall mood, self-esteem, empathy, and even resiliency to suicidal ideation.[271–274]

An easy way to implement a gratitude practice is to think about things you are grateful for before you go to sleep. Once you go to bed, stop for a moment and think about at least two good things that happened to you during the day. It could be as simple as being grateful for the delicious food you ate or the fact that there was less traffic than usual. The more things you can think of, the better.

Have you ever heard about the power of the placebo? People taking sugar pills without realizing it and improving miraculously? Our mind and our body work in ways that we are still trying to understand, but over and over again we have seen scientifically that when the mind believes in something, the body responds accordingly. Recent studies show that self-affirmations activate areas in the brain that lead to feelings of reward, which then facilitate behavior change and new beliefs.[275,276] In other words, self-affirmations have an actual effect on your brain that will promote changes in your behavior. As you refocus your inner conversation and adopt a more positive approach, your behavior and attitude will become more positive as well.

MINDFUL EATING

Nowadays, with our easy access to food (for most of us), people no longer honor the act of eating; they just cram in as much food as they can, as fast as they can, while watching TV. When you eat this way, you overload your digestive system, block the satiety feedback, and end up eating much more than you need. Not to mention that you don't even appreciate how rich and flavorful your food is.

When having a meal, sit for a moment and disconnect from technology, like your cell phone or laptop. If you have people around you, use this moment as an opportunity to connect. If you're alone, put on some Marvin Gaye and enjoy your food slowly. Look at your food, smell it, taste it, and chew it thoroughly so you have enough digestive juices to facilitate the digestion in your stomach. Just the act of chewing has been found to reduce stress, improve mood, and enhance cognitive function and attention.[277,278] Keep eating until you are about 80 percent full and then stop. This is something the Japanese call *hara hachi bu* and is one of the secrets to their longevity. This is a great strategy to avoid overeating. After all, if you want to perform well after a meal, the goal should not be to be full but to no longer be hungry. Can you understand the difference?

Neo Note: Emotional Eating
Sometimes we eat to address feelings of lack. If there is trauma or other forms of emotional distress triggering your "hunger," you will always face a losing battle. Being mindful is also perceiving these hidden issues. It's noticing little things like "opening exceptions" in your diet whenever you are stressed, or grabbing some ice cream when you're lonely, or eating more than you normally would in order to forget about work. Sometimes it could even be something much deeper, like not being able to follow a healthy diet because of childhood traumas. Staying overweight can be an unconscious defense mechanism for some.[280] Try to detect possible emotional patterns triggering your hunger and poor self-discipline. Once you identify them, seek professional help.

SOCIAL CREATURES
During the past decade, with the changes in our lifestyle and the expansion of the web 2.0, another early mortality risk factor has been growing exponentially. Care to guess what it is? It's social isolation, or, in plain English, loneliness. This might surprise you, but according to research, social isolation is worse than obesity and as bad as smoking 15 cigarettes a day in terms of predicting a premature death.[281]

Humans were only able to thrive because of their communities. In a community, we could help each other, hunt bigger animals, protect the fragile, and increase the chances of surviving. As you can imagine, that is something that appeals to our programming, so that information is still in our genes to this day.

A 2010 meta-analysis concluded that people with larger social networks presented about 45 percent lower risk for all-cause mortality.[282] While this information is purely observational, there are other studies with more objective measures that can justify this improved longevity. One study uncovered that elderly who volunteered and spent time with others in their community had lower levels of inflammation (lower C-reactive protein and interleukin-6).[283] Another study suggests that people with pro-social behavior (which favors the community) have better immune gene expression.[284] In other words, if you favor your social networks—the real ones—you may have lower inflammation, a better immune system, and a longer life.

Group relationships are also important to rein in stress levels. It's been shown that women with healthy social support have lower levels of stress hormones after a stressful event.[285] This can be attributed in part to the release of the hormone oxytocin, which is prompted by social interaction. This hormone suppresses the release of stress hormones and keeps you happy. In women, this effect is especially strong because estrogen boosts the effects of oxytocin.[286] However, men obviously still benefit from the effects of social interactions. In fact, researchers concluded that the relationship between social isolation and inflammation was more significant in the dudes.[287] I totally knew that nothing beats some bromance.

Sadly, data is showing that social isolation is getting worse.[288-290] The reason this is happening is complex. Our modern lifestyle doesn't expose us to as much social interaction as before. Furthermore, we have the issue of social media that is turning us into socially awkward people who cannot interact in real life. Finally, the idea of people soon "inhabiting" a metaverse is definitely not making this picture any brighter. Despite how things are progressing, it's up to us to refuse to go with the flow. We need to take the initiative to change our ways of living. Put down this book for a second and go hug someone. Seriously, do it now. I'll wait for you.

ENVIRONMENTAL TOXINS

After the great world wars, with the boom of the chemical industry, our toxic load exploded. As discussed before, toxic chemicals started to be used in food production to increase yields or simply make cheaper foods. But this did not stop with our diet. Harsh chemicals have been used in everything you can think of, from home appliances to food containers, paints, furniture, even to medications, lotions, toothpastes, and the water we drink, just to name a few. Toxic chemicals are everywhere. And, while it is impossible to avoid them all, you should know the worst offenders so you can protect yourself and the people you love.

These toxic chemicals are giving you headaches, causing inflammation, lowering your immunity, and even messing with your hormones. Remember the concept of molecular mimicry? Well, many of these toxins are similar to some of your hormones and bind to their receptors. This can cause impaired development, reproductive issues, hormone-sensitive cancers, thyroid disease, obesity, and metabolic syndrome.[291-293]

What is more concerning is that these symptoms can stay hidden, appearing only later in life, not only affecting you but also being passed down through your family tree.[294] As much as I would love mention them all, I had to be practical here and discuss only the main ones. At the end of this chapter, I recommend some great resources where you can explore this topic further if interested.

THE MOST WANTED LIST
BPA

Bisphenol A, or BPA, is a chemical compound used in many things, but in particular in cans and other food containers. Many health agencies in the world, including the FDA in the United States, still consider it safe in low doses. But the amount of evidence contending that BPA is in fact a concerning endocrine disrupter is becoming hard to ignore. Researchers from the University of Missouri–Columbia performed a meta-analysis of more than 100 studies and concluded that even in low concentrations (sometimes within the safe range), BPA had significant adverse effects.[295] They also noted that some of the studies that did not reveal any adverse effects from BPA were in fact funded by the chemical industry. Interesting!

In a 2020 review of epidemiological studies, the authors concluded that there was a positive correlation between the level of BPA and the risk of obesity.[296] Unfortunately, getting fat may be the least of your concerns. One of BPA's worst effects may be connected with reproductive health. One study concluded that men with the highest levels of BPA had decreased sperm count, vitality, and motility. In other words, BPA can drown your little swimmers, boys.[297] Ladies, another study showed that women with higher BPA levels were the ones less likely to become pregnant when undergoing fertility treatments.[298]

Concerned about this? You should be. BPA is everywhere. It's in most receipts (thermal paper), electronics, plastic toys, baby bottles, dental fillings, water bottles, plastic food containers, and even the lining of canned products. Unfortunately, BPA doesn't just stay there. It leaches out. For example, one randomized study compared people eating fresh soup with people consuming canned soups. They found that the ones eating canned soup had 1,221 percent higher levels of BPA.[299]

The truth is that most of us use these products daily without realizing the dangers. Even worse, we heat our foods in BPA-filled plastics, which further promotes leaching.[300] No wonder the 2003–2004 National Health and Nutrition Examination Survey conducted by the CDC found detectable levels of BPA in 93 percent of the urine samples analyzed.[301]

The good news is that you can reduce your BPA exposure. A trusty rule of thumb is to stay away from everything plastic—at least as much as you can. And, don't be fooled by so-called BPA-free products. Sadly, many of them use other types of bisphenols, like bisphenol S and bisphenol F. Just because there isn't enough research about these alternatives doesn't mean they're safe. Many authors believe that they might have similar effects.

PFAS

Per- and polyfluoroalkyl substances, or PFAS, are a group of synthetic chemicals that help repel oil and water, so they're frequently used in cookware, wrapping paper, food packaging, and also in carpeting, clothing, and car parts. Within this family we have different chemicals like PFOS (perfluorooctanesulfonic acid), PFHpA (perfluoroheptanoic acid), PFNA (perfluorononanoic acid), PFDA (perfluorodecanoic acid), PFHxS (perfluorohexanesulfonic acid), and the famous PFOA (perfluorooctanoic acid) mentioned in chapter 1 with regard to the dangers of microwave popcorn. The good news is that many governments have banned some of these PFAS. The bad news is that not all have been banned, and many products with PFAS are still in circulation. More bad news: it takes a long time for the body to detoxify from these compounds.[302] That's possibly why the CDC estimated that 98 percent of Americans have trace amounts of PFAS in their bodies.[303]

As seen before, this class of chemicals has been associated with endocrine disruption and cancer. Other studies also suggest associations with excess weight, metabolic dysfunction, decreased fertility, kidney disorders, thyroid disease, autoimmune disorders, and cardiovascular and respiratory issues.[304–306]

Just like with the case of BPA, even though you cannot eliminate your exposure to PFAS—since even food crops, livestock, and water contain them—you can substantially reduce it.[307]

Phthalates

Phthalates, which are curiously pronounced "tha-lates" (*you're welcome*), are synthetic compounds used to soften plastics and make them more durable. They are in medical supplies (gloves, medical tubing, and bags, for example), wall coverings, toys, vinyl flooring, plastic wraps for food, and even personal care products like hair spray, lubricants, soaps, and shampoos (because phthalates can act as solvents).

Just like BPA and PFAS, phthalates are powerful endocrine disrupters. In animal studies, phthalates have been seen to induce fertility disorders in both males and females.[308] In humans, similar results have been proposed through epidemiological studies. Different studies have associated high levels of phthalates with sperm DNA damage, low semen quality, reduced testosterone levels, endometriosis, preterm births, and premature breast development in girls.[309–312] Beyond the reproductive disorders, phthalates were also associated with oxidative stress, insulin resistance, type II diabetes, obesity, allergies, and asthma.[313]

Once again, the solution is to be aware of these chemicals and avoid their primary sources in order to decrease your levels.

DEA

If you are like me and watch *Narcos* on Netflix, you might think we are talking about a different DEA. In this case, I am talking about diethanolamine. This DEA is used as an emulsifier and foaming agent in personal care products like shower gels, shampoos, and toothpastes.

Guess what? You got it. DEA has endocrine-disrupting effects. In animal studies, it has been shown to cause reproductive and developmental issues with reduced postnatal growth and survival rates.[314] In human in vitro studies, it has been shown to trigger endocrine dysfunction and even a toxic effect on sperm.[315,316]

The European Union has already banned DEA in cosmetics. However, in the US and many other countries, it is still considered safe.

BHA and BHT

BHA (butylated hydroxyanisole) and BHT (butylated hydroxytoluene) are synthetic antioxidants with a similar chemical structure. They are used as food preservatives in cereal, chips, dehydrated potatoes flakes, chewing gum, and dry processed foods. They are also present in eyeliners, lipsticks, blush, foundation, moisturizers, cleansers, and perfumes.

The FDA considers both BHA and BHT to be safe in limited amounts in processed foods.[317] But when you live in a world where you are bombarded with toxins from all angles, your best option is to avoid them. After all, at higher doses, these two have been shown to be endocrine disrupters that can cause reproductive disorders and even organ toxicity and cancer.[318–326]

These compounds, like others on my list, are still being debated in the science community, since more research is needed. Nonetheless, I think you are better off staying away from them.

Triclosan

Triclosan is a synthetic chemical with antimicrobial properties that is commonly used in hand sanitizers, mouthwashes, soaps, body washes, toothpastes, deodorants, cosmetics, medical disinfectants, dish detergents, kitchenware, furniture, and toys.

Especially in these times of germophobia and virophobia, when people reach for their hand sanitizer dozens of times a day, human exposure to triclosan is increasing.

Although triclosan is great for killing microbes, research shows that it can accumulate in the body and affect immune responses, trigger inflammation, and alter cardiovascular function.[327] Triclosan has also been shown to make *E. coli* antibiotic resistant after sublethal exposures, which can then make it more difficult to fight.[328] If this weren't enough, there are several studies pointing to triclosan's possible endocrine-disrupting effects, causing reproductive, neuroendocrine, and developmental disorders in humans.[329–332]

The good news is that some countries have already taken measures to stop using triclosan, and one of these nations is the USA, where the FDA banned it from over-the-counter antibacterial hand and body washes.[333] However, the chemical is still being used in many other products and in these same products in other countries.

> **Neo Note: Is Bread Giving You Allergies?**
> Azodicarbonamide (ADA) is a chemical substance used as a whitening agent in cereal flour and as a dough conditioner in industrial bread baking.[334] It is also used as a foaming agent and is found in leather products, carpet underlay, and yoga mats.
>
> In 2014, ADA became famous with the news of Subway removing it from the production of its bread. Did people complain that the bread tasted like yoga mats? Nope, the company made this decision because of the studies reporting that ADA is an endocrine disrupter.[335–337] After Subway, other chains adopted the same measure. Please note that countries in the European Union, Australia, and Singapore have also banned ADA from bread.[338] Unfortunately, at the time of this writing, it continues to be used by many industrial bakers in the US, Canada, and Brazil.
>
> Studies have also shown that ADA can suppress the immune system and trigger asthma and allergies.[339–341] As you know, these are symptoms often associated with gluten intolerance—a perfect example of gluten being blamed for a crime it did not commit.
>
> Best way to protect yourself? Stay away from industrial breads and baked goods. Oh, and don't bite into your yoga mat either.

VOCs

VOCs (volatile organic compounds) are chemicals in air fresheners, dryer sheets, and household cleaners, as well as in fragrances, lotions, shampoos, and other toiletries. Considering that VOCs vaporize into air and also dissolve in water, you can imagine how easily they spread. This wouldn't be a problem if they were harmless. But, as you are already guessing, that's not the case. Studies have associated them with migraines, asthma attacks, other respiratory difficulties, neurological problems, and contact dermatitis.[342,343]

As has been the theme so far, it is impossible to completely eliminate contact with VOCs, but a good strategy is to stay away from most products with synthetic fragrances. Opt for natural products that use essential oils instead.

Parabens, SLS, and SLES

To end this list, I just want to make a brief mention of parabens, sodium lauryl sulfate (SLS), and sodium laureth sulfate (SLES). These chemicals are commonly used in shampoos, toothpastes, mouthwashes, body washes, soaps, detergents, and cosmetics. The reason I'm mentioning them is that they are highly regulated or even banned in some countries. This decision is probably because of the existence of animal and in vitro studies suggesting possible toxic effects. To be fair, there is still plenty of controversy about these compounds. Many studies suggest that they are perfectly safe. Nonetheless, I personally prefer to avoid using products with these chemicals. Focusing on more "natural" alternatives is always a wiser choice.

Neo Note: Heavy Metals

Throughout this book, I have mentioned heavy metals, but I haven't explained exactly what they are. Heavy metals are natural compounds present on the earth. They are metals with relatively high densities, atomic weights, or atomic numbers. Some of them are even good for us in low doses, as is the case with cobalt, copper, iron, and zinc. In contrast, some, such as arsenic, cadmium, lead, and mercury, can be incredibly toxic even in tiny doses.

Because of the industrialization of the world, in particular of our food production, heavy metal toxicity is becoming a frequent health issue. Your body can detoxify from these heavy metals, but because most people have overwhelmed their bodies' detox pathways and have heavy metal exposures beyond what is ideal, these sneaky compounds are accumulating in our tissues and causing health problems. Mild poisoning can cause symptoms like abdominal pain, nausea, diarrhea, vomiting, shortness of breath, tingling in your extremities, malaise, and weakness. The more heavy metals you have in your body, the worse these symptoms will become.

Arsenic

The most common cause of arsenic toxicity is the direct or indirect consumption of groundwater contaminated by industrial runoff. While it's improbable that you will get arsenic poisoning from direct ingestion of contaminated water in developed countries, you can get it indirectly. Higher-than-ideal levels of arsenic can be found in rice (think, rice production in fields with contaminated water), grains, and conventionally raised chickens.

Cadmium

Cadmium poisoning is the least common of the four heavy metals I'm listing here. Usually, it results from excessive exposure to tobacco smoke, car emissions, or spray paint. But you can also ingest cadmium through water and soft drinks from dispensing machines with galvanized plumbing, refined wheat flour, canned evaporated milk, and processed foods.

Lead

Lead can make its way into our water because of old lead piping or inappropriate water treatment, like the famous case of lead contamination in Flint, Michigan. Lead can also be found in canned foods or in old dishes, toys, and jewelry, since it was commonly used as an ingredient in paint. (In some countries with less regulation, it still is.)

According to the Agency for Toxic Substances and Disease Registry, adults can detox 99 percent of the absorbed lead, whereas children eliminate only about 32 percent.[344] In other words, even low levels of lead may cause serious issues in children. Studies have reported delays in growth and development, learning impairment, behavioral disorders, hearing loss, speech problems, abdominal pain, anemia, and respiratory infections.[345-348]

Mercury

Mercury exposure can happen through eating fish because of the pollution of our waters and the phenomenon of bioaccumulation mentioned earlier. Then we have mercury exposure from contact with broken thermostats, lightbulbs, batteries, and auto parts. However, there may be another source of mercury most people don't know about. That is processed foods. Research shows that during the production of high-fructose corn syrup (HFCS), this sweetener can become contaminated with mercury.[349] Considering how many foods contain HFCS, this is a mercury source we need to consider. Finally, we have the case of dental amalgams (metal fillings), which can be made up of over 50 percent mercury.

Mercury exposure will lead to an accumulation of this heavy metal in organs like the lungs, the kidneys, and even the brain, since it can cross the BBB.[350] Besides the "normal" symptoms of heavy metal poisoning, mercury toxicity can cause organ failure, cognitive deficits, and serious neurological issues.[351]

LIMITING YOUR EXPOSURE TO THESE CHEMICALS

Let me say this again: you will never be able to entirely eliminate your exposure, because we live in a toxic world. But you surely can minimize this chemical overload. I know I mentioned a lot of chemicals, and it might feel like you can't use or eat anything. In truth, it may be simpler than you realize. You just need to eliminate or pay attention to the following five things:

- Plastics
- Cans
- Processed foods
- Personal and home-care products
- Unfiltered tap water

When you avoid using plastics, you substantially reduce your exposure to BPA and phthalates. Instead of using plastic water bottles, use glass, ceramic, or stainless steel. Then we have the situation of food containers. Most people use plastic ones and even heat food in them. Swap them for glass or ceramic ones. What about plastic wrap and plastic food bags? Easy, use waxed paper and reusable cloth bags. You always have alternatives.

Then there are canned foods. As you know, most times these are lined with BPA. Besides BPA, you also do not need the aluminum that cans can leach into your food. Although canned food is convenient, let's be real here. The toxin contamination largely outweighs the convenience. It's again the question of do you prefer to prepare food fast and get sick, or do you prefer to take five extra minutes and be healthy? Besides, you can find many typically canned foods in glass jars now.

Next on the list are processed foods. Most processed foods get all kinds of chemicals from this list, and more. By avoiding processed foods, you substantially reduce your exposure to toxins like mercury, BHA, BHT, azodicarbonamide, and more. You also avoid plastic and nonstick packaging, protecting yourself from further BPA, PFAS, and phthalates.

Be particularly careful of your personal and home-care products. Start getting in the habit of reading labels and checking for these. Favor brands that use natural raw materials and that are fragrance-free or naturally scented with plant-based essential oils. Use resources like the Environmental Working Group (EWG; ewg.org) to search for safer products. Or search for blogs in your country with recommendations from people who've already done this research for you.

The last of my major categories is unfiltered tap water. Just stop drinking it. You already read an entire section about this, so I'm not going to spend much time here. Using a good filtration system will substantially reduce your exposure to heavy metals and other contaminants.

If you pay close attention to these five categories, you will drastically reduce your toxin exposure. Obviously, there is a lot more that can be done. If you want to go beyond this, just review the substances I mentioned in this section and try to stay away from them as much as possible. But again, don't obsess too much over this. In chapter 16, I'll show you how to boost your detoxification pathways so your body can fight these toxins on a daily basis.

NEO SUMMARY

• Your lifestyle is equally important as your diet to achieve your best health.

• Human beings were designed to be active during the day, with low-intensity exercise or short bursts of high intensity exertion.

• Your cells follow an "internal clock" programming. If you respect it, you your body will encounter less resistance and function more efficiently.

• Sleeping feels like a waste of time but it's one of the most important things you can do to be healthy.

• Humans have a tight bond with nature and being outdoors has many benefits such as improved gut health, immunity, and mental health.

• Progressive sun exposure is the best way to produce vitamin D, which is essential to optimize most systems in the human body.

• Your emotional health has a tremendous impact on your overall health. Learning how to control your emotions and becoming happier is a skill all should pursue.

• We are social creatures and we need social time to thrive.

• The industrial revolution brought the spread of chemical toxins. While it's impossible to avoid them completely, there are many things you can do to substantially reduce your exposure and improve your health.

NEO ACTION

• Try to be active during the day (get up and walk) and workout 3-4 times a week. Do a combination of resistance training and HIIT.

• Get natural sunlight in the morning.

• Skip breakfast.

• Avoid blue light after sunset and dodge late dinners.

• Perform box breathing or meditation before going to sleep.

• Go *forest bathing*.

• Build up your sun tolerance until you reach the goal of 1 hour in the sun daily.

• Adopt mindfulness practices like breath work, meditation, yoga, gratitude or affirmations. Ideally, combine several of these.

• Spend more time with the people you love.

• Stay away from plastics, canned food and beverages, and processed foods. Be selective about your personal and home care products. And, get yourself a water filter.

NEO RECOMMENDATIONS

SCAN ME

- *10% Happier* by Dan Harris
- *Accessing the Healing Power of the Vagus Nerve* by Stanley Rosenberg
- *Biohacker's Handbook* by Olli Sovijärvi, Teemu Arina, Jaakko Halmetoja
- *Boundless* by Ben Greenfield
- *Breath* by James Nestor
- *Eat Dirt* by Dr. Josh Axe
- *Fast This Way* by Dave Asprey
- *Forest Bathing* by Qing Dr. Li
- *Low Tox Life* by Alexx Stuart
- *Paleo Principles* by Sarah Ballantyne
- *Radical Metabolism* by Ann Louise Gittleman
- *Sicker, Fatter, Poorer* by Dr. Leonardo Trasande
- *Sleep Smarter* by Shawn Stevenson
- *SuperLife* by Darin Olien
- *The 4 Hour Body* by Tim Ferriss
- *The Circadian Code* by Dr. Satchin Panda
- *The Genius Life* by Max Lugavere
- *The Immunity Fix* by Dr James DiNicolantonio and Siim Land
- *The Power of When* by Dr. Michael Breus
- *The Stress-Proof Brain* by Melanie Greenberg
- *The Vitamin D Solution* by Dr. Michael F. Holick
- *The Wim Hof Method* by Wim Hof
- *Toxic Free* by Debra Lynn Dadd
- *Why We Sleep* by Dr. Matthew Walker

my.neodiet.co/neorecommendations

Learn How to Get the Most Nutrition out of Your Food

"The food you eat can be either the safest and most powerful form of medicine or the slowest form of poison."
Ann Wigmore

GOING BACK TO THE KITCHEN

Each day, people in the Western world are relying more and more on premade frozen foods, fast-food restaurants, and food delivery services for all their meals. This is probably why some believe that cooking is a dying skill. I do not share that opinion. I feel people are slowly realizing that convenience is costing them their health and that by going back to the kitchen, they can avert this fate. Obviously, not all of us will become Michelin star chefs, nor is that the goal. But we should try to know the basics well enough to prepare our own meals. When you prep your own food, you have full control over the ingredients being used, and you can choose the best preparation methods to make your food more nutritious and less toxic.

I will not teach you how to cook, since that is not the aim of this book. YouTube has thousands of videos from amazing chefs around the world, with everything from the basics to the most advanced cooking techniques. What I will try to do in this chapter is to discuss what food preparation methods and cookware are the best to help you get the most out of your food. The same way a poor lifestyle can ruin your diet efforts, improper food preparation methods can make the very best ingredients toxic.

THE COOKING TRADE-OFF

We cook most foods to kill harmful bacteria, viruses, and parasites. Cooking is also used to break down certain harmful compounds (like antinutrients) or even to make certain nutrients more bioavailable. Some good examples are the beta-carotene in carrots and the lycopene in tomatoes, which are absorbed more efficiently after these plants are cooked.[1]

But cooking can also do the opposite. Boiling, for example, can substantially reduce the content of several micronutrients such as B vitamins, vitamin C, and certain antioxidants.[2-4] During boiling, micronutrients can also be dissolved in the cooking water. This is not too bad as long as you consume the water. Therefore, broths and soups are great ways to get plenty of the much-needed minerals.

Heat can also wipe out digestive enzymes. Some authors believe that when foods are exposed to temperatures higher than 118°F (47.8°C), enzymes get destroyed and certain foods can become harder to break down.[5,6] In saying this, I am not trying to tilt the scale against cooking in any way. Both raw and cooked foods have been part of our evolution and are equally important. We just need to understand that there is always a trade-off, and by knowing this, we can choose which foods do us more good when cooked and which are better raw.

Another important thing to consider is where you are in your health journey. Even though we all can benefit from raw foods because of their higher levels of beneficial enzymes, if you are still fighting inflammation in your gut, these foods with all their intact insoluble fiber can make your symptoms worse. You are better off not getting those enzymes but thoroughly cooking those foods to help with their "predigestion." Later, as you heal, you can slowly add more raw foods to your diet.

Diversity is key. As you heal, combine plenty of raw foods to your cooked dishes so you can get the best of both worlds.

MAKING BETTER COOKING CHOICES

Many raw-food advocates say you should eat all plants raw. While I agree we should eat plenty of raw plants, not all of them make my list because of their antinutrient content, not to mention that many people simply cannot tolerate them because of the digestive issues they cause. Besides, as we just learned, some plants are actually more beneficial when cooked. Lycopene released when tomatoes are heated is a strong anticarcinogenic agent.[7,8] And asparagus, cabbage, carrots, and some mushrooms release more antioxidants (carotenoids and ferulic acid) when lightly steamed or slow-cooked.[9-14] Additionally, trying to eat poorly cooked legumes can be a direct ticket to the hospital, so let's find some middle ground here.

For cooking vegetables, my favorite method is steaming. While dry-heat cooking methods like roasting may preserve the most micronutrients, most vegetables are tastier when cooked with moist heat.[15] Steaming allows vegetables to preserve significant micronutrient content while still making them taste good.[16,17] After steaming, I also like to briefly stir-fry or sauté with some ghee to further boost the flavor and get some healthy fats with my veggies.

Some authors are big fans of the sous vide method. This technique is similar to slow-cooking, but you cook the food in a plastic pouch so it retains all its moisture. While research indicates this is a good way to preserve nutritional content, I don't recommend it. As you already know, plastics can wreak havoc inside your body, so cooking with them is definitely not Neo Diet friendly.

When thinking about eating raw foods, we usually think of vegetables and fruits. However, some animal products can also be eaten uncooked. Obviously, there is a trade-off with the increased risk of pathogenic contamination. But eating certain animal products raw will allow you to get the most nutrition out of those foods. Eating raw fish in ceviche or sushi may be one of the best ways to obtain its vitamins and minerals but also to preserve healthy fats such as the marine omega-3s EPA and DHA. Meat is no different. I understand that beef tartare is not for everyone, but eating steak rare is something I believe we all can learn to enjoy. Not only are you preserving most of the micronutrients in the beef, but you are also keeping your steak tender and juicy.

Word of caution here. While I am the first to recommend eating rare (or at least medium-rare) steak (from cattle grown in regenerative farms), this recommendation does not apply to poultry or pork because of their higher contamination with pathogens. These meats should be thoroughly cooked.

Back to steak . . . a common mistake people make is to overcook meat. Overcooked meat can feel like a rubber shoe sole because of the way the proteins and sugars fuse as a result of the prolonged high heat. The browning of meat can improve its flavor, but it compromises the absorption of protein.[18] Not only that, but when temperatures exceed 355°F (180°C), this reaction produces harmful compounds such as acrylamide, advanced glycation end products (AGEs), HCAs, and PAHs (when using vegetable oils), as we saw earlier.[19-22] Having said that, by cooking meat gently, we can minimize the formation of these toxins, preserve plenty of nutrients, and get a ton of flavor out of it.

Instead of frying, grilling over a flame, or roasting at high temperatures, consider slow-cooking beef or cooking it in a pan with some butter or ghee at a low-to-medium temperature. Another valid option to get some nutritious and juicy meat is to roast at low-to-medium temperatures but keep a lid on the pan to trap the steam. (Remember, do not use aluminum foil. Opt for a Dutch oven or something similar.)

My favorite way to prepare steaks is at medium temperature, with some ghee or lard in the pan. I usually keep my steak rare because that way I can get more micronutrients, preserve more enzymes, and produce fewer toxins. Rare steak is like beer and coffee, an acquired taste. However, if you don't fancy the idea of seeing some pink in your steak, you are probably better off avoiding the expensive cuts and just buying "roast" cuts to slow-cook.

When using a slow cooker or a Dutch oven, don't use lean cuts. Get all the fat, bones, cartilage, ligaments, and skin in there. As discussed in chapter 9, these are great sources of minerals, trace minerals, glycosaminoglycans (especially chondroitin sulfate, glucosamine, and hyaluronic acid), collagen, and gelatin. These will help you have healthy joints, hair, and skin. Researchers have found evidence that our ancestors, even in different parts of the world, used to stew bones and cartilage after they were finished eating the meat so they could get their amazing health benefits.[23,24] Also, as you slow-cook these dishes, you extract more micronutrients, which makes your taste buds perceive an improved flavor experience.[25] Yes, cooking all parts together and slowly improves the nutrition and the taste of your meal.

As a guiding principle, remember that cooking at a minimum of 131°F (55°C) for at least one hour is usually enough to kill pathogens such as *Helicobacter pylori*, *Listeria*, *Salmonella*, and *Trichinella*.[26]

Because of the fat myth, I grew up hearing that one of the best ways to cook was to grill. And while grilling and other dry-heat cooking methods may be good to preserve micronutrients, they can lead to the formation of harmful compounds. Grilling in particular, when done directly over the flame, may produce plenty of these toxins.[27]

Does this mean you need to stop barbecuing? Of course not. I take much pleasure in spending an afternoon around a grill while eating and talking with friends. But I also try to protect myself by taking a couple of preventive measures. One of them is to properly marinate the meats. Research shows that marinating meats for at least four hours in alcoholic beverages like wine or beer, and seasoning it with chili, garlic, ginger, thyme, and rosemary, can reduce HCAs by up to 90 percent.[28,29] As you might recall, Korean red pepper paste, white tea, or lemon can also help reduce HCAs. Regarding AGE formation, as we saw before, marinating in vinegar, tomato juice, or lemon juice substantially reduces these toxins as well. I like to marinate with a combination of different seasonings to minimize the formation of most of these toxic substances. I always go for some wine (or non-GMO, gluten-free beer) and add some lemon juice, chili paste, rosemary, thyme, a bit of balsamic vinegar, and salt, of course. Not only does it make the food taste amazing, but I'm protecting the ones eating this food.

I also focus on turning the meat often to avoid overcooking, and I avoid letting the meat make direct contact with the flames. Additionally, I try to accompany my meat with veggies soaked in olive oil and vinegar to further fight oxidative stress caused by any remaining toxins.

Even though I try to find hacks so I can have some excesses once in a while, there are things you are simply better off without. One of those things is deep-fried food. There is no supplement or marinade that can fix what those vegetable oils will do to you. The only possible hack I can think of is to use healthier fats, like ghee and lard. But deep frying uses really high temperatures that not only will create toxins but also will mess up the proteins and fat in the food. Instead, you can occasionally use an air frier and use some good fats to get your "hit" of fries. But do it on a day when you deserve those carbs. Deal?

Neo Note: Microwave Cooking

I don't consider microwaves to be cooking appliances, but I do know many people for whom this is their only form of "cooking." The only meals you can cook in a microwave are premade meals, and you already know that these are not the best options if you want to be healthy and perform at your best.

What about using the microwave to reheat healthy food cooked previously? Still not a fan. Studies show that microwave heating can distort molecules in food and substantially reduce levels of vitamins and antioxidants.[30–33] To be fair, there are also studies claiming that microwaving does not affect food at all. But as always, I prefer to stay on the safe side.

Finally, we also have to consider the potential effects the radiation might have on our food. Again, the science is murky, but the more I read about it, the less confident I become.

TIME TO HACK THE KITCHEN

What's the point of sharing with you the best foods and the best ways to cook them if you are then cooking them in PFOA nonstick pans and storing them in plastic? That's why I can't finish this chapter without briefly mentioning cookware and kitchen utensils. Don't worry, I'll keep this short and to the point, but at the end of this chapter I recommend great resources in case you want to explore more about this topic.

Let's start with one of the most obvious cookware materials, aluminum. Aluminum is a light metal that can leach into food and then accumulate in the GI tract, liver, kidneys, and brain.[34–37] Unfortunately, this does not turn you into RoboCop. It just makes you sick.[38] Please take action while you can. Chances are that with increased aluminum accumulation, you may lose your cognitive abilities because of the possibility of developing Alzheimer's disease.[39] Parents, or individuals interested in having kids, please know that aluminum has also been associated with autism spectrum disorder.[40]

If you want to protect yourself and your family, please get rid of your aluminum pans and especially aluminum foil. Research shows that meat cooked in aluminum foil showed an aluminum increase of over three times.[41] And the higher the temperature, the more the aluminum levels rose. Want to cover your roast? Use a Dutch oven or an oven casserole with a lid. Instead of baking on aluminum foil, use parchment paper. Want to wrap some food? Use some unbleached paper. There are always safer alternatives.

In terms of pans, you have various options. The best might be high-grade stainless-steel, carbon steel, or cast-iron pans. Yes, these still leach some nickel and iron, but these minerals are less concerning than aluminum. Another strategy is to rotate among the three so you're not always getting the same metal leaching and overloading your body.

There are also several types of ceramic pans. While some are very good indeed, others might have some questionable coatings. Be very careful about any nonstick claims, because when we get into that, things get toxic. If you recall, Teflon, once considered a nonstick miracle, was later found out to have PFOA, which can still be detected in the blood of nearly every single person in the United States.[42] More concerning is that PFOA has been linked by researchers to endocrine dysfunction, infertility, miscarriages, and cancer.[43–48] Do your research or simply choose one of the three metal options I gave you.

What about food containers? Very simple: choose glass and stay away from plastic. This way, you protect yourself from all the harmful effects associated with BPAs and similar compounds. While we're on the topic of staying away from plastic, please also consider this in other cooking appliances. For example, I highly recommend that everyone have a slow cooker. But please don't use those plastic liners to keep food from sticking to the bottom. Some convenience is not worth undermining your health. Pay a bit more and get one with a removable pot, which makes it a lot easier to clean. Another common mistake I see is people using those fancy multilevel plastic steamers. While they are practical and cheap, they are made of plastic. A much better option is an old-school steamer pot, or a glass or stainless-steel steamer.

Another replacement to consider is to use a countertop toaster oven instead of a microwave. The newer ones have different settings and allow you to roast, toast, slow-cook, warm, and even dehydrate. For smaller food portions, this is your best choice.

Let me finish this section with three more appliance recommendations. First one is a high-speed blender. I think this is something everyone should have. Smoothies can be incredibly healthy and are a phenomenal way to get decent nutrition when you have little time to prepare a proper meal. Next on the list is a seed grinder or a small food processor. This can save you time chopping things like garlic and onions and can also be used to prepare different herbs and spices. It's also a wonderful tool to grind fresh flaxseed and avoid letting it get rancid. And my last suggestion is a pressure cooker. This is essential for cooking legumes and getting rid of most of their lectins.

Neo Diet Kitchen Suggestions:
• Ovenproof baking dishes and casseroles with lids, or a Dutch oven
• Aluminum-free, Teflon-free pots and pans (favor high-grade stainless steel, carbon steel, or cast iron)
• Parchment paper and unbleached paper
• Glass containers
• Slow cooker (with removable ceramic pot)
• Glass, stainless steel, or pot steamer
• Smart oven or toaster oven
• Food processor or seed grinder
• High-speed blender
• Pressure cooker

NEO SUMMARY

• Cooking is the best way to control your nutrition and exposure to food toxins.

• Cooking kills pathogens but can it can also destroy enzymes and decrease the number of micronutrients in your food.

• Cooking may help lower antinutrient content and improve nutritional availability of some foods.

• Both raw and cooked foods are important for a healthy life.

• Steaming is a fantastic way to cook your vegetables while preserving most nutrients.

• Cooking with high temperatures can produce harmful compounds such as acrylamide, AGEs, HCAs, PAHs.

• Marinating meat with alcoholic beverages, herbs and spices substantially reduces the production of these harmful substances.

• Microwave radiation may distort molecules in food and reduce the levels of vitamins and antioxidants.

• Aluminum, plastic, and teflon cookware may leach harmful compounds that can make you ill.

NEO ACTION

• Favor longer cooking times at lower temperatures.

• When grilling, marinade the meat to reduce toxic compound formation.

• Use all the parts for your meat stews.

• Review your kitchen appliances and utensils, and replace the ones that may be putting you at harm.

NEO RECOMMENDATIONS

• *Clean 7* by Dr. Alejandro Junger
• *Low Tox Life* by Alexx Stuart
• *Radical Metabolism* by Ann Louise Gittleman
• *The Bulletproof Diet* by Dave Asprey
• *Toxic Free* by Debra Lynn Dadd

my.neodiet.co/neorecommendations

SCAN ME

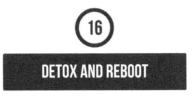

DETOX AND REBOOT

Unleashing the Body's Innate Ability to Heal

"The best and most efficient pharmacy is within your own system."
Robert C. Peale

HEALING MACHINE

After reading these past 15 chapters, you are probably realizing the unintentional damage most of us have inflicted on our bodies over the years. Many of the symptoms you may be experiencing right now are the product of the accumulation of these toxins—toxins that are compromising your body's ability to perform at its best. You might even be thinking, *No way will I ever be healthy. I've already caused too much destruction. Even if I stopped now, my body would never recover from all I've done!*

Splash!

Yes, I just threw an imaginary bucket of ice-cold water at your face. Snap out of it!

Would I spend a year of my life writing this if there were no hope? Of course not. Let me tell you, friend, you are a goddamn healing machine! You've just been disconnected from your power source for a while. But we'll take care of it. I promise!

I know it may seem difficult to believe right now. But you need to understand that even with all those toxins and clogged-up detox pathways, your body is still regenerating itself. Consider the following examples: Every four to five days, your entire intestinal tract gets lined with a new group of epithelial cells.[1] The epidermis (the outermost layer) of your skin is replaced every two months.[2] On average, you get a new batch of red blood cells every three months.[3] And even your entire skeleton is replaced roughly every 10 years.[4]

The only problem is that as all these cells are being replaced, everything else remains the same. Between the lousy diet we've been told to eat, the sedentary and stressful lifestyle we follow, and the harsh chemicals all around us, we keep overwhelming our bodies with "poison."

Although we will never be able to eat 100 percent "pure" foods or avoid all the chemicals around us (at least until Elon creates the colony on Mars), there is plenty we can do. We should focus on decreasing our toxin exposure, building a stronger line of defense, and upgrading our detoxification pathways to get rid of the trash inside us. This, my friend, is antifragility, and it is what I'm going to show you in this chapter. Ready to kick some toxin ass?

REPAIR THE HOLES FIRST

You are probably excited to learn how to detox like a pro. I am also eager to show you. But if I went straight to that, I would be doing you a huge disservice. After all, what is the point of learning how to bail the water from a sinking boat if you haven't plugged the holes? Fixing your digestion is the equivalent of repairing the holes in the boat. A strong digestion is going to keep most toxins outside your body. Only then can you think about removing the ones that already got in. Fixing your digestion is the first and most important thing you can do to detox and heal yourself. Period.

STOMACH ISSUES

The main stomach issue that affects most people is low acid. This happens due to improper diet, use of antacids, stress, and even normal aging. Without enough acid, we cannot properly break down food, kill parasites, or even promote the right environment in the small intestine to fight off SIBO, for example. The first, and most obvious, step is to eliminate processed and other toxic foods, as discussed before. After that, we have to consider things like stopping antacids, managing stress, chewing well, and avoiding large amounts of cold beverages with meals. Only after these basics are taken care of can we think about the strategies to physiologically boost acid production.

Hydrate Your Stomach

One reason you might not be producing enough stomach acid is because you are dehydrated. According to Ayurvedic teachings, water is essential to hydrating the lining of the stomach. If the stomach is "prehydrated," it will produce more acid to digest food.

Stay hydrated during the day and, 15 to 30 minutes before a meal, drink a big glass of water at room temperature (or, if you can tolerate it, drink it hot). This simple trick has been shown to improve digestion and even trigger weight loss.[5]

Want to make this technique even more efficient? Add a pinch of salt and squeeze in half a lemon or one tablespoon of apple cider vinegar (ACV). While the water hydrates your stomach lining, the lemon or ACV will signal your stomach to produce hydrochloric acid (HCl).

346 THE NEO DIET – CHAPTER 16

Neo Note: The Importance of Appetizers
Here is an easy trick to implement. To start off your meal, order a salad with olive oil and vinegar. The vinegar will increase HCl production, and the oil will stimulate bile flow from your gallbladder. Another easy "home hack" is to eat a tablespoon of a fermented food like real pickles, kimchi, or sauerkraut before your meal. The acid in the fermented food will boost your digestive power.

Bitters

Bitters are herbs, roots, bark, fruit, seeds, or flowers that, as suggested by the name, have a bitter taste. Many times, they are used in combination to create an infusion that can be added to cocktails or as a digestive tonic. Our bodies detect the bitter taste as a protective mechanism, because several toxic and poisonous things are highly bitter tasting. If it tastes bad, we tend not to eat it. And that's how the body protects us. Another way the body tries to protect us is by substantially ramping up the production of acid and other digestive juices so we can neutralize the "bitter threat." This is the part we can use to our advantage. By ingesting bitters at the start of a meal, you will get your juices flowing and improve your digestion.[6,7]

Please note that these effects on our digestion do not seem to be present if the bitters are taken in capsule form.[8] It appears that you have to taste them in order for them to work.

Some of the best bitters for digestion are *Angelica archangelica*, *Angelica sylvestris* root, burdock root, Jerusalem artichoke, gentian root, and wormwood. Many times, these are formulated together in infusions and herbal tonics. There are also bitter greens you can have in your appetizer salad, like arugula, dandelion greens, radicchio, and watercress.

Nutrition

The same way we discussed the importance of having a hydrated stomach lining for proper HCl production, your body also needs the right raw materials to produce acid. Please make sure you are getting plenty of HCl-supporting nutrients, such as B vitamins, iodine, sodium, and zinc. Some of the best sources are red meats, seafood, and salt.

Supplements

Many authors I follow and respect recommend taking HCl supplements to boost your "digestive fire." They advise taking as much as you can tolerate and doing it constantly. While there are things I recommend long term, there are very few supplements I believe should be taken this way. HCl capsules are not one of them. As discussed before, there are reasons for the low acid production. If you just take HCl supplements, you're putting a Band-Aid on the issue. The Neo way is not about easy fixes. It's about real fixes. After all, the easy fix will cost you down the line.

Consider this. If you take HCl supplements, your body will not see the need to naturally produce more HCl. As we've heard in high school biology, what is not used atrophies and dies. It's like the example of bodybuilders who do poorly planned, long-term testosterone replacement therapy. Many of them end up with testicular atrophy (a.k.a. tiny balls) because their testicles are no longer required to produce testosterone.[9] By the same principle, we should not do long-term HCl "replacement" (supplementation).

But if you are really struggling to digest right now, you might need an initial boost. And that is okay. Start strong, and over a period of a month or two, cut back on how much of this supplement you're taking, until eventually you no longer need it.

GALLBLADDER ISSUES

We cannot talk about fixing digestion and boosting detox pathways without talking about the gallbladder. As you know, bile is essential to breaking down the healthy dietary fats, and also to flush out toxins and metabolic waste products. You develop gallbladder issues when your bile gets too thick. This will cause a sluggish gallbladder and can even lead to clogged bile ducts. If bile doesn't flow as it should, it can't do its job, and digestive, detox, and metabolic problems arise.

In chapter 2, I mentioned that the gallbladder can be compromised by the increased toxic load in our diet. Another common issue is the excessive consumption of processed carbs, which can progress to metabolic syndrome. Research shows that metabolic syndrome is a risk factor for gallstone formation.[10] Then we have the fact that most people eat too much of oxidized fats and too little of good fats. The oxidized fats make your bile thicker. And the deficit in good fats causes a lack of raw materials to produce new bile. Thus, the body is forced to reabsorb used bile and continue to use it over and over again.[11]

Many doctors believe that once the gallbladder is compromised, the only thing left to do is to remove it. While in some acute situations this procedure is needed, most times there is a lot that can be done conservatively to turn things around. Everyone is different, but on average it's believed that you can recover this small but mighty organ in three to six months.

Nutrition

First and foremost, we have to remove the bad stuff. Stop eating processed foods full of sugar and oxidized oils. Once you eliminate these bad foods from your diet, you need to focus on nutrients that will help clean up your gallbladder and ducts, and also create fresh bile. Fats like olive oil, coconut, ghee, and grass-fed butter will give you the raw materials needed for new bile.

Fiber will help dispose of the old bile. Then, eating vitamin-C-rich foods like camu camu, amla berries, acerola, kakadu plums, and sea buckthorn (i.e., in powder form in your smoothies) can help prevent the formation of gallstones.[12,13]

Iron deficiency is also associated with gallstone formation.[14,15] If you eat meat, you don't have this problem. If you follow a vegan diet, though, you need to compensate by eating more of the vegetables and nuts rich in iron and boosting your vitamin C, since it helps increase the absorbability of nonheme iron.[16]

Another reason gallstones appear is because of bile not having enough bile salts (or bile acids). Without enough bile salts, bile gets too thick due to a higher concentration of cholesterol, which then can cause gallstones (cholelithiasis). But if we have enough bile salts, this won't happen.[17]

Choline and taurine have been shown to boost bile salt production. In other words, if you get enough choline and taurine in your diet, you substantially decrease your chances of cholelithiasis.[18-21] Some great sources of choline are egg yolks, organ meats, beef, shiitake mushrooms, almonds, and cauliflower. For taurine, as you know, the best sources are animal foods. Nonetheless, there is some research stating that edible red algae are a suitable alternative.[22]

Bitters

As I said before, bitters get the juices flowing. This also applies to your bile. So, by incorporating bitters to help with HCl production, you are automatically improving your bile health. That's a nice two-in-one combo.

Supplements

In the beginning, there are some supplements that can be helpful. Supplementing with bile salts, for example, can help immediately change the consistency of your bile and get things moving.

If you want to cover all your bases, there are also supplements that combine bile salts, bitters, choline, taurine, and digestive enzymes. These can be of great help in the beginning but should not be taken forever. The one exception here is individuals who have had their gallbladders removed. In that case, one of these supplements may be something to consider long term.

Also, if you are not getting enough vitamin C in your diet, consider supplementing with a whole-food vitamin C extract.

Neo Note: Forgive

According to the teachings of traditional Chinese medicine, the liver and gallbladder are directly connected with the emotion of anger. Anger will affect your energy pathways and compromise the function of these two organs. While I don't have any research to show this link, I believe we know enough to understand that our emotions have a big impact on our health. Forgiving may or may not heal your liver and gallbladder. Nonetheless, I'm sure that at the very least, it will make you a happier person. Worth trying, don't you think?

DIGESTIVE ENZYME DEFICIENCY

You are not what you eat; you are what your body can digest and absorb. We've already discussed the importance of stomach acid and bile in this equation, but we are still missing a third component, digestive enzymes. These enzymes are proteins that, as the name suggests, help you digest food. They help you break down complex carbohydrates, proteins, and fats into smaller, easier-to-absorb molecules.

Your body naturally secretes them in the salivary glands, stomach, pancreas, and small intestine. Unfortunately, because of common dietary and lifestyle choices (and also genetic conditions), many of us are not producing sufficient digestive enzymes. This is causing improper food breakdown, which has been associated with GI symptoms such as abdominal pain, flatulence, constipation, diarrhea, and steatorrhea (floating stools).[23] As we've seen, if these digestive issues persist, they can lead to obesity, gut dysbiosis, autoimmunity, food allergies and intolerances, fatigue, brain fog, and mental health issues.

How do you know if you have a digestive enzyme deficiency? There are stool tests that can be done, but for most of us, just paying attention is enough. Do you experience GI discomfort after meals? Do you feel full after just a couple of bites? Do you feel like your food is just sitting in your stomach for hours? Do you have frequent floating and "oily" stools? Chances are that you have a digestive enzyme deficiency.

In order to fix this, many authors recommend taking digestive enzyme supplements with every meal. While I think these supplements are excellent and I even recommend them in the book's resources, I don't like the idea of having to rely on them forever—largely because this is not addressing the root cause of the issue. Sure, if you have a genetic condition or exocrine pancreatic insufficiency (EPI) from chronic pancreatitis, cystic fibrosis, or pancreatic cancer, you definitely should take your digestive enzyme supplements long term. Nonetheless, I still believe that by improving your diet and lifestyle, you can improve your digestive performance even with these conditions.

Nutrition

Cleaning up your diet is probably the most important thing you can do. As you already know, diets high in processed foods and refined carbohydrates are associated with the development of metabolic syndrome. Metabolic syndrome can in turn affect the health of your pancreas, which is an important producer of digestive enzymes.[24]

Nutritional deficiencies are also a cause of digestive enzyme deficiency. If the body does not have the raw materials and catalysts, it cannot make the enzymes. Enzymes are proteins, so proper protein consumption is essential. Beyond protein, studies suggest that vitamin B_6 and zinc seem to be essential as well.[25,26]

The good news is that by following the Neo Diet, you will optimize your metabolic health, decrease inflammation (inflammation also lowers digestive power), and get all the nutrients you need.

Eating raw foods is also a great way to boost your digestive power, since raw foods still have digestive enzymes in them. While this does not address the cause of the deficiency, it is a good dietary way to boost digestive enzymes.

One last thing to consider is to season your foods with cardamom, coriander, cumin, fennel, and ginger. These spices are known for boosting digestion and may even help step up digestive enzyme production.[27-31]

Mindful Eating

Eating in a rush or in a stressed state will cause insufficient chewing and digestive juice secretion. If you don't get enough juice, you don't get enough enzymes. Follow the steps we already discussed and aim to eat in a relaxed state, really trying to enjoy your food. Also, avoid having a big meal right after a tough workout. This type of physical stress will also weaken your digestive power.

Gallbladder Fix

Gallstones can block the bile duct and reduce the flow of the digestive-enzyme-rich pancreatic juices. By fixing the gallbladder, we also prevent this issue. This is just a small reminder of how everything is connected and that by fixing one thing, you may be able to fix several distinct problems at once.

Lifestyle

Your digestion might just be overwhelmed by frequent eating. Practicing intermittent fasting is a great way to give your digestive system a well-deserved break. Sometimes that is all we need. Smoking, alcohol abuse, and excessive consumption of analgesic medications are also known for affecting pancreatic health.[32] Poor pancreatic health, poor digestive enzymes. These three are big no-nos. Finally, there is stress. I already recommended not eating in a stressed-out state. But it's not just about eating. Stress boosts inflammation and makes all systems, including the digestive system, perform poorly. Adopt practices to manage your stress, like the ones we discussed in chapter 14.

Supplements

There is no question that digestive enzyme supplements work. Several studies show their efficacy in boosting food breakdown and fixing issues associated with poor upper digestion.[33-41] But most people should not exclusively rely on these. Easy fixes do not make you antifragile; they make you dependent. Am I saying you shouldn't take them? Not at all. They are essential in the beginning, especially if your digestive ability is substantially compromised. Taking a couple of capsules at the beginning of each meal can tremendously boost the chances of your food being fully digested. The trick is to wean your body off them as your digestive capacity improves. Eventually, you just want to use them as a biohack. For example, any time I go to a Brazilian steakhouse and I know I'm going to eat way too much, I always take my digestive enzymes to compensate for the ridiculous amount of meat I'm going to eat. I suggest you do the same with any excesses. As always, I have recommendations in the book's resources.

GUT ISSUES

As we go down the digestive tract, we eventually reach the intestines, or, as most like to call them, the gut. By now, you clearly understand how important the gut is to defend the body from the aggressors in our food and environment. By healing and sealing a leaky gut, you build yourself a fortress that will keep you incredibly healthy from gut to brain.

When we remove the toxic foods from our diet, we have to actively start repairing the damage we caused over the years. Depending on how damaged you are, this might take weeks or even months. Nonetheless, it's worthwhile. After you have healed your gut and upper digestion, you will be able to reintroduce some of the hard-to-digest foods and still feel great. Heck, you'll even be able to eat some crappy food with friends once in a while without thinking about the consequences, because your gut will be able to handle it. That's the beauty of becoming antifragile.

Dysbiosis Fix

Let's start by thinking about your gut as a garden. If you want to replant a garden, what do you do first? You remove the weeds. There is no point in planting new flowers or adding natural fertilizer if the garden is still covered in weeds. The weeds will continue to steal nutrients, compete for space, and eventually kill the "good" plants you are trying to grow.

This same scenario applies in your gut. Instead of recommending all the foods and herbal supplements that help heal intestinal inflammation, I recommend starting the healing process by removing your "gut weeds." In other words, the first step is to heal your gut dysbiosis by going full John Wick on your pathogenic bugs and parasites.

As you are going through an elimination stage and removing all the bad foods from your diet, you are already working toward cleaning up your gut. As you know, these pathogenic bugs feed on processed foods and refined sugars. So, by removing their favorite foods, you start to starve some of them. Unfortunately, at times this is not enough. Since your microbiome population may be completely out of control, we might need to do like Thanos (where are my Marvel fans?) and substantially reduce the population so it's easier to manage and heal.

Just by fixing your stomach acid and increasing your GI motility with the consumption of bitters and the elimination of inflammatory foods, you will actively clear the bugs from your small intestine. As you know, they have no business in there, and just by depopulating that region of your gut, you will feel better immediately.

Besides eliminating the bad foods, it's important that you also eliminate some good foods in the beginning. You won't be able to fix SIBO and SIFO if you keep feeding the masses ample amounts of food. For a short period, it is essential to starve everyone (even the good guys) to stabilize the overgrowths and balance the microbiome ecosystem. You can do this by temporarily eliminating (or substantially decreasing) foods from the FODMAP list. Please note that I wrote "temporarily." As discussed before, many FODMAP foods are essential for our health. But if you recall, I also mentioned that research had shown that a temporary low-FODMAP diet was very effective with many conditions like dysbiosis, SIBO, and IBS. This is because it helps balance the microbiome. Remember, we are first killing the weeds so we can then grow a strong and healthy garden.

Biofilm Fix

In chapter 5, we learned about biofilms. These protective coatings can form over bacteria and fungi, shielding them from antimicrobial and antifungal treatments.[42] There isn't much science behind biofilm treatment, because this is still a fairly recent discovery. Nonetheless, there are some interesting studies on "anti-biofilm" foods and supplements that appear to be effective in dealing with this issue. Research shows that acetic acid from apple cider vinegar is effective at destroying biofilms.[43] ACV has also been recognized for its antimicrobial properties, which makes it a good two-in-one bad-bug killer.[44–46] ACV is also great for promoting stomach acid, and it may help improve insulin sensitivity.[47–50]

Because of all the above, I recommend using ACV to season your salad. And if you're brave enough do a shot of it in the morning, and before going to bed (if you can tolerate it).

In terms of supplements, there are three that seem to be the best biofilm busters. Two of them, you may be already consuming as you heal your digestion. I'm talking about digestive enzymes and probiotics. A combination of digestive enzymes and probiotics (in particular *Saccharomyces boulardii*, *Lactobacillus acidophilus*, *Lactobacillus rhamnosus*, and *Bifidobacterium breve*) have been shown to be powerful destroyers of biofilm.[51–55]

The final one is N-acetylcysteine (NAC). NAC is a powerful supplement traditionally used to fight oxidative stress and inflammation, stabilize blood sugar, boost detoxification, improve immunity, relieve symptoms of respiratory diseases, promote fertility, and enhance brain health.[56–73] If this weren't enough to make it a super supplement, research also suggests that it has anti-biofilm properties.[74] Despite its recognized safeness, as of 2021 NAC is getting more difficult to purchase in the US because the FDA is considering "promoting" it to a prescription drug, following the lead of some European countries. Depending on where in the world you live, it may be easier or harder to get. Just google it. Either way, a combination of probiotic and digestive enzymes should be enough to do the trick.

Parasite Fix

The idea of having worms, protozoa, and other bugs inside us seems more like a sci-fi movie than real life, but they do exist, and they live inside many of us. When I say many of us, I'm not just referring to people living in tropical and subtropical regions of the world. I'm also talking about Europe, Oceania, and North America.

In a study published in 2002, researchers analyzed fecal samples from 2,896 patients in 48 states of the US.[75] This might surprise you, but 32 percent of them were found to have parasites. That's right, practically one-third of the individuals tested had parasites living inside them. While this small study is in no way, shape, or form a direct representation of the entire population of the US or any other "developed" country, it shines a light on how bad this issue may be. As the authors of a 2019 study conclude, "parasitic diseases are one of the world's most devastating and prevalent infections, causing millions of morbidities and mortalities annually."[76] This is another epidemic barely anyone is talking about.

Parasites steal your nutrients, produce toxic waste, trigger your immune system, spread viruses, and make you sick. Sadly, there is very limited research on the effects of parasites in humans. Many medical experts suggest that some of the common symptoms of a parasitic infection are anal itching, abdominal pain, insomnia, changes in appetite, mood swings, fatigue, brain fog, migraines, allergies, and rashes.

How do you get parasites? You can get them by drinking improperly treated tap water, eating in restaurants, eating raw or undercooked foods (especially pork or sushi), eating contaminated fruits and vegetables, swimming in lakes, being bitten by an insect, or being in contact with animals (yes, even your adored pets). Considering this, it's easy to understand that it is not a matter of if, but a matter of when. Exposure to parasites is inevitable. Once again, the idea is not to live in a bubble but to become resilient and learn how to fight off these aggressors.

If you have a combination of the symptoms listed earlier, it's probably a good idea to do an intensive cleanse for a month or so. However, even if you don't have reason to believe you currently have a parasitic infection, I suggest taking some natural supplements against parasites for a week every three months. It's an easy way to keep them at bay.

Some of the best natural supplements to get rid of these sneaky bastards are allicin (from garlic), berberine, black walnut, clove oil, *Mimosa pudica*, neem, oregano oil, papaya seeds, sweet wormwood, and vidanga (*Embelia ribes*).[77-90] There are many brands that combine several of these extracts.

Microbiome Diversity

After the cleanup comes the selective repopulation of the gut. By staying away from the foods that promote pathogenic bacteria and slowly adding the foods that support the growth of the good bugs, you create the foundation for a healthy and thriving microbiome. As you incrementally add fiber, resistant starches, polyphenols, fermented foods, and probiotics, you ensure that your beneficial bacteria stay strong. In return, they maintain your gut, produce postbiotics to boost your health, and keep you protected against bad bacteria and even some toxins.

The goal is not to pick one or two prebiotic foods and eat crazy amounts of them. The goal is to eat a variety of these foods. Consuming a wide mix of prebiotics will ensure that you can feed the different species of good bacteria and will promote microbiome diversity. As you know, microbiome diversity is a predictor of good health, and it should be something always to aim for.

Another way to do this is to make an effort to eat more seasonal foods. These will support the right microbes at the right time of the year. Plus, it's a good way to change up your diet and challenge yourself to eat different things.

Also, don't forget about getting a variety of fermented foods. These are phenomenal to increase your microbiome diversity.

Probiotics

We cannot talk about repopulating the gut without mentioning probiotics. As you know, I don't believe in taking probiotic supplements forever, but I do believe in their occasional use, especially when healing the gut. Right after the food elimination period, your body is still not ready to handle a bunch of prebiotics and fermented foods. During this time, taking probiotics is an awesome hack to boost your gut health, even if most probiotics have only transient effects.

When shopping for probiotics, look for respected brands with a variety of strains. Remember, diversity is key. Some of the important strains to look for are *Bifidobacterium breve*, *Bifidobacterium lactis*, *Lactobacillus acidophilus*, *Lactobacillus plantarum*, *Lactobacillus rhamnosus*, and even the yeast *Saccharomyces boulardii*.

Another potent type of probiotics is spore-based or soil-based organisms (SBOs). In short, these are microorganisms found in the soil. While they seem to be a new trend, we have been consuming SBOs for thousands of years. Humans have been getting SBOs from working their land and eating their vegetables and roots with dirt residues on them. While our modern lifestyle has decreased our exposure to SBOs, we can still make a conscious effort to go outside, get dirty, and of course take SBO probiotic supplements.

SBO probiotics have a higher survival rate because they tolerate stomach acid, and even exposure to heat and cold during storage and processing.[91] Besides their resilience, research has shown that they possess antioxidant, antimicrobial, immunomodulatory, and pathogen-fighting effects.[92] There are several species and strains of SBOs, but when choosing your supplement, look for the *Bacillus clausii*, *Bacillus coagulans*, and *Bacillus subtilis* strains. These are the ones that seem to be the most beneficial to humans.

Neo Note: SBOs to Fight LPSs

SBOs may also heal your gut unexpectedly. They seem to be a powerful tool to fight the nasty lipopolysaccharides (LPSs). According to a 2017 study, 30 days of supplementing with SBOs led to an incredible 42 percent reduction in LPSs.[93] Another great reason to "eat some dirt."

Gut Lining Fix

The next step in our healing journey is to patch the holes and strengthen the walls. Just by taking care of your microbiome dysbiosis and removing all gut lining aggressors (such as lectins and toxins), you are halfway there. Without causing further damage and by reducing the inflammation, the gut lining will finally have the chance to heal. In this section, I am going to focus on the other half—the half that comprises eating the foods or taking the supplements that can speed up your recovery by patching the holes and decreasing intestinal inflammation. So, let's do this!

Some of my favorite gut-healing foods are mushrooms, coconut oil, bone broths, meat stews, onions, capers, radicchio, asparagus, and carrots.

Research shows that mushrooms improve gut barrier integrity.[94] They are also recognized as being able to help reverse dysbiosis, increase microbiome diversity, and stimulate immune cells.[95]

We've already discussed the antimicrobial and anti-inflammatory properties of coconut oil. As researchers have demonstrated, it has the ability to reduce intestinal inflammation, especially in people with Crohn's disease.[96]

Then we have bone broths and meat stews. The slow cooking process allows us to extract important gut healing nutrients such as glutamine, collagen, glycine, proline, and healthy fats.[97]

Next on the list are onions, capers, radicchio, and asparagus. These are excellent sources of the polyphenol quercetin, which has been found to reduce gut permeability and boost the activity of the gut lining.[98–101]

And finally, carrots and fresh carrot juice have been used as an Ayurvedic remedy for healing GI inflammation for hundreds of years. To be honest, most of the authors who suggest carrots for this were relying on anecdotal evidence, since there aren't many studies exploring this treatment. Nonetheless, there is one study from 2020 that indeed links a carrot-derived polysaccharide with decreased inflammation and improved gut wall integrity.[102] I would love to see more research to support this ancient Ayurvedic practice.

Before getting into supplements, there is one more thing you can do. Go outside and get some sunlight on that skin. Not only does a nice tan look good on you, it has been discovered that vitamin D helps reduce intestinal hyperpermeability.[103,104]

Neo Note: Rebuilding the Mucous Layer

Protecting the gut lining, you have a layer of mucus. The healthier the mucous layer, the harder it is for lectins and other aggressors to cause leaky gut and invade your insides. This mucous layer also provides nice real estate for your microbiome. As you can surely guess, the problem here is that because of years of poor diet and lifestyle, most people have a very thin mucous layer that quite honestly is not protecting much. One way to reverse this situation is to feed your gut bugs. If you provide them with prebiotics, they produce the postbiotic butyrate. Butyrate will then feed the cells from the intestinal lining and boost their mucus-producing ability.[105]

Besides the intestinal mucus-producing cells, researchers have uncovered a type of microbe in our gut that seems to be a mucus-secreting beast. Its name is *Akkermansia muciniphila* (let's just call it Akke). Studies have shown that when mice were fed Akke supplements, their gut linings became strong and there was a substantial decrease in inflammation.[106] Good job, guys!

The bad news is that your Akke population tends to decline with age.[107] Once way to fight this is to supplement with them (although there aren't many brands yet and they're not very affordable) or to make sure you provide your existing Akke with plenty of their favorite foods so they can continue to thrive and grow. Research has suggested that pu-erh tea promotes the growth of this population of microbes.[108] The prebiotic inulin present in many vegetables is also a beloved meal.

Last but not least, we have supplements. Supplements can be used at the beginning of your gut-healing journey because they can exponentially speed up your body's ability to fix your leaky gut. Some of the best supplements to produce mucus, tame intestinal inflammation, and promote gut lining integrity are L-glutamine, colostrum, silica, deglycyrrhizinated licorice, marshmallow root, slippery elm bark, aloe vera, and the Ayurvedic supplement triphala (a combination of amalaki, bibhitaki, and haritaki).[109-122] With the exception of triphala, which is usually sold separately, you can find several brands of supplements with a combination of many of these gut-healing agents.

Neo Note: Dr. John Douillard's Gut-Healing Decoction[123]

I learned about this gut-healing decoction from Dr. John Douillard's book *Eat Wheat*, but you can also find it on his website, lifespa.com. This has been his go-to remedy for healing guts for almost 30 years, so that says a lot. And the herbal agents used are all well studied for their gut-healing properties. So, without further delay, let me share it with you.

- 1 tablespoon chopped (not ground) licorice
- 1 tablespoon chopped (not ground) slippery elm bark
- 1 tablespoon chopped (not ground) marshmallow root
- 2 quarts (about 2 liters) filtered or spring water

In a large pot, soak the chopped herbs in the water overnight. In the morning, boil the mixture down to 0.5 quart (0.5 liter). Filter the mixture, saving the liquid and discarding the herbs.

You should have about 2 cups of decoction to sip on throughout the day. Take 1 tablespoon every two hours on an empty stomach for one month. Some cases may benefit from two months. Monitor your improvement and decide.

LYMPHATIC ISSUES

As you know, the lymphatic system is your second line of defense. It is there to catch toxins that have passed through your GI tract and escort them out of the premises. We cannot talk about healing and detoxing without mentioning how to fix the lymphatic system. Although the first step is to improve the first line of defense, you also need to cleanse and decongest your lymph so it can work like it's supposed to.

Not only will a decongested lymphatic system allow you to catch and expel toxins, it will also help you with cleansing other harmful agents, like amyloid plaques in your brain.[124] Think of your lymphatic system as your drainage system. If this system gets clogged, toxins build up in different organs and can cause a myriad of symptoms. As we've seen, lymphatic congestion has been associated with digestive issues, inflammation, autoimmunity, depression, and other brain dysfunctions. On the other hand, if your pipes are clean and everything is moving, you will be a toxin-expelling machine and will feel like a superhuman.

While Western medicine does not have much on healing the lymphatic system, this is one of the pillars of Ayurveda, and we will explore some of its treatment practices.

Rehydration Therapy

As discussed in chapter 12, many of us are prone to suboptimal hydration levels. Considering that lymph is made of water, it's easy to understand the importance of staying hydrated in order to keep our lymph flowing. In fact, lymphatic system performance is directly connected to hydration levels.[125]

Rehydration therapy is just a fancy name for proper consumption of water during the day. For most people, just following the recommendations in chapter 12 is enough to maintain proper hydration levels and decongested lymph. But for others, this might not be enough.

If you feel you are hydrated but still have symptoms of lymphatic dysfunction, it's probably best to consider Rehydration Therapy 2.0. To do this, boil filtered water and carry it in a thermos throughout the day. Every 10 to 15 minutes, drink two or three sips of this hot water. Do this for about two weeks. This is a practice that comes from the Ayurvedic "playbook." While the water helps hydrate you, its temperature cause vasodilation, which will boost your circulation and improve your lymphatic function. Hot water is also believed to be more effective at detoxifying. Think about it. When you wash your dishes, it's a lot easier to get the grease off with hot water than with room temperature or cold water. Hot water will be more efficient at getting the grease out of your drains.

Nutrition

Traditionally, lymphatic congestion was often treated with foods that stain. Think of berries, cherries, beets, chlorophyll-rich plants, saffron, and turmeric. What these plants have in common is their powerful antioxidant properties. Considering that congested lymph gets thick because of the excess of toxins and oxidized fats it carries, one can see how a powerful antioxidant may help reverse this situation.

Citrus fruits should also be considered since they have vitamin C and flavonoids, which are known for promoting healthy lymphatic vessels.[126-128] Additionally, apples, berries, cherries, and grape skins have a class of flavonoids called procyanidins that may be boosters of immunity and lymphatic activity.[129]

Then we have one of my favorite cure-alls, apple cider vinegar. Research shows that ACV is effective in blocking oxidation of fats and cholesterol, which in turn works as a strong antioxidant for the lymphatic system.[130]

In the actual apple (and also in cranberries and tart cherries), there is an organic compound called malic acid that is known for inducing systemic alkalinization and treating calcium oxalate stones.[131] Although there are no studies on malic acid and improvements in lymphatic function, in Ayurveda, alkalinization is associated with a more free-flowing lymph. Opt for tart apples. Not only will they have less sugar, but they'll also pack more malic acid.

Lastly, I would like to recommend fenugreek tea. For starters, it's pretty tasty. Second, fenugreek is known for its lymphatic cleansing properties and for helping remove toxic wastes, dead cells, and trapped proteins from the body.[132]

Lifestyle

Unlike the cardiovascular system, which has the heart, the lymphatic system does not have a dedicated organ to pump its fluids. Lymph relies on muscular contraction to move. Therefore, exercise is essential to getting lymph moving. You already have plenty of reasons to stay active, and the health of your lymphatic system is another one.

Massages are also great for boosting the lymphatic system. The manual pressure will encourage lymph to move and will help drain any lymphatic swelling you may have. Another option is dry skin brushing. This technique can be done independently, and besides encouraging lymphatic movement, it revs up blood circulation and exfoliates the skin.

One more thing to consider is breath work. Deep breathing will help you de-stress, which by itself already helps the lymphatic system. On top of that, by activating your entire rib cage with these deep breaths and activating your abdomen during your exhalations, you squeeze the lymph from the interstitial spaces and push it toward the exit ducts.[133]

Supplements

All the supplements I am about to recommend can come from your diet, since they are all herbs, roots, or spices. But, to be practical, it's a lot easier to consume most of them in supplement form. There are dozens of herbal remedies that have been used in ancient traditions with the goal of decongesting the lymphatic system. Unfortunately, not all of them are supported by modern science. Some of the ones with the most evidence supporting their antioxidant, detoxifying, and lymph-decongesting abilities (and also my favorites) are astragalus root, gotu kola (a.k.a. *Centella asiatica* and brahmi), graviola, manjistha root (*Rubia cordifolia*), fresh red root extract, and turmeric (combined with an oxalate binder because of its high content of this antinutrient).[134–143]

DETOXIFICATION NEEDS TO BE FACILITATED

As *New York Times* best-selling author Dr. Alejandro Junger has stated, we are experiencing an evolutionary paradox. In the past 100 years, our lifestyle and the world around us have changed drastically, but we have not physiologically adapted to these changes.[144] Our ability to fight the toxins in our food and environment is the same as it was 100 or even 1,000 years ago. We are not on a level playing field. Sadly, within the medical community, many professionals and experts haven't woken up to this reality. They haven't realized that we direly need to level the playing field. They still operate under the assumption that the body can cleanse itself and doesn't need any help. If this were 200 years ago, I would be clapping in support, but we both know that is not the case anymore. If we were so good at naturally detoxifying, why are toxins still making us sick?

Detoxification and cleansing have gotten a bad rap. This is in part because some of the supplement companies selling cleansing powders, teas, and programs know nothing about how the body works. They just follow the trends and try to profit from them. Then we have a bunch of social media influencers who, instead of doing their research, just look at the affiliate commission plan and promote the hell out of these trendy cleanses. What happens next? People think this is all a scam, since they don't feel any different or, worse, they get sick.

We cannot let this be the perception. Detoxification is real, and it's happening in your body right now. But you need to boost it once in a while so your organism can catch up with the overload of toxins. Think about it. If the place where you live suddenly had a 20-fold increase in its population, that would lead to 20 times more trash. But let's say that the trash collection services could not hire anyone else and were still operating with the same team. Soon you would start seeing trash piling up everywhere. Roads would be filled with litter, and you could no longer move. Bugs and animals would invade the streets and would start spreading disease. This is what's going on inside the body. There is a lot more trash, but our biology hasn't evolved to send out more trash collectors. That is why it's necessary to occasionally give it a push and force it to hire some part-time workers in order to catch up.

Boosting your detoxification pathways is not a myth. It's an essential tool for anyone who aims to survive in this toxic world and be healthy. Don't fool yourself, thinking you don't need a good detox boost. I'm sure that at a certain point in your life you have consumed fast foods, processed beverages, and pesticide-contaminated vegetables and fruits; have taken pharmaceuticals; and have been exposed to cigarette smoke, inhaled industrial fumes, and so on. Even when you are born, you are already packing toxins. In a 2005 EWG research article, it was uncovered that the umbilical-cord blood of American babies contained on average about 200 industrial chemicals and toxins.[145] Obviously, your body can take care of some of these substances, but as they accumulate, this becomes more and more difficult. Therefore, everyone should follow a detox program a couple of times a year.

WHO SHOULD BE CAUTIOUS WITH A DETOXIFICATION PROGRAM?

Engaging in a detox facilitating program is something that is safe and recommended for most of the population. But there are some people in whom the prioritization of the detoxification system may compromise other functions of the body or be a bit too much if they are in a fragile condition. For example, I do not recommend engaging in a detox program for people who are pregnant or breastfeeding, because the released toxins may end up in the baby. And if a woman is pregnant, her body should be focusing on building and developing the baby. Nothing else.

Then we have the case of individuals with advanced diseases that require constant medical care. Depending on the stage of the disease, a detox program can be too much for the body to handle. In these cases, attempting a detox program should occur only under direct physician supervision.

Finally, I would like to mention that a detox program may affect the way the body absorbs certain medication. If you need to maintain a stable level of certain antiarrhythmic meds, antiepileptics, anticoagulants, hormones, or chemotherapy agents, talk with your physician first.

UNDERSTANDING TOXIN ACCUMULATION AND DETOXIFICATION

In broad brushstrokes, when toxins enter your body, the lymphatic system is supposed to handle them. But as it gets congested, fat-soluble toxins find their way back to the liver, where they are held. As the liver gets overloaded, they are being released back into the bloodstream, where, best case, they end up being put away in the body's fat cells. Sometimes the worst happens and they end up in more dangerous places, like the organs.

Most detox programs focus on weight loss and on the release of these stored fat-soluble toxins. The goal is to release them and hope they get excreted from the body. Unfortunately, if things are not done properly (which is the case with most programs), you incur the risk of having those toxins just move from one fat cell to another. Or, worse, having them move from your fat cells and end up in your heart or brain.

There is a reason why I have been guiding you through these different stages before the actual detox. You need to improve your digestion and your lymphatic system in order to actually expel these toxins out of your body. Additionally, you need to eat the right foods and/or take the right supplements to neutralize the toxins in their way out. Remember that these toxins are full of free radicals that act almost like lava, burning and corroding everything in their path. Some have the power of molecular mimicry and can compromise your endocrine system and mess up your gene expression before they get excreted, if they're not neutralized properly. So, it is essential to understand all phases of the detoxification process so we can support them.

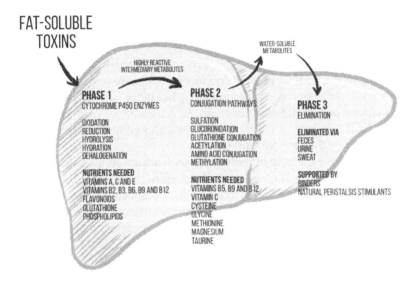

PHASE 1 AND PHASE 2 DETOXIFICATION

During phase 1, toxins are released and then suffer several enzymatic reactions such as oxidation, reduction, hydrolysis, hydration, and dehalogenation. To keep things simple, let's just say that these reactions are the first step in transforming fat-soluble toxins into water-soluble molecules (a process that only ends in phase 2) so they can be more easily excreted from the body.[146] In case you're wondering, this process occurs in the liver, and it is intermediated mostly by the cytochrome P450 (CYP450) enzymes.[147]

Phase 1 can be dangerous, since the enzymatic reactions cause the release of free radicals. Additionally, these reactions produce intermediate metabolites that can be even more toxic than the original toxins. These intermediate metabolites have been shown to alter gene expression, which can lead to mutations, autoimmune responses, and even cancer.[148] So, it's essential to activate phase 2 as quickly as possible so we can neutralize these toxins, avoiding harming the liver and causing DNA damage and systemic inflammation. Therefore, sometimes it's better to go through phase 1 slowly, so as not to cause a toxin overload.

Can you see how so many of those aggressive cleansing programs on the market can make us worse?

Phase 2 is known as the conjugation pathway, because the liver adds another molecule to (or *conjugates*) the intermediate metabolite to make it less harmful and more water-soluble for excretion.[149] While I am putting this in a very simple way, phase 2 is quite complex and may require several steps to get toxins ready to leave your body.[150] Just in case you want to know more, the main steps are sulfonation, glucuronidation, glutathione conjugation, acetylation, amino acid conjugation, and methylation.[151,152] As you can imagine, to perform this complex detoxification process, the liver requires energy and a consistent supply of antioxidants, vitamins, minerals, and other micronutrients.

Finally, there is phase 3, which is basically the elimination part, but let's skip that for now.

Main Nutrients to Support Phase 1:
• Vitamins B_2, B_3, B_6, B_9, and B_{12} – found in almonds, asparagus, avocados, beef, beets, broccoli, cauliflower, dark leafy greens, eggs, mushrooms, organ meats, and shellfish.

• Vitamins A, C, and E – found in almonds, acerola, avocados, beet greens, camu camu, carrots, celery, dairy, eggs, guavas, organ meats, red palm oil, sea buckthorn, and sunflower seeds.

• Flavonoids – found in berries, broccoli, brussels sprouts, cabbage, citrus fruits, and parsley.

• Glutathione – found in asparagus, avocados, cruciferous vegetables, green beans, liver, walnuts, and watermelon.

• Phospholipids – found in eggs, fermented soybeans, fish, lean meats, and organ meats.

Main Nutrients to Support Phase 2:
• Vitamins B_5, B_9, and B_{12} – found in almonds, asparagus, avocados, beef, beets, broccoli, cauliflower, dark leafy greens, eggs, mushrooms, organ meats, and shellfish.

• Vitamin C – found in acerola, camu camu, guavas, and sea buckthorn.

• Cysteine – found in beef, broccoli, brussels sprouts, dairy, eggs, garlic, onions, poultry, and seafood.

• Glycine – found in bone broth, gelatin, organ meats, and poultry.

• Glutamine – found in beef, organ meats, parsley, poultry, and seafood.

• Methionine – found in beef, eggs, and seafood.

• Magnesium – found in almonds, avocados, dark chocolate, dark leafy greens, and green bananas.

• Taurine – found in beef, dairy, eggs, and shellfish.

To Avoid during Phase 1 and Phase 2:

• Glyphosate-contaminated fruits and vegetables. Focus on organic, at least during the detox program.

• Caffeine, alcohol, and over-the-counter meds.

• Grapefruit, starfruit, black pepper, and turmeric. Although the science is not clear, some research suggests that these foods and spices may inhibit phase 1 detox. [153-156] Out of caution, I recommend staying away from them at this stage.

Supplements to Boost Phase 1 and Phase 2

In my opinion, the most important thing to do is to focus on your diet. As you can see from the food list shared earlier, many of the foods are the same in both phases. So, making sure you eat plenty of these detox-boosting foods is a must.

Since a detox program should be controlled and timed, I feel that the use of supplements can be a great tool. If you go camping, you can try to roll a stick in your hands to start a fire, or you can just take a lighter with you. The supplements here act as the lighter. They help you activate and speed up your detox pathways while protecting your liver from the increase in toxic activity. Every practitioner has their favorite detox supplements, and I realize I am ignoring some good ones. But I had to keep this simple and concentrate on the ones I believe can simultaneously help phase 1 and 2 while setting up the body for a successful phase 3. Here are my picks.

Burdock Root Tea + Dandelion Tea + Holy Basil Tea

These teas are some of my favorite supplements (you can also take them in capsule form if you prefer), because they can be purchased in many health stores (or from online retailers) at very affordable prices. Besides that, they are phenomenal to assist your body during the detox program.

Burdock root, along with the other roots and herbs on this list, has been used as health tonic in many traditional medicines across the world. Science now shows us that it is a potent blood purifier, lymphatic system strengthener, and natural diuretic. [157] It purifies the body by helping the liver detoxify, while protecting it with an increased production of glutathione (essential for phase 1 and phase 2). [158,159] The fact that burdock root helps lymph move and makes you pee is just an awesome bonus for phase 3 detoxification.

Dandelion root is rich in the vital liver-supporting B vitamins. It also has anti-inflammatory and antioxidant properties that have been shown to protect the liver. [160-162] This herb is also known for being a good diuretic that helps flush toxins out of the liver. [163]

The last one on this list is another powerhouse, and one you will always find in my pantry. Holy basil (or tulsi) is one of the best detoxifiers out there. It increases the activity of antioxidant enzymes such as superoxide dismutase and catalase, boosts glutathione levels, and enhances the activity of the CYP450 enzymes.[164] It's also a tea you can drink regularly to protect yourself from food and environmental toxins. Studies show that it can protect cells from industrial chemicals, heavy metals, pharmaceuticals, and even the effects of radiation and chemotherapy.[165]

My recommendation is to cycle these teas during the day. Take one in the morning, another in the early afternoon, and another at night. Please pay a bit more and purchase them from companies with good practices, preferably with organic farming.

Milk Thistle

We cannot talk about liver detox without talking about milk thistle. This is definitely the Michael Jordan of the detox plants. You can also ingest it in tea form, but I prefer to take a more concentrated approach by using a supplement. The main active ingredient in milk thistle is silymarin. This substance has been linked to liver cell renewal and regeneration, liver oxidative damage protection, decreased inflammation, and increased toxin elimination.[166,167] Basically, all we want for a successful detox.

D-Limonene

D-limonene, which is the predominant chemical form of limonene, is extracted from the peels of citrus fruits. This is another great short-term detox supplement. D-limonene has strong anti-inflammatory and antioxidant properties, shown to protect the liver.[168–172] Studies also show that this substance activates phase 1 and phase 2 liver detox enzymes, which will boost the liver's cleansing ability.[173,174] Last but not least, D-limonene stimulates the secretion of bile, which is essential for digestion, lymphatic function, and detoxification.[175]

Indole-3-carbinol (I3C)

Indole-3-carbinol (I3C) is a natural compound obtained through eating cruciferous vegetables. But you would need to eat buckets of them to get the therapeutic dose needed to support our detox protocol. That's why I recommend taking I3C in supplement form. In a nutshell, I3C supports the liver detoxification processes by inducing the activity of the CYP450 enzymes while protecting the liver with its anti-inflammatory and antioxidant properties.[176–178] I3C is also a precursor to diindolylmethane (DIM). Researchers suggest that DIM may stimulate fat breakdown (and release the fat-soluble toxins), enhance estrogen metabolism (possibly removing the toxic xenoestrogens), and potentially have anti-inflammatory, and anticarcinogenic effects.[179–182]

Magnesium

As you are noticing, I keep recommending magnesium. It is one of the most depleted minerals in the soil, which makes it hard for us to get enough just from fruits and vegetables. Magnesium is essential to many physiological processes, and liver detoxification is no exception. Magnesium is an important cofactor for the production of several compounds involved in phase 1 and phase 2 detoxification, and it may bind to some heavy metals.[183,184]

Neo Note: Coffee Enema for Liver Detoxification

Yes, you read that right. I am talking about squishing coffee up your anus. Before you say I'm crazy, let me just state that I'm not the one who invented this stuff. It's believed that this "technique" was "created" by German physicians in the early 1900s but then made popular by Dr. Max Gerson and his famous Gerson Therapy.

Side note: I wonder how the German physicians came up with this. Was it after some lab experiments, or was this the result of an intense night at Oktoberfest?

The truth is that there isn't much research on the subject. Nonetheless, there is a lot of anecdotal evidence, with people describing this practice as almost miraculous for digestive disorders, constipation, IBS, dysbiosis, parasites, liver disease, and even cancer. The healing properties seem to come in part from the induction of the detox pathways. In theory, coffee would stimulate the release of toxins from the liver, boost the levels of glutathione, and make your bowels move. But as I said, we need more research to support this.

PHASE 3 DETOXIFICATION

Phase 3 detoxification is what I like to call "bind and release." This is the stage at which toxins get neutralized and escorted out of your body through sweat, urine, feces, and even your breath. It's my opinion that this is neglected in most detox programs. People assume that as long as the toxins are released and made water soluble, the body will automatically and effortlessly excrete them. Meanwhile, because of the sheer quantity of toxins being put in circulation, your body may become overwhelmed and not move things out as fast as necessary. We need to go all *Fast and Furious* here. It should be a drag race to see how fast you can get these toxins out of your system. After all, if we don't get rid of them quickly enough, they will cause inflammation and may hide again in your fat and organs.

You are going to change your diet to promote kidney activity and induce peristalsis (GI motility) so you can start clearing like a pro. You will also adopt some simple lifestyle changes to promote lymphatic drainage, sweating, and fat loss, to make this even more efficient.

Neo Note: Phase 2.5 Detoxification

A few years back, I heard the term *phase 2.5 detoxification* from Dr. Kelly Halderman in a podcast interview she did. According to her, phase 2.5 detox is where the toxins from the liver enter the bile to be removed by the lymphatic system. Many people feel worse during or after a detox program because the gallbladder and the lymphatic system were not properly addressed. When these are compromised, toxins don't have anywhere to go, and end up being reabsorbed. According to Dr. Halderman, high levels of inflammation can also cause the 2.5 detox phase to come to a halt. This is one reason why, in the Neo Diet, we focus so much on bile and lymph health, and also concentrate on eating plenty of anti-inflammatory and antioxidant foods.

Nutrition

Besides eating all the amazing foods I already mentioned during Phase 1 and 2 of your detox, at this stage it's important that you ramp up your water and fiber game. You need that extra water to transform yourself into one of those old-school "boy peeing" fountains. The extra fiber is for you to sit in the bathroom until you don't feel your legs when you get up. Get the idea?

Please follow the recommendations in chapter 12, increase your water intake, drink some smoothies, and if you're up to it, drink some celery juice. Celery juice not only will help you hydrate, but it will also promote intestinal motility.

The addition of more fiber to your diet not only will add more bulk to your stool, but also help bind to toxic bile and encourage toxin excretion. Of course, fruits and vegetables have plenty of fiber, but you can add some psyllium husk, aloe vera, or acacia gum supplements to your smoothies to throw in a fiber boost. Another well-tried and tested hack is to soak a pitted prune in a big cup of water overnight. Before your first meal, cook the prune in that same water and gulp down the puree. Plan on being next to a bathroom, because this works incredibly well for most people.

Neo Note: Fasting for Detox

As I discussed before, sometimes it's not about what you eat but the time you spend without eating. Fasting takes you out of the "feasting" state and allows your body to burn fat, release toxins, and recycle damaged proteins and cells. Fasting also allows your body to stop spending energy on digestion. This energy can then be allocated to the intense detox process going on inside you.

During a well-designed detox program, fasting can be a catalyst to make the detox process more efficient and get better results in less time. Please note that I am referring to intermittent fasting, because during the detox program, it is essential that you have nutrients coming in to support all phases of this cleansing process.

Binders

Binders are compounds that attach to toxins (pathogenic bacteria, mold, heavy metals, and other chemical toxins), neutralize them, and take them out of your body. It's important to note that there is no universal binder. There is no single substance that will bind to all toxins. Therefore, it is imperative to consume a combination of different binders to increase your chances of getting all the junk out of you.

Some of the best binders to consider are activated charcoal, bentonite clay, chitosan, chlorella, silica, and zeolites.

Activated charcoal

This is not your typical grill charcoal. The raw material is the same, but it is processed much differently, so please do not save the leftovers from your next barbecue.

Activated charcoal, like most binders, goes through your gut undigested and ready to do its work.[185] Its porous texture and negative electrical charge attract positively charged molecules such as toxins and gases, "traps" them (what's known as adsorption), and escorts them to the end of the tunnel.[186] Research shows that activated charcoal is efficient at absorbing pesticides, herbicides, mold toxins, endotoxins, and inflammatory molecules.[187–191]

This supplement is one that I always carry with me on my trips, because it is great to fight food-poisoning symptoms like gas and diarrhea.[192,193] Activated charcoal is also effective in treating overdoses of prescription drugs and over-the-counter medications.[194,195]

Bentonite Clay

You've probably heard of bentonite clay face masks, but this substance has also been used as an ingestible detox aid for centuries. Bentonite clay is a phenomenal binder for mold toxins, pesticides, herbicides, and heavy metals.[196–203] Research has also uncovered that it can be used to get rid of cyanotoxins from swimming in lakes polluted by algal blooms.[204] Bentonite clay may even help balance your microbiome and improve symptoms of IBS, food allergies, and food poisoning.[205]

Chitosan

Chitosan is a supplement made from chitin, a substance in the exoskeletons of insects, shellfish, and the cell walls of fungi.[206] In your GI tract, chitosan turns into a gel-like substance and attaches to toxins as it journeys inside you.[207] Studies show that this supplement can bind to toxins in your bile, heavy metals, PCBs, BPA, and phthalates.[208–213] Chitosan has also been found to promote the growth of good bacteria, which may be connected to some weight-loss benefits also linked to this substance.[214–217] But if you're allergic to shellfish or mushrooms, you should avoid chitosan supplements.

Chlorella

Along with spirulina, chlorella is one of my favorite algae. Besides being incredibly nutritious, it may also help us detox from heavy metals, dioxins, and radioactive particles from chemotherapy and radiation.[218–223] Chlorella has notorious antioxidant effects and studies support that it also helps protect the liver.[224–228]

Silica

When you look for silica supplements, you will notice that many of them do not mention anything about detox or binding properties. Many silica supplements you find in the market (as of this writing) are marketed for bone health and collagen production.[229–232] But silica is also used therapeutically to detoxify heavy metals, particularly mercury.[233–235] Silica-based gel supplements have also been shown to be effective against food poisoning.[236,237]

Zeolites

The word *zeolite* comes from the old Greek *zéō* (boiling) and *líthos* (stone). These minerals form when volcanic lava comes in contact with water. *Boiling stone, get it?* There are several unique forms of zeolites, and they're composed of different elements such as aluminum, oxygen, silicon, titanium, and zinc.[238,239] Similarly to activated charcoal, zeolites have a porous form and negative electrical charge that attracts and binds to toxins.[240] Research shows that these powerful minerals can help the body detoxify from heavy metals, pathogenic bacteria, viruses, histamines, cellular metabolites, radioactive elements, and industrial toxins.[241–251] Zeolites also have a strong antioxidant effect that has been shown to protect vital organs such as the liver and brain from oxidative damage.[252–257]

Zeolites are so powerful that they're even present on the battlefield. Several studies show they have been used successfully in dressings to stop heavy bleeding and improve clotting in severe injuries and accidents.[258–262]

Natural Peristalsis Stimulants

It's been quite a detox journey, hasn't it? Now, the last step is to get all those nasty toxins out of your body. Everyone should have regular and consistent bowel movements, but during a detox program, it is essential to ensure that you have a "code brown" at least three times a day. Your diet will be essential here. By consuming more fiber and staying hydrated, you will make everything move along. Adding a supplement like psyllium husk, aloe vera, or acacia gum to your smoothies will also do wonders not only to promote intestinal motility but to soothe your gut.

To make my detox protocol even more efficient and reduce the possible side effects, I like to add two "intestinal tonics": triphala and ashwagandha.

I briefly mentioned triphala before, when I recommended it to heal the gut. Besides being a powerful gut healer and adaptogenic, it's also a great peristalsis stimulant (or prokinetic).[263] Ashwagandha is another Ayurvedic supplement that may stabilize GI distress and treat constipation.[264] However, I like to use this supplement to help fight the stress associated with the detox protocol. Ashwagandha is known for lowering cortisol levels, bringing down inflammation, reducing anxiety, and boosting immunity.[265-271] To me, these are essential to balancing the organism during the final stages of the detox program. Instead of feeling drained and debilitated, ashwagandha and triphala will help you feel strong and full of energy.

Neo Note: When You Really Need to Go

Following the dietary and supplement recommendations here, 99 percent of people will experience the intestinal motility needed for this detox. If you are part of the 1 percent still having some difficulties, you might benefit from a natural laxative. One of the best natural laxatives on the market is Swiss Kriss. The active ingredient is the herb senna, which is commonly used in numerous laxatives. There is a good reason it is used in different formulations. This stuff works!

If you feel you need this boost, take it the night before you begin the detox program. This will get everything moving, and then my other recommendations will help you keep the pace. Please read the label and follow the instructions, because taking too much Swiss Kriss can be a real shit show. Literally!

Lifestyle

During the detox program, it is important to add some light exercise. The keyword here is *light*. You do not want to overexert yourself, because most of your energy should go toward the cleansing process. But some exercise will be crucial to promoting lymphatic movement. Opt for long walks, stretching, Pilates, or yoga (inverted poses are particularly good for lymphatic drainage).

This type of exercise most likely will not be enough to make you sweat, so we will need to find alternatives, since sweating is a great way to get rid of heavy metals, phthalates, BPA, and mold toxins.[272] One of the best ways to induce sweating is to use a sauna. Yes, I know, most people don't have saunas at home. I also don't have one, but I use the one at my gym. Please check whether you have a gym near you that offers one. If not, maybe you can book one or two spa days during your detox program. It's a worthwhile investment. Alternatively, consider springing for an infrared sauna blanket. They are becoming more affordable, and using one is something you can do consistently at home. If you live in a tropical region or are planning to do your detox during the hot summer months, go outside, get some sun on you, and sweat like there's no tomorrow.

P.S. Don't forget to replenish your body with water and electrolytes during and after your sweat sesh.

BEFORE THE DETOX PROGRAM

You need to know what to expect and be in the right state of mind before you throw yourself into a detox program. That will make your experience more enjoyable and successful. I know this was a long chapter with a lot of information. I'll even hazard a guess that you got a little overwhelmed because it feels like you *have* every problem I listed. Let me assure you, you are not a "freak" who has everything. Remember, in the body, all is connected. What started as a stomach acid issue could have developed into leaky gut, parasites, food allergies, and depression. The great news is that if you fix just the stomach acid, the rest will also get better.

Not sure what is the actual cause of our problems? Let me tell you a secret. Ready? Not even the best functional medicine doctor in the world will know for sure. The body is so complex that the cause can be many things. Just start from the beginning and follow the sequence of steps laid down in this chapter. I promise, things will get much better and you will overturn whatever you are going through now.

The first detox program will produce insane results for most people, but for some, they may feel only slightly better. And that is okay. Let's face it. The first time you follow this program, you might still be facing severe digestive issues that did not simply disappear in the first days of the program. Your liver, gallbladder, lymphatic system, and kidneys may not yet be in a position where they can be efficient with detoxification. But in your next detox, three months from now, your body will be in a completely different position. By then, you will have been following the Neo Diet formula for a while, and you won't be the same person. That next detox will be life-changing. Mark my words.

There is one last thing I want you to know. You may feel worse in the beginning. This may occur because you are releasing toxins and also because you will have pathogenic bacteria being eliminated. The toxin elimination and bacteria die-off reactions may cause fatigue, headaches, irritability, or flu-like symptoms. That's normal and will go away in a day or two.

DETOX PROTOCOL

If you search online, you will find several intensive detox programs of three or four days. Without being a hater, let me just say that I prefer (and see better results with) a less-aggressive two-week detox program. During the first two or three days, we focus on phase 1 detox foods (and optional supplements) to ignite the fire. Then, it is essential that we neutralize the toxins and expel them. This is when we add phase 2 foods, light exercise, and sauna time. During this entire period, we stay hydrated, take binders, and promote phase 3. After you're finished with the protocol, we slowly start adding back other foods to our diet and assess how we feel.

In chapter 18, I provide you with my Jumpstart Blueprint, in which I will guide you step by step on how to complete the best detox program out there.

Whether or not you follow the Jumpstart Blueprint, or any other program, I recommend completing a detox protocol three or four times a year.

NEO SUMMARY

• We live in a contaminated world and our bodies have not evolved to handle this excess of toxins.

• Detoxification is a natural process that occurs in your body all the time.

• Detoxification programs should occur during the year to assist our toxin-overwhelmed bodies.

• Detoxification is more than just taking liver-supporting supplements. It's fixing the digestive and lymphatic systems, boosting liver function, and facilitating the "evacuation routes".

NEO ACTION

• Eliminate toxic foods and reduce your chemical exposure.

• Follow the recommendations to heal your digestion and lymphatic system.

• Complete a detox program 3 or 4 times per year.

NEO RECOMMENDATIONS

• *Boundless* by Ben Greenfield
• *Clean 7* by Dr. Alejandro Junger
• *Detox for Life* by Dr. Dan Nuzum & Gina Nuzum
• *Eat Wheat* by Dr. John Douillard
• *Guess What Came to Dinner?* by Ann Louise Gittleman
• *Happy Gut* by Dr. Vincent Pedre
• *Patient Heal Thyself* by Jordan Rubin
• *Radical Metabolism* by Ann Louise Gittleman
• *The Wahls Protocol* by Dr. Terry Wahls
• *Toxic* by Dr. Neil Nathan

my.neodiet.co/neorecommendations

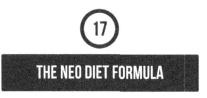

THE NEO DIET FORMULA

This Is Not a Diet, This Is a New Way of Living

"As to the methods there may be a million and then some, but principles are few. The man who grasps principles can successfully select his own methods. The man who tries methods, ignoring principles, is sure to have trouble."
Harrington Emerson

THE NEO DIET FORMULA

Stand tall, stand proud. You just graduated with my imaginary degree in Advanced Nutrition. But on a serious note. What you've learned here certainly defied many of your long-held beliefs. And yet you remained open-minded and kept going. You are awesome! Before we pop the champagne (or the kombucha), I have to remind you of something. As self-help guru Tony Robbins always says, "Knowledge is *not* power. Knowledge is only *potential* power. Action is power."

Knowing all the material in this book will do nothing for you unless you put it into practice. You have to follow it and make it part of your routine. You have to live it.

Obviously, I am not expecting you to memorize all I've written here. Heck, I wrote this entire book, read it a couple of times, and I still don't know every single detail by heart. Use this book as a guide. Whenever you're uncertain about something, open that chapter and review it. No sweat.

There is one thing I'd like you to memorize, though. It's the word *Hordil*.

What is Hordil? Glad you asked. Hordil is the acronym I created to describe the six fundamental pillars the Neo Diet is built around. It's the foundation of your superhuman health.

HORDIL
- **H**eal the Digestive System
- **O**ptimize the Microbiome
- **R**egain Metabolic Flexibility
- **D**ecrease Inflammation and Boost Cellular Performance
- **I**mprove Detox Pathways and Minimize Toxic Exposure
- **L**ive a Neo Lifestyle

Here is an easy way to always remember. Think about the similar-sounding word *ordeal*. An ordeal is a difficult or painful experience, right? Well, Hordil is just the opposite. It's the health foundation that will allow you to have an easy and thriving human experience.

The Neo Diet Formula is the map I created so anyone can follow the Hordil strategy without having to think about it. It's your step-by-step guide. In this chapter, we're going to put all the pieces from previous chapters together and organize them in an easy-to-follow manner. I am even going to give you my **Food Matrix**, which you can print and keep on your fridge door so you never have doubts about what foods to eat. Then, in the following chapter, I will share the **Jumpstart Blueprint,** which is my detox and elimination plan. This protocol is equivalent to pressing the reset button on your body. It will help you go back to factory settings so you can correct the more severe issues that you have going on. After that, we will discuss your **Neo Lifestyle**. I will also guide you on how to personalize your nutrition and lifestyle to match your bioindividuality (your unique physiology) and to achieve your desired health goals.

Let's do this!

DETERMINE YOUR BASELINE

To get where you're going, you have to first know where you are. You need objective data to determine your baseline and to assess how much you have progressed. Relying solely on gut feelings and on the subjective perception of how you look in the mirror any random morning will not do you any favors. That's how people get discouraged and give up.

I am 100 percent confident that the Neo Diet will work for you. But I cannot promise you will lose X number of pounds or that your brain fog will disappear in X number of days. Everyone is starting at a different point and has a unique set of issues. Promising specific results is nothing more than a marketing stunt. What I can promise is that you will become a lot healthier. Better yet, I'll show you!

Here is my challenge for you. Before you adopt any of my recommendations, and especially before you start the Jumpstart Blueprint, please take some time to determine your starting point. I want you to fill out the Baseline Sheet I'm about to share with you. In this sheet you will write your weight, percentage of body fat (most modern scales tell you this), and key body circumferences. Ideally, I also recommend that everyone go to their physician and have some blood work done. This is one of the most objective ways to determine whether you are getting healthier. In the Baseline Sheet, I share some of my favorite markers.

Finally, you are also going to take your "before" pictures. Ask someone you trust to take pictures of your entire body, preferably in underwear, from the front, back, and sides. Shoot them against a plain wall and with good lighting. Save the pictures next to your Baseline Sheet.

Then, do not measure a thing for a while. Don't even look at your scale. I'm serious. People get too anxious about results, and that stress can really slow down progress. Ideally, you would reassess all the Baseline Sheet's points only after 90 days. Three months is a good time frame to see big health changes. I realize most of my readers won't wait that long. That being said, please reassess at the end of the Jumpstart Blueprint. I'm certain you will see the difference even in such a short period.

You can access your Baseline Sheet in the book's resources: my.neodiet.co/resources

Oh, and if you're proud of your results, brag about it. Share your pictures and your Baseline Sheet data points with our tribe.

NEO HACKS FOR INSANE RESULTS

Preparation is one of the key factors that will determine how successful and enjoyable this experience will be. Like Abraham Lincoln said, "Give me six hours to chop down a tree, and I will spend the first four sharpening the axe." In other words, before you change your diet and lifestyle, I want to set you up for success. By following a couple of easy steps, you will exponentially increase your chances of reaching your goals, and you will make this journey a fun one to be a part of.

Here are my favorite Neo Hacks for insane results.

Clean the Pantry

Would you go to a rehab facility located in front of a liquor store? No way! Even if you could resist the temptation, you would be miserable the whole time you were there. Trying to clean up your diet while having your pantry full of processed food is the same. If temptation is there, you might sin. Put on some rock or EDM music that pumps you up and hit the pantry. It's time to get rid of all the junk that has been making you sick.

Get rid of all processed foods. I'm talking about cereals, chips, crackers, cookies, sugary snacks, pizzas, industrial breads, wheat products, margarines, buttery spreads, cooking sprays, vegetable oils, commercial salad dressings, processed cheese spreads, processed meats, juices, sports drinks, sodas, coffee creamers, ice creams, jellies, sugar, artificial sweeteners, frozen packaged foods, etc. If you have read this far, you know the stuff I'm talking about.

I recognize there is an ethical dilemma between throwing food away or giving it to someone, knowing that it is bad for them. This decision is on you. If you prefer to trash it, do it. If you prefer to give it away, go to a food bank or other local institution in your area. What's important is that you get it out of your house.

Clearly, you will not clear the pantry and leave it empty. Hit the grocery store and buy some of the amazing wholesome foods we have discussed in the book. Shortly, I'll share with you the Food Matrix you can use as a guide.

While you're raiding the kitchen, go through all your toxic cookware and utensils and toss them out. I know buying new cookware is an investment, but your health is worth it. Like they say, pay the grocer (in this case it's more the retailer) now or pay the doctor later. Go back to chapter 15 and review the must-go's and the must-haves.

Plan Ahead

During the Jumpstart Blueprint and even when you're following the Neo Diet principles on your own, although you will have a Food Matrix to use as inspiration, I am not assigning you meal plans with exact recipes to follow. I recommend taking a weekend day, every single week, to review the Food Matrix and plan the meals you are going to cook during the week to come. Not only that, but also to create a grocery list so you have everything you need when the time comes. By doing this, you don't give yourself any excuses to fail. You'll always know what meal to eat each day. This is particularly important for your evening meals, because at that time of the day you are in a state of decision fatigue and have less willpower.

Remember the words of Benjamin Franklin: "If you fail to plan, you are planning to fail!"

Trust the Process

This is just another reminder to forget about old dogma. Do not worry about calories or eating too much salt or butter. Forget about all those myths and stop overthinking. Overthinking will cause stress and anxiety, which will elevate your cortisol levels. I don't need to tell you the consequences of that, do I?

While we're on the subject of anxiety, please forget about your scale. Hide it somewhere. When the time comes, you will check your weight. Until then, don't worry about weight fluctuations. Focus on adapting your body to your Neo way of eating and trust the process.

Beware of Friendly Fire

Your friends and family (some members, at least) are people who love and care about you. But when they see you changing your life, they may question and even try to sabotage your decision. They might do this because they don't know any better and are genuinely concerned about you. They might also discourage you because your new position is going against their beliefs and even their identity. Or they might simply get jealous about your determination to change. It's just human nature. The point is that some of the people you love will not understand why you are doing what you are doing and will make a point of letting you know.

My advice is, share this only with people who are also interested in getting healthier. Share your book or gift them a copy so they can follow this journey with you. To all others, reveal nothing. If they ask, don't give much information and change subject. Later, as they see how much healthier you look, they will want to follow and they will ask about what you're doing. Until then, leave them in the dark.

The Power of a Community

It's a known fact that if you want to adopt a new habit, the act of surrounding yourself with people who already have that habit will substantially increase your odds of long-term success. A supportive community will have immense power in your transformation. We all have bad days, and on those days, all we need is to hear others share their victories to inspire us. Or we might just need some tough love and a reality check. At times, we might feel super excited about reaching a health goal and need to share it with someone who will understand and cheer. This is all possible by being part of a community that has the same values and goals.

Nowadays, the easiest place to find such a community is on the Internet. Do your research. Alternatively, I have created the Neo Hacker Tribe for all my readers. I would love to have you and be there to support you when I can. Please join here: my.neodiet.co/neohackertribe

Also consider going to health conferences, fitness studios, spas, healthy cafés, and juice bars to find like-minded people. Nothing beats in-person interaction.

Accountabilibuddy

This term was originally coined in an episode of *South Park*. An accountabilibuddy is someone (a buddy) who holds you accountable for what you said you would do. You have higher chances of completing a goal if you commit to it with someone. That's why I am asking you to find an accountabilibuddy. Someone who will hold you accountable and someone for whom you are going to do the same.

The idea is to share your goals, timelines, routines, pictures of meals, and even results of your most recent blood work. It's having someone you can talk to when you are feeling discouraged, or when you're happy about your victories. It's having someone who is following the same path as you and absolutely understands what's in your mind.

Community and support groups are great, but having a go-to person who has your back is a game changer. Feel free to look for an accountabilibuddy in your group of friends, if they are also reading the book, or just go to the

Internet and say that you are looking for one. I'm sure there will be other Neo Hacker Tribe members looking for you as well.

Mindset

The most important thing that will dictate your success is your mindset. In his book *Eat Smarter*, Shawn Stevenson says, "you can't bring the old you to the new results."[1] And I could not agree more. During this journey, your body will change, and your mind will need to evolve as well. If it doesn't, you will eventually revert to your old conditioning.

I've made a point of busting several of the nutrition myths holding you back, and have supported my claims with more than 2,500 scientific references, so you can change your beliefs about food. You need a healthy relationship with your diet. A relationship of nourishment and joy, not of restriction and lack.

It's essential to understand why you are choosing to let some things go. You are letting them go because they are the same things making you fat, dumb, tired, and sick. Instead, you are choosing other foods that will empower you to meet your health goals and make you feel amazing. Knowing and thinking about your "why" daily will be essential to "brainwashing" your mind into your new self. Or, as I like to call it, your Neo Self.

Let me be honest. Some days, it will not be easy. All those years of improper conditioning will give you some fight. You will be breaking addictions and patterns, even emotional ones. And your body and mind will play tricks on you. You will have days when you just want to eat a spaghetti sandwich with french fries and ice cream. But it's on those days that you have to make a conscious effort to remember why you are doing this. The best way to remember it is to write it down. Think about all the reasons that made you want to be healthier and write them down.

"I am doing because I am tired of feeling brain fog. I am doing this because I want to have energy. I am doing this because I want to stop having pain every time I eat. I am doing this because I want to look good."

You need to be clear about your why. Whatever it is. It is your why that is going to keep you on course on the tough days.

Last mindset piece of advice: Start slow. Don't try to radically change your entire life in one day. That will cause a ridiculous amount of stress, and, without a doubt, it's a recipe for disaster. Incorporate small changes into your diet weekly. Aim to find healthy replacements instead of just eliminating foods, so you don't feel deprived.

If you eat something that goes against your goals, don't stress too much about it. Feelings of guilt and shame only trigger more relapses. Instead, remember, every meal is an opportunity to do better. Next meal, you are back on track. At the end of the day, you won't be perfect. No one is. So don't get discouraged. Take one step at a time and value every little bit of progress.

Routine Beats Motivation

Knowing your why and staying motivated are important, but there is one thing that beats all of that. Having a routine.

Do you know how many times I feel like skipping the gym and just lying on my couch watching movies? Frustratingly, it's a lot. But you know what happens? I go to the gym because it's part of my routine. I have a commitment to myself (and to others) to do certain things on a daily or weekly basis.

Same with this book, for example. Many days, I did not feel like writing, but because I had planned to write every single weekday, I forced myself to do it.

In the beginning, it's more of a mental effort, but as a routine becomes a part of you, it becomes the natural thing to do.

Remember: Excuses keep you where you are. Routines make you move forward.

Set Goals

It has been known for years that people who set goals are more likely to achieve them. Goals use your brain's reward system to favor compliance. Once you set a goal to run 30 minutes and you do it, you feel good about yourself, and that rush of dopamine will make you want to do it again.

Writing the goals down is even more effective. When they're written, they're real. They're not just "wishes" wandering through your mind. Writing down your goals will promote clarity and will force you to confront the discouraging voice inside your head saying that you can't do it. Just let that hater "talk to the hand" and write those health goals.

There are many approaches to setting and writing goals. Some authors believe you should be incredibly specific and define timelines. While I get the idea behind it, I also know that it can be frustrating if you end up setting a too-ambitious goal and fail. That is why I prefer to break down bigger goals into smaller "task goals." Instead of just writing a goal like *I will lose 20 pounds in four months*, I focus on the tasks necessary to achieve it. The truth is that I don't have full control over the exact amount of weight I can lose (in a healthy way) in a determined timeline. But I can control what I will do to achieve it. And those goals are always ones I can achieve.

While my initial goal may be to lose 20 pounds in four months, I'll try not to hold on to the specifics. It might take me six months or it might take two. Instead, I keep an open timeline for this goal and focus instead on specific task goals like:

   - *I will lose 20 pounds.*
      - *I will do an intermittent fast of 16 hours daily.*
      - *I will meditate for 10 minutes daily to lower my stress levels.*
      - *I will go to the gym 3 times a week.*

Take a few minutes to think about what you want to achieve and write it down. Visualize and feel how good it will be once you achieve it. Get yourself all pumped up.

One trick that helps many people is to keep a notebook. This will work almost like a diary, but you use it to write your goals, track your progress, note how you felt after eating certain foods, and even record your daily tasks. Do something that works for you. You can also get my template in the book's resources: my.neodiet.co/resources

These simple but effective tricks will be a game changer, I promise. I know you are excited about starting the program, but don't skip these. I would not have written them if they were not important.

Now that the preparation is done, it's finally time to put together everything we've learned and go crush those goals. It's game time, baby!

THE HORDIL STRATEGY

The Hordil strategy represents the six fundamental pillars I built the Neo Diet around. It's the concept that consolidates everything we have discussed so far. Although they are expressed in different ways, they are all connected. As you work on one pillar, you influence the other ones as well. Let's briefly review them and see how we are incorporating them in the Neo Diet.

HORDIL
- **H**eal the Digestive System
- **O**ptimize the Microbiome
- **R**egain Metabolic Flexibility
- **D**ecrease Inflammation and Boost Cellular Performance
- **I**mprove Detox Pathways and Minimize Toxic Exposure
- **L**ive a Neo Lifestyle

As you follow the principles of the Neo Diet and guide yourself using the Food Matrix, you will eliminate the toxic foods that have been damaging your gut and causing inflammation and disease. Simultaneously, the Food Matrix will promote the consumption of foods with healing properties that will allow you to reverse any upper and lower digestion issues and build up that digestive fortress you're supposed to have.

As you heal your GI tract, you start setting up the right environment for your microbiome. Pathogenic bacteria, fungi, and parasites find it hard to live inside you, and the good guys take over. As the good guys take over, they further improve your digestion, modulate your immune system, and produce the incredible postbiotics that will soothe inflammation from head to toes. You will also notice that you can start eating things you were intolerant to before. If you have an autoimmune condition, it will get better.

An optimized microbiome and a diet (and lifestyle) that promotes insulin sensitivity will finally give your body the chance it needs to leave the anabolic state, and to heal, recycle damaged cells, and burn off those extra pounds of fat. Not only will you be losing fat, but your energy levels and stamina will improve. Your cellular metabolic rate will go up, and every organ in your body will work better.

All the symptoms associated with metabolic disease will slowly start to fade, and your probabilities of developing problems like heart disease, strokes, Alzheimer's, Parkinson's, and even cancer will drastically decrease. If you already have any of these diseases, you may notice the symptoms getting better.

As your body finally has the opportunity to eject years of accumulated toxins, inflammation will continue to diminish and your cells will work like never before. All your systems will run more smoothly, and you will feel a vitality that you never expected to feel. Remember the energy you had as a kid? It will slowly come back. Your mind will get clear, and suddenly words and thoughts you used to struggle to remember will naturally pop into your head. Your work performance will skyrocket. Heck, your performance will improve not only at work but in all facets of life.

Your body will gain more muscle, even without changing your workouts. Your hormones will make you feel confident and strong. Anxiety and depression will be things of the past.

Your lifestyle will change. You will spend more time outdoors and more time with the people you love. This will make you happier and will further reinforce these habits.

All will work as it should be, and you will finally feel like the superhuman you were designed to be.

WELCOME TO THE FOOD MATRIX

When I initially designed this book, I planned to describe the most common foods in detail. The idea was to create a small food glossary in which I would share nutritional profiles, antinutrients, and other interesting facts. Unfortunately, as I got to that stage of my writing, I realized my plan would easily take this book to 800-plus pages, and that was completely out of the question.

What I did instead was to create a food ladder system you can use to guide yourself, without having to read about each food individually. I still plan on one day building that food glossary and sharing it on my website, but for now, I believe a food ladder system is the easiest and fastest to implement. And we want easy and fast, don't we?

Foods were assigned to the different levels of the ladder according to their level of digestive complexity, metabolic impact, antinutrients, and other toxins. But please keep in mind that just because one particular food is absolutely benign for most people, it may not work for you depending on your current food sensitivities or allergies. Please remember, this is just a guide, not a one-size-fits-all program.

I call this ladder system the Food Matrix. The food ranking system was inspired by Dave Asprey's Bulletproof Diet Roadmap, and the Food Matrix's name was actually borrowed from Paleo superstar Robb Wolf—*it was just the perfect name to use in this book*. Thanks, guys!

The Food Matrix assigns the most common foods to four different levels:
A—Awesome Foods
B—Best to Test
C—Can Try after Healing
D—Definitely Avoid As Much As Possible

"A Foods" are some of the easiest to digest because of their lower antinutrient ratios. These are the ones you should eat the most.

"B Foods" should also be an important part of your diet but may be more reactive for some people. That's why I recommend seeing how you do with these foods. In general, B Foods also should not be eaten as much as A Foods.

"C Foods" are foods that should not be eaten until you have stabilized your digestive health. While they may have some important nutrients, they are harder to digest and may cause food intolerances. Even after healing, these foods should be eaten in moderation.

Finally, we have "D Foods," the ones you should aim to avoid. These are the foods with the most antinutrients, synthetic chemicals, toxins, and oxidized oils, or the ones that are not metabolically friendly.

Use the Food Matrix as your guide to choosing the best ingredients for your meals. Experiment with them and be creative.

What about recipes? Unfortunately, you won't find them here. I don't believe in plans that give you exact meals to eat. That one-size-fits-all approach is one of the big issues of the nutrition industry. Not only do we react differently to different ingredients, we also have different flavor preferences and different metabolic goals. While one reader wants to lose fat and revert a metabolic syndrome, another reader may want to fix their gut and pack on some muscle. Obviously, their meals will have to be different.

My advice is to keep things simple. Pick a good source of protein, some fat, and lots of vegetables. Boom! You've got a meal!

Nevertheless, in the book's resources, I share some recipes you can use as inspiration. There, you will also find a downloadable, full-size Food Matrix poster. I keep one in my kitchen and recommend you do the same.

For now, let's review the less-colorful "book version" of the Food Matrix.

	PROTEINS	VEGETABLES
A-FOODS	pasture-raised beef, lamb and other grazing animals; eggs from pastured poultry; collagen protein; gelatin; hemp protein or seeds; organ meats; spirulina;	arugula; bamboo shoots; bok choy, broccoli; brussels sprouts; cabbage; cauliflower; celery; chives; fennel root; kohlrabi; lettuce; lemongrass; watercress; nopales; radishes; scallions; shallots;
B-FOODS	bone or beef broth from pastured animals; pastured heritage pork and bacon; pastured poultry; hemp tofu; wild-caught anchovies, cod, herring, mackerel, pollock, sardines, salmon and trout; clams, mussels, oysters and scallops from regenerative aquacultures;	artichokes; asparagus; carrots; endive; garlic; green beans; green onions; hearts of palm; leeks; mushrooms; onions; radicchio; radishes; fresh sprouts; cooked collards and kale; traditionally made and unsweetened tomato paste; traditionally fermented pickles and ketchup; kimchi; sauerkraut; peeled and deseeded cucumbers, squash and zucchini; bull kelp; dulse; hijiki; irish moss; kombu; nori; sea grapes; sea lettuce; wakame;
C-FOODS	low-sugar beef or offal jerky; crab; any large fish; lobster; natto; octopus; squid; tempeh; wild-caught shrimp; whey from pastured animals;	dandelion greens; okra; cooked spinach; peeled and deseeded eggplants, peppers, and tomatoes;
D-FOODS	processed meats; fake meats; farmed seafood; soy protein (including tofu); textured vegetable protein; conventional whey and plant protein powders;	corn; canned vegetables; soy; cherry tomatoes; tomatillos; regular (with seeds and skin) cucumbers, eggplant, peppers, pumpkin, squash, tomatoes and zucchini; raw chard, collards, kale, and spinach;

	OILS & FATS	SEASONINGS
A-FOODS	avocados; bone marrow; coconut oil; lard and tallow from pastured animals; MCT oil; olives; extra virgin olive oil;	high quality natural salt (i.e. Celtic, Himalayan, Redmond, etc); apple cider vinegar; balsamic vinegar; basil; cardamom; coriander; cilantro; cumin; dill; fennel; ginger; oregano; rosemary; thyme; white pepper;
B-FOODS	algae oil; cooking grade argan oil; black seed oil; cod liver oil; perilla oil; red palm oil (RSPO-certified); dark chocolate (at least 70%); home-made guacamole;	coconut vinegar; bay leaves; black pepper; capers; cloves; fenugreek; garlic powder; marjoram; mint; mustard seed; nutmeg; paprika; parley; peppermint; sage; tarragon; traditionally prepared mayonnaise and mustard; miso; coconut aminos; wasabi; pure vanilla extract;
C-FOODS	other cold-pressed seed oils;	turmeric; ceylon cinnamon; organic 100% cocoa powder; organic tamari;
D-FOODS	margarine; canola, corn, cottonseed, peanut, safflower, sunflower, and other vegetable oils;	conventional table salt; artificial flavorings and seasonings; commercial seasoning mixes; commercial dressings and sauces; MSG;

	DAIRY	NUTS & SEEDS
A-FOODS	butter from pastured animals; ghee;	baru nuts; macadamia nuts, pili nuts; pistachios; hemp seeds;
B-FOODS	coconut kefir; coconut yogurt; colostrum;	peeled almonds; walnuts; basil seeds; flaxseeds; sacha inchi seeds;
C-FOODS	raw A2 milk from pastured animals; cheese, kefir and yogurt from A2 milk (e.g. buffalo, goat, sheep, cows from Switzerland and Southern Europe); whey cheeses (e.g. Ricotta, Gjetost, Primost and Mysost);	brazil nuts; chestnuts; hazelnuts, pecans; pine nuts; tiger nuts; sesame seeds;
D-FOODS	fake butters, spreads and dairy; condensed or evaporated milk; conventional ice cream; pasteurized milk or yogurt;	cashews; peanuts; nut butters (except unsweetened macadamia, pistachio and walnut butter); chia seeds; poppy seeds; pumpkin seeds; sunflower seeds;

	STARCH & LEGUMES	FRUITS & SWEETENERS
A-FOODS	organic basmati rice; lupini beans;	açaí berries; acerola berries; blueberries; cranberries; coconuts; lemons; limes; raspberries; chicory root; monk fruit; raw yacon syrup;
B-FOODS	organic white rice; baobab; cassava; jicama; konjac root; parsnips; potatoes; rutabaga; sprouted mung beans; sweet potatoes; tapioca; taro; yams; green bananas; green plantains; green mangos; green papayas;	bananas; blackberries; bilberries; grapefruits; lingonberries; pineapples; pomegranates; strawberries; tangerines; tart apples (e.g. Reinette, Granny Smith, Golden Delicious, Gala, Red Delicious) watermelons; organic honey; organic 100% maple syrup; erythritol; stevia;
C-FOODS	organic black, wild and red rice (ideally pressure-cooked); amaranth; millet; sorghum; traditionally-made sourdough bread; beets; turnips; pressure-cooked adzuki beans, black beans, mung beans, lentils, black-eyed peas, chickpeas, green peas and quinoa;	apricots; cherries; dates; figs; grapes; guavas; kiwis; lychees; mangos; melons; nectarines; oranges; papayas; passion fruits; peaches; pears; persimmons; plums;
D-FOODS	conventional bread and baked goods; cereal; chips; cookies; conventional pasta; pastries; popcorn; oats; canned legumes; edamame; hummus;	goji berries; star fruit (carambola); raisins; canned fruit; fruit jams and jelly; candy and other types of sweets; all types of sugar; agave; conventional honey or maple syrup; high-fructose corn syrup; aspartame; acesulfame; lactitol; mannitol; saccharin; sorbitol; sucralose; xylitol;

	BEVERAGES
A-FOODS	filtered water; natural mineral water; spring water; tea;
B-FOODS	natural coconut water; unsweetened coconut or macadamia milk; coffee; kombucha; kvass; water kefir;
C-FOODS	high-quality wine, champagne and distilled spirits;
D-FOODS	tap water; almond milk; oat milk; soy milk; fruit juices, sodas and other processed drinks; liqueurs and sugary alcoholic drinks and cocktails;

Neo Note: The Logic behind Some Choices

While I can't take the space to explain why every single food was organized and ranked the way it was, here are some things you should know.

Some foods are not in the "right" category.

You will find that I have baobab, green bananas, green mangos, green papayas, and green plantains as starches, although they are fruits. I did this on purpose because we can use them as a prebiotic food like any other in that category. Beets are not a typical starch but were also added here due to their higher sugar content. Olives and avocados are technically fruits. And peanuts are really legumes and not nuts.

These are just a few examples. The whole idea was not to organize foods only by type but also by how they're usually seen and consumed.

Food categories are not mutually exclusive.

Many foods in one category could easily belong in another one. Though they're mostly seen as one thing, that doesn't mean we can't use them for another purpose. For example, many of my protein sources, dairy foods, and nuts are also great sources of fat.

Know your fats.

I listed many oils and fats, but that doesn't mean you should cook with all of them. You already know that you should use saturated fats like coconut oil, ghee, tallow, and lard for cooking, while EVOO, MCT, and other oils should be consumed "cold."

Conventional is still better than processed food.

As you know, I am a big advocate of eating pasture-raised animals, not only due to their superior nutritional profiles but also because it is the right thing to do for our planet. I also believe that if you are flexible and resourceful, you can do this without increasing your food budget. But if you cannot find these products near you or can't make them fit your budget, please don't let that stop you from improving your health. Conventionally raised animals are still better than eating processed foods. Just try to avoid fatter cuts, because it's in the fat that most toxins accumulate, and favor butter, eggs, and plant fats.

Don't stress over Organic

Ideally, we would eat organic produce all the time, but I also understand that we have to work our budgets. Please use the EWG's Clean Fifteen and Dirty Dozen lists to guide you there.

Why I downgraded Fermented Foods

Earlier in this book, I mentioned that fermented foods are powerhouses of nutrition and probiotics. But they also are high in histamines, and some people may not tolerate them (at least in the beginning). This is the only reason I've categorized them as B or C Foods. But as you heal, they should be an important part of your diet. This also applies to A2 dairy products.

Are they Superfoods or "Super-Foes?"

Some may find it strange that I have placed foods like Ceylon cinnamon, 100 percent cocoa powder, and turmeric as C Foods. While they can indeed be powerful when used therapeutically, they also contain high levels of antinutrients and are commonly contaminated with toxins and heavy metals. You should aim to buy these products from reputable companies and consume them only occasionally.

Don't be afraid of Spices and Herbs

I am well aware that many of the spices and herbs I recommend may have high levels of antinutrients, but because they are being used in such small quantities, I believe they are safe to use. Who wants to eat food without proper seasoning?

Am I Missing Foods?

Is there a food you want to eat that's not in the Food Matrix? Go for it. Eat it and see how you feel. The only thing I suggest is that if this food is something you intend to eat frequently, do some research about possible antinutrients and other toxins. It's always good to know what you are putting inside you.

NEO FOOD REPLACEMENTS

Changing your diet can be overwhelming. All of a sudden, you are learning about how the foods you eat every day are making you sick, and you feel lost, not knowing what to eat. Besides that, having to give up on those foods can cause feelings of lack, which will only make things worse. Therefore, I recommend finding replacements for some of the "less-healthy" food you eat now. That way, you're not losing something; you are replacing it with a healthier version. Here are a few suggestions.

Bread: This is a tough once, since it depends on what the bread is for. If you are looking to have a sandwich, you should consider a wrap instead. Use cassava or coconut wraps. You can also try to do a lettuce wrap, but that one can be messy. If you're looking for toast, you are probably better off making a gluten-free, keto version at home. There are plenty of recipes online using coconut or almond flour. Eventually, as you heal your gut, you can reintroduce bread as an occasional treat. Just make sure it is sourdough bread made from organic ancient grains.

Cereal: I have some great news. You will get used to skipping breakfast, and you won't have a place for cereal in your life. *#byyyee*. But if the cravings hit and you really want some cereal, go for nut granola from sprouted almonds, walnuts, pecans, pistachios, and coconut flakes instead.

Chia seeds: Easy! Basil seeds.

Chips: You will lose your snack craving, but until then, you can replace your chips with carrots, celery, jicama sticks, and dehydrated vegetables from A and B Foods.

Milk: Best options are coconut milk and macadamia milk. Eventually, as you heal your gut, you can go for raw A2 milk if you can find it.

Pasta: Replace traditional pasta with vegetable noodles from beets, carrots, radishes, squash, and zucchini. Another alternative is to eat shirataki noodles. These Japanese noodles are made from the konjac plant and are low carb. Whenever you are more metabolically flexible, you may also consider eating pasta made from amaranth, millet, or sorghum.

Peanut butter: If you want your nut butter fix, grab butters made from pistachios, macadamias, or walnuts.

Rice: The best low-carb replacement is riced cauliflower. It's definitely not the same, but it does the trick. Another higher-carb alternative is to cook millet or sorghum.

Salad dressing: Nothing beats the old-school salad seasoning. Grab some EVOO, ACV, or balsamic vinegar.

Sodas: Ideally, you lose that habit. However, if you are really craving something bubbly, consider sparkling water with berries, lemon, lime, or mint for flavor. You can also drink some kombucha, but in moderation.

Soy sauce: Need some soy sauce? Go for the real deal, the traditional, organic, and fermented tamari. Consume sparingly.

Vegetable oils: Use some good saturated fat like ghee, lard, tallow, or duck fat. Despite not being rich in saturated fat, olive oil is also a good option because of its high content of antioxidants.

Yogurt: Stick with coconut yogurt initially. Later, find yourself some A2 milk yogurt or kefir.

NEO DIET SUCCESS PRINCIPLES

Here are my 15 guiding principles for massive success in achieving your best health.

1. Start your day with one or two big glasses of water and a teaspoon of salt.
2. Focus on two meals a day.
3. Eat protein, vegetables, and good fats daily.
4. Combine cooked and raw foods.
5. Eat small amounts of fermented foods daily.
6. Eat organ meats and other offal at least once weekly.
7. Eat stews or drink bone broths at least once weekly.
8. Eat algae or seafood at least once weekly.
9. Perform intermittent fasting most days and adopt a 24-hour fast once a week.
10. Do some sort of physical activity daily.
11. Engage in social activities at least once a week.
12. Aim to get 1 hour of sun exposure daily if possible.
13. Go outside and be exposed to nature at least once a week.
14. Adopt a daily mindfulness practice, even if it's just five minutes a day.
15. Enjoy an occasional "bad" food, but always aim for a healthier version if possible.

THE JUMPSTART BLUEPRINT

Your Journey Starts Here!

"I'm trying to free your mind, Neo. But I can only show you the door.
You're the one that has to walk through it."
Morpheus

UNDERSTANDING THE JUMPSTART BLUEPRINT

The Jumpstart Blueprint is the program I created to help bring your body back to its "factory settings." It's a comprehensive detox and metabolic reset program that will initiate or optimize your health journey following the Hordil pillars.

This is not mandatory. Heck, nothing is mandatory in the Neo Diet. However, I highly recommend that you complete this blueprint now and even every four months, to help your body cleanse and to get you to your health goals faster.

Before you start your Jumpstart Blueprint, I advise that you do a two-week preseason. In sports, the preseason is the time before competition when athletes prepare their bodies and minds for what's coming. This allows them to be even more successful during the regular season. During our preseason, I want you to implement all that you learned in the previous chapter. Weigh yourself, take measurements and pictures, get some blood work done, clean up your pantry, go grocery shopping, grab some supplements, prepare your notebook, find a community and an accountabilibuddy, set up your goals, and most importantly, start following the Food Matrix. Following the Food Matrix before you start your first Jumpstart Blueprint will allow you to remove all the bad stuff from your diet and start shifting your metabolism. This will make the program much more effective and enjoyable.

After your preseason, you will be more than ready to crush your 28-day Jumpstart Blueprint. Why 28 days, you ask? I realize I would sell a lot more books if I promised a quick 7 or 14-day program. We all want fast results. But you deserve better. You deserve something that can cause a real, significant (and safe) change.

I did not come up with the 28 days randomly. Research supports that it takes around 28 days for the microbiome to adapt to dietary changes.[1]

Additionally, this period will give you enough time to boost your detox pathways safely and start the digestive healing process, allowing you to slowly reintroduce harder-to-digest foods. Finally, between the preseason and the actual program, enough time will have passed for you to integrate these changes and make them a habit, which will exponentially increase your chances of succeeding.

After those four weeks, you will feel an incredible difference. Obviously, more complex issues will require more time, but in the next chapter, I'll discuss how you will use the Neo Diet Formula to continue your healing and optimization journey beyond the blueprint.

Here is some great news. This program is flexible and gives you plenty of options. Even though I will advise you on what to do, when to eat, and what to eat, I will give you options and will not instruct on portion sizes. Everyone is different, and I don't want anyone hungry during this blueprint. You eat what you prefer and as much as your body tells you to eat, as long as you follow the guidelines I'm suggesting.

I also have some less-than-good news. Your first week or so, you may not feel your best. Your body will go through significant metabolic changes, and you may go through a withdrawal stage because you'll be eliminating some of the toxic foods your body was so used to. This is one reason I recommend the preseason (to spread this withdrawal over time) and some optional supplements to reduce or even clear up these symptoms. During that one or two weeks, you may question yourself. But let me assure you of one thing. Give me those two weeks, and I promise you will get the taste of what health and high performance feels like. After those two weeks, you won't want to stop!

THE JUMPSTART BLUEPRINT OVERVIEW

The Jumpstart Blueprint was designed to incorporate all the pillars of the Hordil strategy. We will start the healing of your digestive system, boost your detox pathways, optimize your microbiome, and provide you with the all-important metabolic flexibility. In doing this, we will decrease inflammation, improve cellular performance, and cement the habits of your new lifestyle.

Week 1: Eliminate and Reboot

During week 1, we will focus on eliminating the most common dietary triggers. These are the foods that are causing dysbiosis, inflammatory reactions, hormonal imbalances, metabolic issues, and low performance. By removing them, not only will you start to get better, but you will be able to assess which foods are causing issues when you later reintroduce them. During this stage, we will also be getting rid of the "weeds" in your gut so it can finally heal. We will achieve this through the elimination diet and also with easier-to-digest meals. These meals will also help shift your digestive energy toward the detox pathways.

Week 2: Detox

In week 2, we will shift all our attention to the detoxification mechanisms. You will detox like you never have before. We'll start with intermittent fasts to lower the digestive burden and also to trigger fat breakdown so more toxins can be released. This is the week when you might experience the most significant weight loss. Despite that, all will be done in a perfectly safe and controlled manner.

Week 3: Rebalance

During week 3, you will continue to experience significant detoxification, but we'll shift our focus toward metabolic optimization and cellular repair. We will favor low-carb, high-fat meals and increase fasting time. This will trigger metabolic changes that will allow for cellular renewal and lower systemic inflammation. Energy levels will go up, and you will start performing much better, both physically and mentally.

Week 4: Expand, Build, and Conquer

Lastly, in week 4, we will start reintroducing more fiber and some carbs. This will help you build a stronger microbiome, continue to heal your gut, and balance your endocrine system so that you can maintain a high-performing but flexible metabolism in the long term. We will also start to wean you off supplements and integrate lifestyle changes that will allow for an easy transition into your post-blueprint life and help you conquer your health goals.

WEEK 1: ELIMINATE AND REBOOT

	DAY 1	DAY 2	DAY 3
EARLY MORNING	- Neo Juice	- Neo Juice	- Neo Juice
MID-MORNING	- Tart apples, celery stalks or carrots - Tea and water	- Tart apples, celery stalks or carrots - Tea and water	- Tart apples, celery stalks or carrots - Tea and water
LUNCH	- Solid Meal	- Solid Meal	- Solid Meal
MID-AFTERNOON	- Tart apples, celery stalks or carrots - Tea and water	- Tart apples, celery stalks or carrots - Tea and water	- Tart apples, celery stalks or carrots - Tea and water
DINNER	- Neo Soup	- Neo Soup	- Neo Soup

	DAY 4	DAY 5	DAY 6	DAY 7
EARLY MORNING	- 2 large glasses of water -1 tsp of salt	- 2 large glasses of water -1 tsp of salt	- 2 large glasses of water -1 tsp of salt	- 2 large glasses of water -1 tsp of salt
MID-MORNING	- Neo Juice	- Neo Juice	- Neo Juice	- Neo Juice
LUNCH	- Solid Meal	- Solid Meal	- Protein Smoothie	- Protein Smoothie
MID-AFTERNOON	- Tea and water - 1 tsp of salt	- Tea and water - 1 tsp of salt	- Tea and water - 1 tsp of salt	- Tea and water - 1 tsp of salt
DINNER	- Neo Soup	- Neo Soup	- Neo Soup	- Neo Soup

Ready for your first week?

As you probably noticed, I did not assign days of the week to the plan. I did this on purpose because we all have unique lives and different preferences. If you don't have a preference, I actually suggest you start the blueprint on a Tuesday. Mondays tend to be more stressful days, and we don't want that less-than-positive energy on the first day of the blueprint.

Next, let me address the elephant in the room. I am recommending that you not drink any coffee during this week. I know this may sound impossible for many people, but if you want to reboot your system, you really need to take a small break from the java. Trust me, it will be worth it. And the next time you have your coffee, you will enjoy it even more. As an alternative, you can get your caffeine from tea or even some matcha.

If you look at the plan, you'll notice that we progress through the week preparing you for the last two days, when you will consume only liquid meals. This was designed in order to decrease the digestive burden and allow your body to shift its focus toward the healing of the GI tract and detoxification.

Every day of the week, your first meal will be the Neo Juice. This powerbomb is guaranteed to wake you up even though you're having no caffeine. Ideally, you prepare it using a juicer. If you don't have a juicer, add some water and do it in a high-speed blender. At the end, please use a cheesecloth or a nut-milk bag to strain it, because we want to skip the fiber at this stage of the blueprint. Ideally, follow the Neo Juice recipe as it is. But if you really can't drink it without some sweetener, I'll close my eyes and let you add some monk fruit or stevia. Don't tell anyone.

Neo Juice
- 3 celery stalks;
- 1 carrot;
- 1 cucumber (peeled and deseeded);
- 1 deseeded small tart apple or 1 cup of jicama;
- 1 peeled lime or lemon;
- 1/2 cup of chopped fresh mint leaves;
- Fresh ginger (size of your thumb) or 1 tsp of powder ginger;
- 1 tsp of monk fruit or stevia (optional);

Although you may question my juice ingredient selection—*it's certainly not the typical sweet and flavorful juice you may be used to*—I want you to know that the recipe was conceived to take advantage of all the benefits of these ingredients. Together they will bring down inflammation, boost your digestive power, and start fighting pathogenic bacteria, mold, yeasts, and viruses. So, drink it and put a smile on that face!

Throughout the day, you can have small snacks if you want, but if possible you should aim to get used to not snacking. I also recommend drinking plenty of tea. In the morning, you can opt for some green or black tea to get your beloved caffeine, but then I recommend going for Dr. John Douillard's Decoction Tea. Also, remember to have some salt throughout the day. This will help replenish your body's minerals and keep your cravings low.

Earlier in the book, I shared the original version of this remedy. For the blueprint, I am recommending the "lighter" alternative, because it's easier and faster to prepare. You just have to fill a tablespoon of a mix of the gut-healing plants licorice, slippery elm, and marshmallow. Let it brew for a couple of minutes and then filter it. Discard the plants and drink the tea. This is phenomenal to heal the GI tract.

Dr. John Douillard's Decoction Tea[2]
- 1/3 tbsp chopped licorice;
- 1/3 tbsp chopped slippery elm bark;
- 1/3 tbsp chopped marshmallow root;
Steep this mixture in hot water for 5-10 minutes. Filter and drink it.

For lunch, you will eat a Solid Meal. It's okay to eat a bigger meal here. I know liquid meals can be a bit unfulfilling. The only thing I ask is that you keep your meals simple. Pick a good source of protein and some well-cooked vegetables, and drizzle a generous dose of olive oil on top. Please note that I am asking for cooked vegetables. Other than in the Neo Juice (from which we remove the fiber), we are avoiding raw fruits and vegetables. Raw fruits and vegetables require a strong digestion to break them down and absorb them.

And because this week we are letting your digestive system rest, we will focus on cooked, "predigested" meals.

Here are your options for your Solid Meal this week:

PROTEINS	SIDES	SEASONINGS
pasture-raised beef, lamb and other grazing animals; eggs from pastured poultry; organ meats; wild-caught anchovies, herring, mackerel, pollock, sardines, salmon and trout;	arugula; avocado; bamboo shoots; bok choy, broccoli; brussels sprouts; cabbage; carrots; cauliflower; chives; fennel root; kohlrabi; lemongrass; watercress; nopales; radishes; scallions; shallots; organic basmati rice (ideally pressure-cooked);	salt; ghee; ACV; organic balsamic vinegar; basil; cardamom; coriander; cilantro; cumin; dill; EVOO; fennel; ginger; lemon; lime; oregano; rosemary; thyme; white pepper;

About 15 minutes before your Solid Meal, do a shot of ACV or take a bitter tonic. This will get your juices flowing to better digest the meal. Optionally, you would also take your digestive enzymes right before (or during) the meal to really help you break down that Solid Meal.

On your last two days, you are going to replace this Solid Meal with a protein smoothie. This smoothie will have good sources of fat and protein so you will fill satiated even while on liquid meals. You can be creative with your smoothie as long as you follow the guideline of avoiding too much fiber and sugar, and making sure you add healthy fats and protein. I like to keep it simple. Usually, I'll just add one full glass of coconut milk, two to three scoops of collagen or beef isolate protein (hemp is also okay), half a cup of blueberries, one teaspoon of camu camu or acerola (for the vitamin C), and a couple of drops of pure vanilla extract. Put everything in the blender and add some water if it gets too thick. Easy and delicious!

This week, your daily dinner will be the gut-healing Neo Soup. Whenever you prepare it, make enough for the entire week. That way you don't have to spend much time in the kitchen. The quantities shared in the recipe should be enough for the whole week, but if you want more, please just adjust accordingly.

Besides being delicious, this soup is full of nourishing and gut-healing ingredients. You are getting plenty of nutrients, such as choline, collagen, glutamine, glycine, proline, taurine, minerals, and healthy fats.

About 15 minutes before eating your soup, do a shot of ACV or take a bitter tonic.

Optionally, add one teaspoon of L-glutamine to your soup bowl and stir it in. This extra dose can really boost your leaky gut healing efforts.

Neo Soup (6-10 servings)
- 10 cups of organic bone broth from pastured animals or organic chicken/vegetable broth;
- 4 cups of chopped daikon radish or turnip;
- 2 heads of cauliflower;
- 8 cups of sliced leeks or scallions;
- 6 cups of watercress or arugula;
- Juice from 1 lemon;
- 2 tbsp of ghee or $\frac{1}{4}$ cup of EVOO;
- Fresh ginger (size of your thumb) or 1 tsp of powder ginger;
- Salt to taste;
- 1 cup of chopped dulse (if you can find it);

Bring the broth to a simmer. Add all the ingredients, except the watercress, and let it cook for 20 minutes. Then, blend the soup, add the watercress, add more water or salt to adjust consistency and flavor, and let it simmer for another 5 minutes. Blend it again and it's ready to serve.

Lifestyle

In terms of lifestyle changes, I think this is the perfect time to start creating the habits you want to implement in this new version of yourself. Although it's not written in the planner, I would love for you to be more active during the day. Find excuses to walk and get up several times to move throughout your workday.

Other practices to implement are sun exposure and your daily 5-to-10-minute mindfulness practice. I know that sun exposure will depend on where in the world you live and when you decide to start this program. In any case, always keep this goal in mind to get your daily vitamin D when possible. Additionally, every day before you go to work or start your normal day-to-day, take 5 to 10 minutes to meditate or simply sit still and enjoy some music.

These practices should be integrated into your daily routine and continued beyond the blueprint.

For this week, what I really want you to focus on is some breath work. This will lower your stress and also promote greater lymphatic activity. Breathe deeply, activating your entire rib cage and squeezing your abdomen during your exhalations. Do this for 5 minutes, either in the morning or at night.

The same way you did for this week, please work on forming the habit of checking the planner and reading the upcoming week's section, so you have all your meals planned and your routine defined. Repeat this every week. By the way, I created a grocery list suggestion (and blank template) for each week. To download and print the grocery lists, recommended tools, and calendars, please go to the book's resources at my.neodiet.co/resources.

Last note: Because you will be saving so much energy that is usually channeled to your digestion, it's normal to get to the end of the day still firing on all cylinders, not being able to sleep. This is typical. Just do some breathing exercises and drink some chamomile tea to relax. That should do the trick.

WEEK 2: DETOX

	DAY 8	DAY 9	DAY 10
EARLY MORNING	- 2 large glasses of water -1 tsp of salt	- 2 large glasses of water -1 tsp of salt	- 2 large glasses of water -1 tsp of salt
MID-MORNING	- Light Meal	- Light Meal	- Tea and water - 1 tsp of salt
LUNCH	- Solid Meal	- Solid Meal	- Pre-meal - Solid Meal
MID-AFTERNOON	- Tea and water - 1 tsp of salt	- Tea and water - 1 tsp of salt	- Tea and water - 1 tsp of salt
DINNER	- Solid Meal, Protein Smoothie or Neo Soup	- Solid Meal, Protein Smoothie or Neo Soup	- Solid Meal, Protein Smoothie or Neo Soup

	DAY 11	DAY 12	DAY 13	DAY 14
EARLY MORNING	- 2 large glasses of water -1 tsp of salt	- 2 large glasses of water -1 tsp of salt	- 2 large glasses of water -1 tsp of salt	- 2 large glasses of water -1 tsp of salt
MID-MORNING	- Light Meal	- Tea and water - 1 tsp of salt	- Tea and water - 1 tsp of salt	- Tea and water - 1 tsp of salt
LUNCH	- Solid Meal	- Pre-meal - Solid Meal	- Pre-meal - Solid Meal	- Pre-meal - Solid Meal
MID-AFTERNOON	- Tea and water - 1 tsp of salt	- Tea and water - 1 tsp of salt	- Tea and water - 1 tsp of salt	- Tea and water - 1 tsp of salt
DINNER	- Solid Meal, Protein Smoothie or Neo Soup	- Solid Meal, Protein Smoothie or Neo Soup	- Solid Meal, Protein Smoothie or Neo Soup	- Solid Meal, Protein Smoothie or Neo Soup

Week 2 will be our most intensive detox week. For this reason, coffee is still not recommended. If you are really desperate for your coffee hit, you may drink one on the first day of the week. But try not to make this a daily exception, because it will compromise your detox efforts. Next week, I promise you can go back to your beloved elixir.

This week, we will continue to train your body to be fed in a shorter window of time. This will promote your metabolic adaptation and the release of toxins in the fat you'll be burning.

I'm sure you already noticed that this week we will introduce two new types of meals: Light Meals and Pre-meals. In fact, they are very similar, being slightly different only in timing and quantity. These are being introduced because once you increase your fasting times, you may not have enough digestive power to go straight to a complex meal. To avoid any digestive distress, we first feed the body something light and easy to digest. Later, after we've woken up your digestive system, you can have a more complex meal.

For a Light Meal, you might choose a small bowl of Neo Soup; a small protein smoothie; a basil seed pudding; a coconut yogurt with hemp seeds, blueberries, blackberries, or raspberries; a handful of nuts (macadamia nuts, pili nuts, pistachios, or sprouted walnuts); or even some eggs. Consider this your "get used to not having breakfast" meal.

For a Pre-meal, I recommend an appetizer like a small bowl of Neo Soup or bone broth, or a small salad with some bitters, olive oil, and vinegar. This mini-meal will have the function of activating your digestion and should be eaten 15 to 30 minutes before your main meal. Please also continue with your habit of taking your shot of ACV before the meals.

This week you will also add Solid Meals at night, and you'll have more options in terms of what to eat. Here is your list for Week 2.

PROTEINS	SIDES	SEASONINGS
pasture-raised beef, lamb and other grazing animals; eggs from pastured poultry; organ meats; wild-caught anchovies, herring, mackerel, pollock, sardines, salmon and trout; clams, mussels, oysters and scallops from regenerative aquacultures; hemp protein; lupini beans;	arugula; asparagus; avocado; bamboo shoots; bok choy, broccoli; brussels sprouts; cabbage; cauliflower; celery; chives; fennel root; green beans; kohlrabi; lemongrass; mung bean sprouts; nopales; parsnips; radishes; scallions; shallots; watercress;	salt; butter from pastured animals; ghee; red palm oil (RSPO-certified); ACV; organic balsamic vinegar; basil; cardamom; coriander; cilantro; cumin; dill; EVOO; fennel; ginger; garlic; lemon; lime; oregano; parsley; rosemary; thyme; white pepper;

This week, it's important that you eat generous portions of meat (including some organ meat if possible), eggs (avoid cooking the yolks if you trust their quality), and cruciferous vegetables. These are filled with essential detox nutrients, as you already know. Also, at least twice this week, try to make a smoothie. You can follow my recipe suggestion from last week. This is a great way to take in some vitamin C (from extracts like camu camu and acerola), get some extra L-glutamine (in case you used it in week 1) in your gut, and even mix in one or two raw egg yolks so you don't compromise them with cooking. Just make sure to drink your smoothie immediately so it doesn't spoil.

Optionally, you can also add half a tablespoon of chlorella to your smoothie to take advantage of its binding and lymph-moving properties.

Your tea selection will expand this week. You can continue with the Decoction Tea but should also add burdock root, dandelion, fenugreek, and holy basil teas. These are phenomenal to get your lymphatic system moving and to boost your detox pathways. Keep changing teas throughout the day so you drink one cup of each most days. This is also a great way to augment your water intake, which is key for an effective detox protocol.

As you probably noticed, this week I recommend several supplements. As always, supplements are optional, but there are two that I consider essential: magnesium and a good binder. Magnesium is essential for many physiological processes, including detoxification, and unfortunately it is challenging to get enough through diet alone. Please take your magnesium first thing in the morning and before you go to bed.

Then, I also think a binder is essential because if you don't have binders in your system, most of the released toxins will not find their way out and will just move to other places in your body, possibly making you feel even worse. The other supplements will boost detoxification even further while minimizing symptoms, but are completely up to you.

During this week, in between meals (twice a day) you are going to take a good binder composed of activated charcoal, bentonite clay, chitosan, silica, and zeolites, or at least most of these. The ones I find more important are activated charcoal and zeolites. So, if you can't find a good comprehensive binder where you live, please aim for these two.

If you are interested in the other supplement recommendations, please take them according to the instructions on the label. If you are working with a tighter budget but are still considering these herbal remedies, milk thistle and triphala (in this order) are the ones that are going to give you more bang for your buck.

Lastly, ensure that you are having frequent bowel movements this week. These are essential in order to get all the toxins out. In the rare event of constipation, please follow my recommendations in chapter 16 and take a laxative.

Lifestyle

During week 2, we will maintain the lifestyle changes introduced last week and will include a few more for this week alone. Twice this week, try to find a spa or a gym where you can use a sauna for 10 to 30 minutes. Forcing your body to sweat will help you flush out a ton of toxins through your skin. Also, do some yoga (gyms have classes or you can just watch a YouTube video) or some full-body stretches to help lymph mobilization and further facilitate detoxification. Finally, do some dry skin brushing (plenty of tutorials on YouTube) or get a massage, either by a professional or from someone willing to give you one. Similarly to yoga, this will help get your lymph moving and boost the detox pathways.

WEEK 3: REBALANCE

	DAY 15	DAY 16	DAY 17
EARLY MORNING	- Light Meal (optional)	- 2 large glasses of water -1 tsp of salt	- 2 large glasses of water -1 tsp of salt
MID-MORNING	- Coffee, tea and water - 1 tsp of salt	- Coffee, tea and water - 1 tsp of salt	- Coffee, tea and water - 1 tsp of salt
LUNCH	- Pre-meal - Solid Meal	- Pre-meal - Solid Meal	- Pre-meal - Solid Meal
MID-AFTERNOON	- Tea and water - 1 tsp of salt	- Tea and water - 1 tsp of salt	- Tea and water - 1 tsp of salt
DINNER	- Solid Meal, Protein Smoothie or Neo Soup	- Solid Meal, Protein Smoothie or Neo Soup	- Solid Meal, Protein Smoothie or Neo Soup

	DAY 18	DAY 19	DAY 20	DAY 21
EARLY MORNING	- Light Meal (optional)	- 2 large glasses of water -1 tsp of salt	- 2 large glasses of water -1 tsp of salt	- 2 large glasses of water -1 tsp of salt
MID-MORNING	- Coffee, tea and water - 1 tsp of salt	- Coffee, tea and water - 1 tsp of salt	- Coffee, tea and water - 1 tsp of salt	- Coffee, tea and water - 1 tsp of salt
LUNCH	- Pre-meal - Solid Meal	- Pre-meal - Solid Meal	- Pre-meal - Solid Meal	- Coffee, tea and water - 1 tsp of salt
MID-AFTERNOON	- Tea and water - 1 tsp of salt	- Tea and water - 1 tsp of salt	- Protein Smoothie or Neo Soup	- Tea and water - 1 tsp of salt
DINNER	- Solid Meal, Protein Smoothie or Neo Soup	- Solid Meal, Protein Smoothie or Neo Soup	- Solid Meal	- Pre-meal - Solid Meal

Week 3 is my favorite because it marks the turning point in the blueprint. You just finished the most restrictive weeks and are now ready to reap the rewards of your effort. Your body will feel five years younger, and your mind will have a sense of clarity you probably haven't experienced in some time.

And that's not all. This is also the week when we are going to upgrade your cells. We will increase your fasting time, dabble in ketosis, and promote autophagy. This will allow your cells to repair themselves and become more efficient. At the end of this week, you will finally get a taste of what your body can feel like when it's healthy and working without limitations. You will love it!

Ideally, I would prefer that you try 16-hour intermittent fasts every day of this week, and then finish the week with a 24-hour fast. However, I understand some people may be starting at a more metabolically challenging position and may experience more physical and emotional symptoms when attempting these daily fasts. That's why I've added 2 days when you have the option of having a light meal for breakfast. Everyone is starting at different stages, so don't be hard on yourself if you feel you need these optional meals.

On your fasting days, eat all your meals within that 8-hour window. Also, try to have your last meal around 7 p.m. so you can respect your circadian rhythm and reap the benefits of your glymphatic system's nightly "brain wash."

On day 21, the goal is to complete a 24-hour fast. Your last meal will be dinner on day 20, and then you will eat again only at dinnertime on day 21. If this is your first 24-hour fast, you certainly will be happy to eat when the time comes. Take it easy and start with something light so as not to overwhelm your digestive system. If at any moment you feel you cannot do the whole 24 hours, chances are these feelings are emotional and not actually physiological ones. Try to go for a walk. Get your mind busy with something. Eat some salt and drink some tea. Most times, this will be enough to overcome the food cravings. If this fails and you are really desperate for some food, eat some healthy fats and nonstarchy vegetables. Avoid protein and starches until you reach the 24-hour mark. Then go for it.

Not sure if you noticed, but I have added coffee to the planner. *Yaaaaaay!* It doesn't appear in the early morning slot because I prefer you to wait 60 to 90 minutes from the time you wake up. Hydrate yourself first and go through your morning rituals, and only then have your coffee. If you want, you can follow Dave Asprey's suggestion and perform a modified fast by drinking coffee with MCT oil (preferably C8) and grass-fed butter or ghee. This "fatty coffee" will keep your hunger in check while not significantly affecting your insulin levels. If you are just starting with longer fasts, this hack makes them a lot more enjoyable and easier to sustain.

Since we are lengthening our fasting times and eating low carb, insulin levels will be lower, which will cause your kidneys to excrete sodium. Therefore, you really want to increase your salt intake to avoid the famous "keto flu."

Overall, most of last week's recommendations on Light Meals, Pre-meals, and protein smoothies still apply. In terms of the Solid Meals, please follow the same principles but make sure to eat some healthy fats with every meal.

Here are your expanded options for this week.

PROTEINS	SIDES
pasture-raised beef, lamb and other grazing animals; eggs from pastured poultry; organ meats; wild-caught anchovies, herring, mackerel, pollock, sardines, salmon and trout; clams, mussels, oysters and scallops from regenerative aquacultures; Hemp protein; Lupini beans;	arugula; asparagus; avocado; bamboo shoots; bok choy, broccoli; brussels sprouts; cabbage; cauliflower; celery; chives; fennel root; green beans; kohlrabi; lemongrass; mung bean sprouts; nopales; parsnips; radishes; scallions; shallots; watercress;

SEASONINGS	FATS
salt; ACV; organic balsamic vinegar; coconut vinegar; basil; bay leaves; black pepper; capers; cardamom; cloves; coriander; cilantro; cumin; dill; fennel; fenugreek; ginger; garlic; lemon; lime; marjoram; mint; mustard seed; nutmeg; oregano; paprika; parsley; peppermint; rosemary; sage; tarragon; thyme; white pepper;	avocado; bone marrow; butter from pastured animals; coconut oil; ghee; lard and tallow from pastured animals; MCT oil; olives; EVOO; red palm oil (RSPO-certified); baru nuts; macadamia nuts; peeled almonds; pili nuts; pistachios; walnuts; basil seeds; flaxseeds; sacha inchi seeds;

Besides choosing some healthy fats, we are also going to eat foods rich in mitochondria-boosting substances such as melatonin and phospholipids. You can get melatonin from pistachios, mushrooms, mustard seeds, EVOO, and coffee. Phospholipids can be found in egg yolks, clams, mussels, oysters, and scallops. Try to add these to your diet this week as much as possible.

In terms of supplements, you may continue with the supplements you started these past 2 weeks. Optionally, you can buy some MCT oil to add to your coffee, smoothies, and salads. This will help you transition to states of ketosis, boost energy levels, and make this week even more powerful. Word of caution: please start slowly with MCT, because your body may take some time to get used to it. Too much too soon can lead to some time sitting in the bathroom.

Lifestyle

Our focus last week was on boosting your detox pathways and adding sauna time and dry skin brushing or massage to your routine. This week you may interrupt these practices (or continue if you can fit them in your day-to-day) and add some resistance training to your week. You need to continue to stay as active as you can during the day, but I would also recommend adding at least 2 gym days for some weight training. Unless you have bodybuilding goals, 30 minutes is more than enough to work on your major muscle groups, as seen in chapter 14. Don't forget to finish your training session with some stretching.

WEEK 4: EXPAND, BUILD, AND CONQUER

	DAY 22	DAY 23	DAY 24
EARLY MORNING	- Light Meal (optional)	- 2 large glasses of water -1 tsp of salt	- 2 large glasses of water -1 tsp of salt
MID-MORNING	- Tea and water - 1 tsp of salt	- Tea and water - 1 tsp of salt	- Tea and water - 1 tsp of salt
LUNCH	- Pre-meal - Solid Meal	- Pre-meal - Solid Meal	- Pre-meal - Solid Meal
MID-AFTERNOON	- Tea and water - 1 tsp of salt	- Tea and water - 1 tsp of salt	- Tea and water - 1 tsp of salt
DINNER	- Solid Meal, Protein Smoothie or Neo Soup	- Solid Meal, Protein Smoothie or Neo Soup	- Solid Meal, Protein Smoothie or Neo Soup

	DAY 25	DAY 26	DAY 27	DAY 28
EARLY MORNING	- Light Meal (optional)	- 2 large glasses of water - 1 tsp of salt	- 2 large glasses of water - 1 tsp of salt	- 2 large glasses of water - 1 tsp of salt
MID-MORNING	- Tea and water - 1 tsp of salt	- Tea and water - 1 tsp of salt	- Tea and water - 1 tsp of salt	- Tea and water - 1 tsp of salt
LUNCH	- Pre-meal - Solid Meal	- Pre-meal - Solid Meal	- Pre-meal - Solid Meal	- Tea and water - 1 tsp of salt
MID-AFTERNOON	- Tea and water - 1 tsp of salt	- Tea and water - 1 tsp of salt	- Protein Smoothie or Neo Soup	- Tea and water - 1 tsp of salt
DINNER	- Solid Meal, Protein Smoothie or Neo Soup	- Solid Meal, Protein Smoothie or Neo Soup	- Solid Meal	- Pre-meal - Solid Meal

Congratulations, you have reached week 4. I'm so glad you accepted this challenge and embarked on this journey with me. I'm sure you already feel the positive changes in yourself. But let me not get sidetracked here, because we still have one more week in front of us. As you certainly noticed, the planner looks exactly like last week's. This is the final structure and the one you should aim to follow most weeks going forward. Obviously, you can move things around to fit your schedule, but this should be your guiding template.

This week we will focus on two things: (1) slowly expanding your diet, adding more prebiotics and probiotics to build a strong microbiome; and (2) adding carbs to some dinners to boost your hormonal health.

Starting this week, you can use the Food Matrix to make your meal choices. You may consume any A Food or B Food, but please monitor how you feel when introducing the second category. Aim to eat low carb most times, but eat some starches at night two or three times a week on the days you hit the gym. These refeeds will refill muscle glycogen reserves, help you sleep better, and balance your hormones. Please keep assessing which starches your body seems to do the best with.

If you are overweight or insulin resistant, please continue following a more carb-restricted diet. You may eat some starches but less frequently and in less quantity, at least until you become more metabolically flexible.

You will also introduce fermented foods. Please go slowly with these and let your body get used to them. More is not always better. Take your time and try different fermented foods to see which ones you feel the best with.

Another way to start rebuilding your microbiome without having histamine concerns is by taking probiotics. This is optional of course, but I believe that this is the perfect time to introduce them.

Regarding the other supplements you're taking, please continue with magnesium, since this is one of those you should take several times a year. Please stop taking the binders and save them for your next blueprint three or four months down the road. Same with any other optional detox supplement from week 2. If you're taking digestive enzymes or L-glutamine, slowly wean your body off them. Your digestion will continue to improve, and your gut will continue to heal.

Lifestyle

This final week I suggest simply adding some HIIT to your exercise routine. Increase to 3 or 4 days a week and do a combination of resistance training and HIIT. You will notice that after the blueprint, it will be a lot easier to lose fat and pack on muscle.

Please continue to stay active during the day and aim to spend as much time outdoors as you can.

Final Notes

Once you're finished with this week, pat yourself on the back for completing the blueprint. Better yet, pop some champagne and drink a glass or two. This accomplishment is worth celebrating. You just took a gigantic step toward changing your health and your life. I'm proud of you!

But please remember, this was just the first step. You will continue to improve and to feel even better. In the next chapter, I'll share how you can make these new habits stick and how you can personalize the Neo Diet to your unique biology.

For now, though, take a picture, get your measurements, and compare them with what you have in your notebook from the first day. I'm sure you'll be surprised by how much you've progressed. Enjoy that victory and brag a bit using #NeoTransformation on social media.

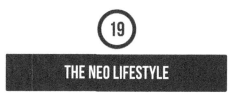

19

THE NEO LIFESTYLE

Don't Let "Perfect" Be the Enemy of "Good"

*"There are lots of people in this world who spend so much time
watching their health that they haven't the time to enjoy it."*
Josh Billings

THE NEO LIFESTYLE

You've completed the Jumpstart Blueprint and have been exploring and testing the different foods in the Food Matrix. Now what? Now it's time to continue. The Neo Diet is not just a trendy short-term diet; it's your new way of eating. Use the Food Matrix as the basis of your diet and explore different recipes using these ingredients. Most importantly, continue to monitor how your symptoms progress and whether certain foods, even in the A and B groups, cause any exacerbation.

As you heal and feel better, it's time to slowly put your body to the test. See if it can handle B Foods more frequently and even C Foods occasionally. We are healing to become antifragile, not to stay inside a bubble forever.

In the beginning, even if your gut is mostly healed, you may still experience some symptoms. That's why I tell you to go slowly. The first time you go to the gym you will be sore, but slowly your body will take it better and better. We follow the same principle here. Try one food at a time and always take notes. We are all different. One food could be harmless for your friend but really trigger your GI tract.

Progressively increase the quantity and variety of B Foods you eat. Quoting Dr. Will Bulsiewicz, "the goal is to hit that sweet spot where your dietary choices are perfectly matched to the strengths and weaknesses of your gut, and then magic ensues."[1] With practice comes perfection. Eventually, you will feel confident in your body's ability to handle different foods, and you'll get to know which ones make you feel the best.

But please remember that things won't be perfect all the time. There will be times when a food you're normally okay with will cause a reaction. It happens to me, and I've been on this path for some time. The point is that this is the exception, not the rule, and you can trust that your organism will take care of it.

If you had serious digestive and metabolic issues before starting the Neo Diet, you might take more time to get here. Don't be impatient. We are all starting at different points. Just continue with a more rigid Food Matrix for longer before you try reintroducing hard-to-digest foods. It might take you two months; it might take you a year. This is not a race. What matters is that you make the journey enjoyable and keep getting better.

> ### Neo Note: Reintroducing Wheat and Dairy
> Probably the most challenging foods to reintroduce for some will be wheat and dairy. They require strong digestive power and a healed gut. As you know, this may take a couple of months to achieve. After reading the sections on wheat and dairy, you know you should be very picky about the products you choose. Industrial grain or dairy products are foods you should avoid at all costs. Their raw materials and the way they are processed make them gut busters with no nutritional value. Instead, once your gut is in a better position, follow the recommendations I gave you earlier and choose organic, traditionally made, fermented products, which will be a lot easier to digest and will have an improved nutritional profile.
> Obviously, the first time you reintroduce these foods, you will not eat 10 artisanal breads with a ton of cheese. You have to train your gut to start digesting gluten and lactose. Even someone who is intolerant has a threshold that needs to be crossed in order to trigger symptoms. So, by starting slowly and each day increasing the quantity, you will microdose your way to success.
> There are several studies showing that your gut can adapt with slow, consistent modifications. It most definitely can be trained to tolerate foods you're sensitive to. You just need to feed it limited quantities to train it. That's it.
> In no time, you'll be able to eat these products consistently without even thinking about it.

PERSONALIZING YOUR DIET
The Neo Diet gives you general guidelines to follow, but it was not designed to be a one-size-fits-all protocol. In truth, there is no such thing, because we all have our unique goals and bioindividuality.

For example, if you want to lose weight, you should probably step up your protein consumption. If you have metabolic syndrome or something more severe, such as cancer, you probably should adopt more of a strict ketogenic approach. If you want to pack a bit more muscle, you probably should consider consuming more carbs, especially after exercise. That insulin peak will trigger muscle anabolism and help you recover faster. That being said, do some carb cycling so you can still keep a high insulin sensitivity. On days when you don't exercise, follow more of a keto approach, and on the days you hit the gym, cut back on your fat intake and bump up your carb consumption.

The point here is that you can play with different ratios depending on your goals. And as your goals change, your diet can also change. See what makes you feel best and what works for you.

Personalizing your diet is the key to long-term success. It will allow you not only to pursue different goals but also to eat the foods that work for your biology. For example, after exercise I can eat a potful of rice and have no issues. But if I eat white potatoes, I feel lousy for the rest of the evening.

In a 2015 scientific article, it was concluded that your glycemic response is influenced not only by the food you eat but by unique biological factors that are part of you, such as body composition, genetics, and microbiome.[2] In the study, the researchers tested the glycemic response of different individuals after the participants ate either a banana or a cookie with the same amount of carbs. One would assume that people would have a worse response to the cookie, since the banana has fiber and it's not processed, right? Not really. Some people had that response, while others reacted a lot worse after eating the banana. This supports the idea of using guiding principles but also personalizing them to how your body responds.

As you test different things, you will notice these patterns and learn from them. So, right after the detox phase of the Jumpstart Blueprint, I guide you to make notes on how you feel with the different foods you reintroduce. This should be something you always pay attention to.

You may never get yourself completely figured out. As time passes and your gut changes, you may be able to eat foods that made you sick three months ago. I think that is the fun part about this. You keep testing and keep hearing what your body has to say.

PERSONALIZED NUTRITION 2.0

In the future, I imagine ordering a testing kit online and having a drone deliver it to my doorstep. Inside the kit, there is a "robot capsule" to swallow. The pill will collect samples of saliva, blood, and feces while inside me. It will also assess the power of my digestive juices and the integrity of my GI tract. And I won't even need to worry about searching for the capsule in my feces. All the data will have been transmitted wirelessly while the capsule was traveling inside me. *Ding!* It's a notification. My personalized diet plan has been created.

While this doesn't exist yet, at least in this exact form, we already have access to several tests that can give us insight into how to personalize our diet according to our genetics, microbiome, and overall digestive health.

If you undergo a DNA test (once in your lifetime), a high-quality and comprehensive GI test (yearly), and blood tests (quarterly), you can have objective data on what you need to focus on, dietwise.

When you do a genetic test, you may learn about the foods that your genes have more history with. For example, if you have South American ancestry,

410 THE NEO DIET – CHAPTER 19

you may be a better metabolizer of high-carb foods like grains, tubers, and fruits. While others will have a high glycemic response to these foods, you can keep your insulin sensitivity. Does this mean you should just eat carbs? Not at all. But you may be someone who does better with more carbs than on a strict keto diet.

Genetic testing will also inform you about possible single nucleotide polymorphisms (SNPs) you may have (as discussed in chapter 2). This is important because it identifies the exact micronutrients you may benefit from the most to compensate for your genetic "limitations."

Usually, the genetic test will group all these different factors and give you a report describing your susceptibility to nutrient deficiencies and tendency to develop certain diseases. It will also give you what the genetic analysts believe to be your preferred macronutrient ratios, and a list of foods that will support your unique micronutrient needs.

These are only estimations because, as you're well aware, epigenetics will regulate and influence your genes. That's why it's important to combine gut tests and blood work to really have an idea of what's happening inside you. The gut test will tell you about your microbiome health and what foods to eat to correct any dysbiosis or GI integrity issues. And your blood work will tell you about your endocrine health and inflammation status. All of this should be assessed by a skilled professional who'll then guide you with a personalized nutrition plan.

Please note that this is not "required." I know very well that some of these tests can be pretty expensive. For most of you, the principles shared so far are more than enough to be pretty effective in personalizing your diet. But if you still have issues, this is something you should consider. Just don't do it alone. Get the guidance of a professional.

Neo Note: 7-Day Carb Test
One trick I learned from nutrition expert Robb Wolf is the 7-Day Carb Test.[3] It's easy to do, and it's a fun way to learn more about how your body reacts to certain carbs.

For 7 days, you will test a specific amount of carbohydrates every morning at breakfast. To do this, you will just need to get yourself a glucometer.
 - Each morning, start by eating 50 effective grams (you can determine this online) of a specific carbohydrate source, and nothing else.
 - Wait two hours, and then use your glucometer to assess your blood sugar.
 - If your blood glucose is between 90 and 115 milligrams per deciliter, it means your body can metabolize that food well. If the number is above this range, please retest that food on a different day at breakfast again, but with half the amount (25 effective grams).
 - If on the second trial, and with only half the quantity, this food still hikes

your blood glucose above 115 milligrams per deciliter at the two-hour mark, this is definitely a food you should avoid.

For more details on this test, please visit my.neodiet.co/7daycarbtest.

INTUITIVE EATING

Another way in which you will eventually personalize your diet is through intuition. That's right. Your body will tell you exactly what to avoid and what to prioritize. I know how this sounds, but it's true. As you clean up your diet, and especially after your first detox program, you'll notice that you've become more sensitive to foods. I don't mean you get sick with the smallest thing. I mean that your perception skills improve, and you become more aware of the effects foods have on you. After eating certain foods, you will rapidly notice how they change your mood, energy levels, or focus, for example. Getting to this stage is a beautiful thing. Immediately, you will be able to tell which foods your body and microbiome are in tune with and which ones they are not. Just by paying attention, you'll make better choices next time.

Because you will no longer suffer from the effects of the hyperpalatable foods that messed up your taste buds and your hormones for the longest time, you will also be able to "hear" hints from your body. Some days, you may experience an intense desire to eat a big, juicy steak. When this happens, it might mean that you are low in B_{12}, iron, or zinc, for example. Other days, you may feel like eating a basket of citrus fruits and berries. Your body is possibly asking for vitamin C. You get the idea.

This is one of those things that come with time and get better with practice. Just focus on healing and be open to listening. Use the Neo Diet as your guide, and then tap into technology and your intuition to personalize it to your unique needs.

THE 90/10 RULE

One important thing I want you to learn from my mistakes is not to obsess over your diet. Some people, when they first learn about proper nutrition and a healthier lifestyle, go all in. And even though "all in" can be good, it is important to know when to hit the brakes so one does not develop orthorexia. Orthorexia is an eating disorder characterized by having an obsession with healthy dieting and consuming only "pure" foods. At this stage, eating healthy becomes a source of stress and anxiety that will cause more harm than if the individual just ate junk food every day.

Besides the stress, orthorexia can also lead to extreme elimination diets. You are so concerned about not eating anything "bad" that you eliminate everything until eventually there is only a handful of meals you can eat. To me, that is not being healthy. Being healthy is being antifragile and eating some "bad" stuff once in a while as a hormetic stressor to make you even stronger. Being healthy is also having a positive relationship with food. You should be excited about eating and not the opposite.

That is why I suggest that we adopt the 90/10 rule.

No, I am not getting confused with the 80/20 rule (also called the Pareto principle). I am purposely using a different ratio and assigning it a different meaning. The 90/10 rule is a reminder to stay healthy 90 percent of the time but to "relax" 10 percent of the time.

I recommend following this rule for various reasons. To begin with, this rule is a great way to prevent orthorexia. Then, it's also an excellent strategy to occasionally put the body to the test and reap the benefits of hormesis. Furthermore, it's a reminder to enjoy life. There will be days you want some ice cream. Go eat that son of a gun. Lastly, it also promotes more social interaction. Several of your friends will not follow a healthy diet but will still invite you for dinner. With the 90/10 rule, you are "allowed" to eat with them without being that person who sends a list of preapproved meals.

Please don't get me wrong. I believe you should focus on being healthy. But once you are more advanced in your healing journey, it's okay to eat that pizza. Don't be in such constant fear of failing that you end up not living and enjoying life.

Let's make one thing clear, though. This is not a get-out-of-jail-free card. If your first thought is that you can use that 10 percent to devour a bucket of wings, two apple pies, and a pint of ice cream, you need to reconsider your goals and your relationship with food. This also tells me you still have further healing to do and that you should not adopt the 90/10 rule yet. All I ask is common sense. Keep your goals in mind and be reasonable.

I leave you with a quote from Dr. Michael Ruscio: "As long as you're feeling well most of the time, don't sweat the small stuff. No one is perfect, and no one is invincible."[4]

DIETARY SUPPLEMENTS

I have said this and will say it again. Diet always comes first. You cannot expect one pill to fix what pounds of bad food are doing to your body. The goal is always to get as much nutrition as possible from whole foods. Supplements are only there to be used therapeutically or to address any dietary deficits.

Back in the day, soils were rich in micronutrients, and everything was organic. The nutrient profile of these foods allowed us to be incredibly healthy if we made the right choices. Sadly, as you are well aware, that's no longer the reality. Soils are depleted, and fruits and vegetables no longer possess the same nutritional power. Even the animals we eat don't get the same nutrition their ancestors did. Therefore, we all could benefit from taking some supplements to compensate for these deficiencies.

Supplements are also a great tool to minimize the effects of some excesses of daily life, optimize performance, and boost and optimize certain bodily systems.

However, before taking any supplement, do your research. Quality is key here. There are plenty of companies selling snake oil. These companies produce cheap supplements that are mostly fillers, and use synthetic nutrients that will do more harm than good. Remember the example of supplements having folic acid instead of actual folate? That's just one of many examples of synthetic alternatives used by some companies.

This could be one reason why some studies have shown that multivitamins present no benefits, and others have even associated them with an increased risk of mortality.[5,6] Another thing research has shown is that some supplements have very poor bioavailability.[7] Meaning, the nutrients do not get to your cells. This has been attributed to the use of synthetic, inorganic raw materials and also to the use of fillers, coatings, excipients, and surfactants.[8]

This is a perfect example of "you get what you pay for." Whenever you're choosing a supplement, go for reputable brands and go all Sherlock Holmes on their websites to see their mission statements and learn more about the ingredients used. The goal is always to pick supplements created with natural ingredients.

In this book, I have mentioned several supplements you can use to speed up the healing of various organs and processes. I won't explain them here again, but you will find them in the book's resources. Please use them therapeutically to address more problematic issues. In this section, I'm just going to share the ones I feel most people would benefit from on a more regular basis.

Magnesium

Magnesium is a mineral that is used as a cofactor in more than 300 enzymatic processes in the body, including production of energy and DNA repair.[9] We don't value magnesium much, but it's a pretty big deal. Unfortunately, studies suggest many of us may be deficient.[10]

Magnesium can be obtained from plants, but because of our agricultural practices, our soils are being depleted of this much-needed mineral.[11] To make matters worse, our environmental pollution is causing acid rain, which further depletes the magnesium content of our soils and produce.[12,13] Unless you get your produce from pristine soils with great agricultural practices, chances are you are at the very least slightly deficient in magnesium. That is why this is my number one recommendation.

Some of the best forms of magnesium are aspartate, chelate, chloride, citrate, glycinate, malate, orotate, taurate, and L-threonate. I recommend cycling through them or taking a combination of different forms.

Vitamin K_2

Vitamin K has two very different forms, K_1 and K_2. We rarely think about vitamin K deficiency because many vegetables have good levels of vitamin K_1. But here is where it gets interesting. First, research suggests that our bodies absorb only about 10 percent of the K_1 from plant foods.[14] Second, K_2 seems to be the form the body can use and benefit the most from.[15-18]

Vitamin K_2 is essential for the absorption of calcium and its deposition in the teeth and bones (where it should be), and not into arteries and kidneys (where it can cause serious issues).[19-21] Besides being important for protecting the cardiovascular system, kidneys, bones, and teeth, studies show that it may also improve insulin sensitivity, promote reproductive health, and protect us from cancer.[22-27]

Some of the best sources of K_2 are emu oil, ghee, gouda, kefir, liver, natto, pasture-raised butter, pasture-raised egg yolks, and sauerkraut. And, although the Neo Diet supports and recommends all these foods, you will probably not eat them in enough quantity to top off your K_2 needs. So, I do recommend supplementing with K_2.

Vitamin D_3

I honestly don't remember the last time I took vitamin D in supplement form, since I spend most of my time in South Florida and make a habit of exposing myself to plenty of sunlight almost daily. But I recognize that a lot of people don't live in places where they can have a routine like mine. This is why I recommend vitamin D_3 supplementation.

As discussed earlier, vitamin D is essential for your immune system, bone health, metabolism, and production of important neurotransmitters and hormones. It's essential for many biological processes, and its deficiency can lead to serious medical issues.

So, if you can't get at least five hours a week of direct sun exposure, please supplement with vitamin D_3, which is the form used in our bodies. Follow the dosage on the label, but get tested to make sure you are within a recommended range. In the book's resources, I share more information about this.

Please note that as you get older, your ability to produce vitamin D diminishes.[28] The older you are, the more you should consider supplementing with it.

Vitamin E

Vitamin E is a fat-soluble vitamin just like A, D, and K. And, like the others, it is essential for optimal health. Some of the foods that contain vitamin E are argan oil, flaxseeds, pecans, pistachios, pumpkin seeds, red palm oil, sesame seeds, and walnuts. Unfortunately, during processing, many of these foods are heated, which can degrade vitamin E.[29] Thus, you should consume these foods raw.

Even so, we may benefit from more vitamin E than we usually get from our diets. As we saw before, this micronutrient is vital to fighting oxidation and to staving off the damage of years of consuming oxidized vegetable oils.[30] It's also great for neuronal health, and it has been studied for the prevention and treatment of various neurological diseases.[31]

Another reason I take vitamin E is because, similarly to vitamin C, it also protects the skin from ultraviolet radiation.[32] And, since I get plenty of sun on my skin, it's a great way to "eat my sunscreen."

Vitamin E is an excellent long-term supplement, especially in the first year of your healing journey, because it will slowly reverse free radical damage and will promote better cellular health.

Look for supplements that contain not only the most studied form, d-alpha tocopherol, but also mixed tocopherols, including beta, gamma, and delta, so you get the full spectrum, as you would in a whole food.

Vitamin C

Similarly to magnesium, vitamin C is an important cofactor for many enzymatic processes in the body. It is essential to producing collagen, boosting immunity, and optimizing the endocrine and cardiovascular systems.[33–36]

Yes, you can get vitamin C from foods like bell peppers, berries, broccoli, cauliflower, citrus fruits, guava, kiwifruit, and papaya, just to name a few. But either I consume loads of the vegetables on this list raw (heat degrades vitamin C) and have GI distress, or I need to eat loads of the fruits and end up getting too much fructose. That's why I've added vitamin C to my list of supplements.

But please note, I don't recommend buying your typical, cheap ascorbic acid supplement. Although more research is needed, some authors believe that the benefits we associate with vitamin C come from its whole food form and not from the isolated ascorbic acid. In its whole food form, vitamin C is accompanied by ascorbigen, J factor, K factor, P factor, rutin, tyrosinase, and other essential cofactors. This is probably why ascorbic acid supplements have been shown to have pro-oxidative effects and even cause GI tract distress, leach minerals from bones, and promote the formation of kidney stones.[37–40]

That's why I recommend that you "supplement" with freeze-dried powder extracts from certain fruits such as acerola, amla berries, camu camu, kakadu plums, and sea buckthorn. These extracts are easy to mix in a smoothie and will give you vitamin C in its whole food form.

Shilajit

Shilajit is a sticky black resin that results from a long process of decomposition of plant matter.[41] In the Ayurvedic tradition, it is recognized as a panacea, which means it helps promote the health of all the systems in the body.[42] Shilajit can be found in high-altitude regions. Traditionally sourced and used by the peoples in the Himalayas, it's also present in regions of Russia, Iran, Mongolia, and even Peru.

Researchers have uncovered that shilajit contains more than 84 minerals, including the powerful humic and fulvic acids.[43] These organic components are believed to play an important role in transporting various micronutrients to their cellular targets, and thus optimizing cellular metabolism and health.[44] They also help remove deep-seated toxins from the body.[45]

Studies have maintained that shilajit may boost cognition and have analgesic, anxiety-reducing, cardioprotective, immunomodulating, antiallergic, antidiabetic, antiulcerogenic, antifungal, antiviral, anti-inflammatory, antioxidant, anticarcinogenic, and antiaging properties.[46-60] Considering all these amazing benefits, I think it's a no-brainer why I recommend this health tonic for long-term use.

FREQUENTLY ASKED QUESTIONS
Is the Neo Diet an alkaline diet?

Alkaline diets are based on the concept that some foods cause your body to produce acid, and so should be eliminated. Even though I agree with the idea of reducing the body's acid load, I still believe that many highly acidic foods are incredibly nutritious and should be part of your diet.

I understand the logic, but I put a "traditional alkaline diet" in the same realm as a carnivore or vegan diet. It's taking the concept to the extreme and has to be very well planned if you want to thrive. But let me explain why I say this.

Our bodies' pH varies depending on the fluid and the tissue, but the common reference is that your blood pH should remain between 7.35 and 7.45. As you probably recall from high school, that's slightly alkaline. If your blood pH were to go outside that range, you would get very sick and die. The great news is that your body does a phenomenal job of keeping you there—so good a job that even if you eat only acidic foods, it will find ways to keep you in that range. But here is where the problems may occur.

If you don't eat enough alkaline foods to neutralize the acid load from animal protein, grains, processed foods, and even most biochemical processes that naturally occur inside us, your body is forced to scavenge minerals from bone and amino acids (particularly glutamine) from muscle, to use as a buffering system. This directly causes osteoporosis (bone loss) and sarcopenia (muscle loss), and also other indirect effects like muscle cramps, headaches, mood swings, inflammation, low energy, and poor immunity.

Does this mean you need to stop eating animal protein, grains, and processed foods? Well, you should definitely stop eating most grains and processed foods. But as we've seen, meat is incredibly nutritious, and if produced right, it can be one of the best and most complete foods one can eat.

We don't need to go to the extreme. It's okay to eat meat, as long as you also eat plenty of vegetables to give you the micronutrients your body needs to balance its pH. Even someone on a carnivore diet can compensate for it by eating plenty of alkalizing organ meats, for example.

In following the Neo Diet, you will eat lots of vegetables (and hopefully some organ meats) that will give your body all it needs so that it never enters a state of increased acidic load.

How fast can I lose weight following the Neo Diet?

I understand this may be one of your primary goals, and that is okay. But if that is your *only* goal, then the Neo Diet is not for you. The Neo Diet is for someone whose main goal is to become incredibly healthy. Yes, you will lose weight and get fit, but this will happen in a sustainable way that will not make you sick or trigger a yo-yo effect.

Aggressive weight-loss approaches will knock down your metabolism. You will lose a lot of weight at first, but then you "eat an apple and gain 20 pounds." Aggressive weight loss is also plain dangerous. While "burning" all that fat, you will release an insane amount of toxins from these fat cells. Your body will not be in a position to effectively detoxify them, and they can move to your vital organs and make you very sick.

I assure you, if you follow the Neo Diet, you will lose weight. Probably even more than you were expecting. But what I won't do is promise you crazy numbers and marketing hype. We are doing things the right, enjoyable, healthy, and sustainable way.

How do I stay compliant during the holidays?

The answer to this question depends on which stage of your journey you're in. If you are in a more advanced stage, give yourself permission to commit some excesses (90/10 rule, remember?). But if you're just starting, you are probably not in a position to indulge in those excesses yet. Does this mean you can't be part of the holiday meals? Far from it. If you're hosting the party, cook healthier versions of the typical dishes you usually eat. Use the foods from the Food Matrix and make substitutions when needed. If you're a guest, offer to bring a new dish you've been playing with. That way, it doesn't look weird. You are just being the nice person who offered to bring something.

And remember what we discussed in chapter 17 about not giving too much info on your new diet. Just keep it casual and say your stomach is a bit upset and you don't want to risk it with the fried turkey or the cheesecake (or whatever else people are forcing upon you). It always works.

How do I stick to the diet when I'm on vacation or traveling for work?

When you're outside your normal routine, you can still follow the Neo Diet pretty efficiently. Just follow one rule I learned from Dr. Steven Gundry: "do what you can, with what you've got, wherever you are."[61]

Ideally, try to do some research to see if there are any "healthy restaurants" nearby. If not, just go to a regular restaurant (not a fast-food chain) and browse the menu for the foods you usually eat. Please remember that the menu is only a suggestion. You can always pick a dish and ask the chef to make a couple of changes to fit your needs, the same way you can ask them not to use peanut oil because you have a nut allergy. You can ask to have your food cooked in butter because you have a "vegetable oil allergy." Most people won't know whether that's true and will just go with it.

The same way you are choosing a better fat to cook your food in, you can also ask to replace the fried potatoes with vegetables, or the salad dressing with olive oil and vinegar, for example. You just have to be willing to ask. Most times, the chef will be more than happy to accommodate you. If they're not, go somewhere else. Easy!

Don't try to be a martyr. If they bring the bread basket, send it back. Don't sit there looking at it and fighting your cravings. Same with dessert. If they ask if you want to see the dessert menu, just say no. There's no point in having to fight your old habits, especially when you're still getting used to this new way of eating.

What do I do if there's no way to avoid a "bad" meal?

Let's imagine the example of someone—let's call her Susan—meeting her partner's parents for the first time. They decide to host Susan for a delicious traditional meal they love. If she wants to make a good first impression, Susan will have to eat the meal and not mention anything, even if it's pure poison. In a situation like this, Susan has to use her biohacker skills.

If you find yourself in a similar situation, here are some things you can do.

- Take with you some digestive enzymes and probiotics to help you break down foods like dairy and grains, and even neutralize some of their effects.

- If you expect a meal rich in lectins or oxalates, take some of the supplements I recommend (in the resources) just for those antinutrients.

- Take some vitamin E to help you fight off the oxidized vegetable oils that may be used.

- Top that off with some activated charcoal to bind to some of the toxins, and you are golden!

Please remember, this is just a short-term trick to protect you on the rare occasion when you really need to eat something "toxic," especially at the beginning of your journey. This is not to be used habitually.

I am experiencing some symptoms. What do I do?

If you've been following the Neo Diet and suddenly you feel one of your old symptoms, it's possible that you simply ate something your body is not healed enough to process. Don't worry, this doesn't mean you just ruined all your progress. It was just an isolated event. But it is important to look at what you ate and assess what possibly triggered the symptoms.

I actually like when this happens. When you eat something that doesn't support your goals, these symptoms are glorious reminders of why you are doing what you're doing. In the beginning of my health journey, all I could think of was eating pasta. A couple of weeks in, I ate this enormous dish of pasta, and I felt groggy and swollen for the next eight hours. After that, my cravings decreased, not only because my body was changing but also because I had that reminder of how that food made me feel.

I'm super excited about the Neo Diet, but some foods you suggest are expensive. How can I make this more affordable?

I won't give you the politically correct answer that you will spend that money at the doctor's office later, because, to be honest, I don't think you will spend more money.

Obviously, organic vegetables are more expensive than "regular" ones. Pasture-raised beef is also more expensive than conventional meat. There is no question about that. But what I want to point out is that you are probably spending a lot more money on other foods that you will avoid by following the Neo Diet. This will give you some wiggle room in your budget to buy the good stuff.

I'll venture to say that most people spend a lot more money on their daily fancy coffees, fast-food deliveries, baked goods, cereals, snacks, cookies, sauces, salad dressings, creamers. and all kinds of lavish sodas than I spend on my entire organic, pasture-raised shopping cart.

Simply comparing prices is not taking in the full picture. You need to do the total math, considering all the crap you won't be eating. I challenge you to do this exercise. Check how much you're presently spending on all the food you eat in a month and then do the math of the estimated cost you'll have when you buy the foods I recommend. You will probably be surprised to learn you will actually save some money.

Do I eat top-quality, pasture-raised Kobe or Wagyu beef with some caviar on the side at every meal? Of course not. Even if I were a Middle Eastern prince, I don't think I would ever spend that kind of money on food.

Depending on your budget, you may need to be more creative. I still eat plenty of pasture-raised ground beef and buy cheaper cuts for stews to save money. I also try to be smart about where and how I buy my produce. If you connect with local farmers, you may discover that some of them follow sustainable practices and offer very competitive prices.

Another trick is to buy in bulk and freeze it. Get yourself a freezer and buy the whole cow from the farmer. It will feed you for a year, and you will spend the same as or even less than you currently pay for conventional meat.

If you can't find any local farmers, search online. Many will ship to your home. Another option is to look for farmers' markets in your region. Often, you'll find farmers selling the "ugly" vegetables and fruits that didn't make the cut to go to the store. Ugly is still nutritious but cheaper. In some countries, there are even membership services that will ship organic ugly vegetables and fruits to your door for a fraction of their normal price. Google it.

While we're on the subject of fruits and vegetables, please note that not all of them have to be organic. The EWG evaluates annually which plants have the most and the least chemical contamination. Use their Dirty Dozen and Clean Fifteen lists to see which ones should definitely be organic and where you may be okay with conventionally grown versions. As of this writing, here is what is suggested:

• **Dirty Dozen** *(buy organic):* Apples, celery, cherries, grapes, hot peppers, kale, nectarines, peaches, pears, potatoes, spinach, strawberries, and tomatoes.
• **Clean Fifteen** *(buy conventional):* Asparagus, avocados, broccoli, cabbage, cantaloupe, cauliflower, eggplant, frozen sweet peas, honeydew, kiwi, mushrooms, onions, papaya, pineapple, and sweet corn.

If you follow these suggestions, trust me, you will be more than able to afford your healthy diet.

I am much better, but I still have symptoms that simply won't go away. What do I do?

As I've said before, I truly believe that just by following my recommendations, most people will be more than capable of fully healing themselves. But if some of your symptoms are still bothering you after you've been on the Neo Diet for some time, the best route is to work with a skilled professional such as a functional medicine specialist.

A skilled professional will correct things you are not even perceiving that you're doing wrong. They will also be able to guide you through the tests needed to uncover hidden problems holding you back, like parasites, mold, genetic predisposition, Lyme disease, or heavy metal toxicity.

Think about it. All the best athletes in the world have coaches. Even though the athlete may be better than their coach ever was, just having someone pointing them in the right direction makes all the difference.

Don't worry. If this is your case, I have your back. In the book's resources, I'll guide you on how to find a professional to work with.

"If you want to do something, go for it—you've got nothing to lose."
Louis Tomlinson

I once read somewhere, "This is the last chapter of this book, but it is the beginning of the next chapter in your life." Never forget that you have an immense power in you. You have the power to heal yourself, to feel younger, to perform physically and mentally beyond your wildest dreams.

Don't settle for less than you deserve. After all, you only live once. So, make it count. Push yourself to do and be the "impossible."

The point of changing your diet and lifestyle is not just to avoid disease and live long. It's to be incredibly healthy so you can have everything else. The fulfilling career, the loving partner, the time with friends and family, the energy to do all that you want, and the happy life we all should go for.

Your decisions will not only improve your life, but will also change the lives of the people around you, and even impact the world. You will inspire people to follow your steps and become better versions of themselves. And your consumer choices will influence the market to produce healthier and more sustainable food. One person at a time, we will have a huge effect on saving our beautiful planet.

By no means does this book hold all the answers. Science is always changing, but we cannot just sit and wait for the absolute truth. We should continue to learn, but act on what we already know. Don't let this book just sit on the shelf. Use the knowledge you've just gained from it and follow this formula with excitement. This is not a "diet"; this is your new way of living. This is the path to your Neo Self!

By following the Neo Diet, you will find a vitality and energy you probably haven't experienced in a very long time. Don't waste it sitting around. Do something meaningful with it. This book may talk about food, but its goal is to empower you to be the superhuman you were designed to be!

I guess it's time to say goodbye. Let's not do one of those *"You hang up first. No, you hang up. No, you hang up."* Let's not hang up. Let's stay in touch. In the "About the Author" section (last pages), you have all the ways we can connect. I can't wait to hear about how this book is helping you kick some ass!

Before you put down the book, can I ask for a tiny little favor?

I am an independent author and do not have the help of a publisher to market my book and share it with the world. If you enjoyed this book, please discuss it with others, recommend it, lend your copy, gift a copy to someone you love, share your favorite piece of knowledge from it on social media, and help me get its message out to the world. That is the only way we can reach and help more people.

It has been an absolute honor to share my work with you. I am humbled that you took the time to read my words. Thank you. You are amazing! 🖤

BOOK REVIEW

"Great opportunities to help others seldom come, but small ones surround us every day."
Sally Koch

Your opinion matters and it would mean the world to me to hear from you.

If there was something you think I could have done better, please email me at hello@neohacker.co. This is my first publication and your feedback is essential for me to correct the next editions and write better books in the future.

If you enjoyed my work, please review it. Leave your sincere feedback in the retailer where you purchased this book and copy it to book review communities like Goodreads, StoryGraph, or others you might be a part of.

Leaving a review will not only help me have a small chance of competing with big publishers, but it's also a way for me to read your success story. One day, I would love to inspire others with your journey.

Many of these retailers allow you to share a review with a picture. Take a picture of yourself holding the book. That way, I can put a face to the name and get to "know" you.

Thank you so much in advance for doing this. You rock!

SCAN ME
my.neodiet.co/review

NEO DIET RESOURCES

Want to know the brands of supplements I've used and recommend? Want to download some of the material I created for you, like the Food Matrix or the Baseline Sheet? Want to check out my kitchenware suggestions? All of that is inside the Resources page I developed just for the readers of The Neo Diet. There, you will find everything I have mentioned inside the book and more.

To access the book resources, please type my.neodiet.co/resources in your browser or scan the QR code on the right.

JOIN MY NEWSLETTER

Please sign up for my newsletter. This is a way for us to stay in touch and is also where I share new articles, health tips, sneak peaks, special offers and even give you firsthand access to my new books and course releases.

To join, please type my.neodiet.co/newsletter in your browser or scan the QR code on the left.

JOIN THE NEOHACKER TRIBE

Being part of a supportive community is essential if you want to achieve your health goals. The Neo Hacker Tribe is the community I created for all my readers. This is where you will ask questions about the book, share your experiences, and is also the place where my team and I can connect with you and post some of our latest discoveries.

Need to find an acountabilibuddy? Hop on the Neo Hacker Tribe and connect with someone. Join us today and introduce yourself!

To join, please type my.neodiet.co/neohackertribe in your browser or scan the QR code on the right.

WORK WITH ME

As you can tell by the size of this book, I really tried to provide as much information and value as possible. Unfortunately, there is only so much that can fit into a book. If you want to dive deeper into optimizing your health, body and mind, please check out my online courses and coaching programs. To learn more, please type my.neodiet.co/coaching in your browser or scan the QR code on the left.

REFERENCES

Throughout this book, I have referred over 2,500 studies and other scientific articles. If I were to add these references here, most people could not hold this book with just one hand. To keep things "lighter", I've put all of my references on the web, organized by chapter, and with direct links so you can check the articles easily.

To access all these references, please visit <u>my.neodiet.co/references</u> or simply scan the QR code below.

ACKNOWLEDGMENTS

Writing this book was one of the biggest and most challenging projects I've done so far. *Pinch me. I still can't believe I did it.* The truth is that I never would have been able to complete *The Neo Diet* if it weren't for the love, support, and guidance of many people.

Foremost, I want to thank my partner in crime, Andreia. Your patience and support gave me the strength I needed to endure the setbacks and keep going. Thank you for always being there for me and for understanding whenever I had to take time to write. You are one reason I took on this project and also why I could finish it. I love you.

I would also like to acknowledge my friends and family. Your questionable diet and lifestyle choices were the inspiration that led me to create this guide. *Ha-ha!* Just kidding, I love you guys!

In all seriousness, I want to give a special thanks to my parents and my inkonas group for believing and pushing me forward. This project was also something I pursued so we can spend more quality time together.

This book would not have been imagined, let alone written, if it weren't for the brilliant work of many authors and researchers who inspired me with their articles and books. During the past 15 years, I have read hundreds of books on diet and nutrition. It was these same books that helped me pursue a healthier life. The research of these amazing people guided me on my healing journey and led me to develop this huge passion for this subject. Because of you, I'm healthier and happier, and I have a purpose. Thank you.

As I'm sure you can understand, I cannot list all of these people here. However, I would like to give a special thanks to some authors whose books were essential in shaping *The Neo Diet*. While many of you have different health ideologies, you all taught me important nutrition concepts that ended up becoming part of my work. I hope one day I'll have the pleasure of meeting you and thanking you in person.

I'd like to show my particular respect and appreciation for Dave Asprey, Dr. Josh Axe, Sarah Ballantyne, Benjamin Bikman, Dr. Will Bulsiewicz, Dr. Dana Cohen, Dr. Will Cole, Dr. James DiNicolantonio, Dr. John Douillard, Tim Ferriss, Dr. Jason Fung, Dr. Mahmoud Ghannoum, Ann Louise Gittleman, Ben Greenfield, Dr. Steven Gundry, Dr. Mark Hyman, Sayer Ji, Dr. Alejandro Junger, Chris Kresser, Siim Land, Max Lugavere, Dr. Ben Lynch, Darin Olien, Brad Pilon, Diana Rodgers, Dr. Michael Ruscio, Dr. Paul Saladino, Dr. Catherine Shanahan, Mark Sisson, Shawn Stevenson, Nina Teicholz, and Robb Wolf.

Last, but certainly not least, I would like to thank you, and every single person who has been supporting my work. I may not know you personally, but I appreciate every single one of you.

Thank you for reading *The Neo Diet*!

A SPECIAL THANK YOU

I could not finish this book without thanking four amazing human beings that took their time to help me. Not only did you help me catch several mistakes, but your feedback was also crucial to helping me make *The Neo Diet* a better book.

Ana, Andreia, Sage, and Sam, I cannot thank you enough for your kindness and support.

You are the best!

ABOUT THE AUTHOR

Kevin Aventura is an author, entrepreneur, and human optimization coach. Growing up, he always felt like no matter what he did, his less-than-optimal health never allowed him to achieve the best version of himself. This was the reason he obtained his physical therapy degree and pursued further studies in naturopathy. Kevin believes that everyone deserves to feel like the superhuman they were designed to be. As a way to follow his vision, he created the NeoHacker community. An online resource where he shares evidenced-based research on biohacking, debunks health misinformation, and empowers others to achieve their health and performance goals.

Kevin is also passionate about traveling and photography, having even created content for several renowned brands on his social media channels. He spends his time between Portugal and South Florida (USA).

To connect with Kevin and learn more about his work, please check the following links, or scan the QR code at the bottom:

- Community Instagram: my.neodiet.co/instagram
- Personal Instagram: my.neodiet.co/kevin
- Facebook Page: my.neodiet.co/facebook
- Twitter: my.neodiet.co/twitter
- NeoHacker Tribe: my.neodiet.co/neohackertribe
- Website: neohacker.co

It's Time to Become Your Neo Self!

Please note that all these templates (and a couple of extra ones) can be downloaded inside the Resources section (my.neodiet.co/resources).

NOTEBOOK TEMPLATE

DATE: / /

MEAL TRACKER | HOW IT MADE ME FEEL

WATER INTAKE   How many bottles

MOOD TRACKER   Grade 1 - 5

TOP GOALS

_____

_____

_____

VISUALIZE

DAILY ROUTINE

☐ _____

☐ _____

☐ _____

GRATITUDE: WINS OF THE DAY   TODAY'S TASKS   WHAT TO PRIORITIZE FOR TOMORROW

_____   _____   _____

_____   _____   _____

_____   _____   _____

OTHER NOTES

BASELINE SHEET

NAME:

BASICS	VALUE	MEASUREMENTS	VALUE
WEIGHT		CHEST	
FAT WEIGHT		WAIST	
MUSCLE WEIGHT		HIPS	
FAT PERCENTAGE		ARM	
		THIGH	

BLOOD WORK	REFERENCE	RESULTS
FASTING GLUCOSE LEVEL	70-100 mg/dL	
FASTING INSULIN LEVEL	2-20 mIU/mL	
HEMOGLOBIN A1C	4 - 5.6%	
HDL	> 60 mg/dL	
TRIGLYCERIDES (TG)	< 150 mg/dL	
TG/HDL check the values and do the math	< 2	
LP(A)	< 30 mg/dL	
APO B	< 100 mg/dL	
LIPO-PLA2	< 200 ng/mL	
HOMOCYSTEINE	4-15 µml/L	
FIBRINOGEN	200-400 mg/dL	
C-REACTIVE PROTEIN (CRP)	< 1.0 mg/dL	

PAIN CHART

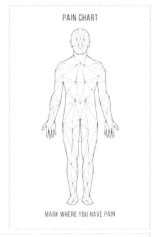

MARK WHERE YOU HAVE PAIN

NOTES ABOUT YOUR PAIN

MAKE NOTES ABOUT YOUR MOOD, ENERGY LEVELS, DIGESTIVE SYMPTOMS, BRAIN PERFORMANCE, AND ANY OTHER SYMPTOM YOU MAY BE EXPERIENCING RIGHT NOW

TAKE A PICTURE
IN YOUR UNDERWEAR

BODY MEASUREMENTS
TUTORIAL

SCAN ME

PROGRESS SHEET ①

NAME:

BASICS	START	AFTER 28 DAYS	AFTER 90 DAYS	AFTER 6 MONTHS	AFTER 1 YEAR
WEIGHT					
FAT WEIGHT					
MUSCLE WEIGHT					
FAT PERCENTAGE					

MEASUREMENTS	START	AFTER 28 DAYS	AFTER 90 DAYS	AFTER 6 MONTHS	AFTER 1 YEAR
CHEST					
WAIST					
HIPS					
ARM					
THIGH					

PICTURE EVOLUTION	START	AFTER 28 DAYS	AFTER 90 DAYS	AFTER 6 MONTHS	AFTER 1 YEAR

	START	AFTER 28 DAYS	AFTER 90 DAYS	AFTER 6 MONTHS	AFTER 1 YEAR
DIGESTIVE SYMPTOMS	☆☆☆☆☆	☆☆☆☆☆	☆☆☆☆☆	☆☆☆☆☆	☆☆☆☆☆
ENERGY LEVELS	☆☆☆☆☆	☆☆☆☆☆	☆☆☆☆☆	☆☆☆☆☆	☆☆☆☆☆
MOOD	☆☆☆☆☆	☆☆☆☆☆	☆☆☆☆☆	☆☆☆☆☆	☆☆☆☆☆
BRAIN PERFORMANCE	☆☆☆☆☆	☆☆☆☆☆	☆☆☆☆☆	☆☆☆☆☆	☆☆☆☆☆
OVERALL WELLBEING	☆☆☆☆☆	☆☆☆☆☆	☆☆☆☆☆	☆☆☆☆☆	☆☆☆☆☆

PROGRESS SHEET

NAME:

BLOOD WORK	START	AFTER 90 DAYS	AFTER 6 MONTHS	AFTER 1 YEAR
FASTING GLUCOSE LEVEL				
FASTING INSULIN LEVEL				
HEMOGLOBIN A1C				
HDL				
TRIGLYCERIDES (TG)				
TG/HDL				
LP(A)				
APO B				
LIPO-PLA2				
HOMOCYSTEINE				
FIBRINOGEN				
C-REACTIVE PROTEIN (CRP)				

I recommend giving yourself 90 days for more radical blood work differences. That is why I have skipped that mark on this second sheet. Nonetheless, if you want to check your blood after 28 days, please do. I am confident your results will still please you

SHARE YOUR TRANSFORMATION
#NeoTransformation
#NeoHacker
#NeoDiet
Every month we prize the best transformation

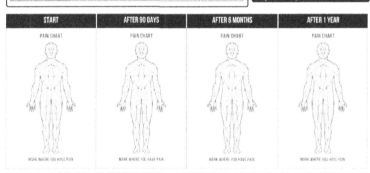

START	AFTER 90 DAYS	AFTER 6 MONTHS	AFTER 1 YEAR
PAIN CHART	PAIN CHART	PAIN CHART	PAIN CHART
MARK WHERE YOU HAVE PAIN	MARK WHERE YOU HAVE PAIN	MARK WHERE YOU HAVE PAIN	MARK WHERE YOU HAVE PAIN

FINAL REMARKS: DESCRIBE YOUR PROGRESS THROUGHOUT THE PAST YEAR